BASIC MEDICAL MICROBIOLOGY

BASIC MEDICAL MICROBIOLOGY

PATRICK R. MURRAY, PhD

Senior Worldwide Director, Scientific Affairs
BD Diagnostics Systems
Sparks, Maryland;
Adjunct Professor, Department of Pathology
University of Maryland School of Medicine
Baltimore, Maryland

ELSEVIER

ELSEVIER

1600 John F. Kennedy Blvd.
Ste 1800
Philadelphia, PA 19103-2899

BASIC MEDICAL MICROBIOLOGY
ISBN: 978-0-323-47676-8

Notices

Knowledge and best practice in this field are constantly changing. As new research and experience broaden our understanding, changes in research methods, professional practices, or medical treatment may become necessary.

Practitioners and researchers must always rely on their own experience and knowledge in evaluating and using any information, methods, compounds, or experiments described herein. In using such information or methods they should be mindful of their own safety and the safety of others, including parties for whom they have a professional responsibility.

With respect to any drug or pharmaceutical products identified, readers are advised to check the most current information provided (i) on procedures featured or (ii) by the manufacturer of each product to be administered, to verify the recommended dose or formula, the method and duration of administration, and contraindications. It is the responsibility of practitioners, relying on their own experience and knowledge of their patients, to make diagnoses, to determine dosages and the best treatment for each individual patient, and to take all appropriate safety precautions.

To the fullest extent of the law, neither the Publisher nor the authors, contributors, or editors, assume any liability for any injury and/or damage to persons or property as a matter of products liability, negligence or otherwise, or from any use or operation of any methods, products, instructions, or ideas contained in the material herein.

Library of Congress Cataloging-in-Publication Data
Names: Murray, Patrick R., author.
Title: Basic medical microbiology / Patrick R. Murray.
Description: First edition. | Philadelphia, PA : Elsevier, [2018] | Includes bibliographical references and index.
Identifiers: LCCN 2016058724 | ISBN 9780323476768 (pbk. : alk. paper)
Subjects: | MESH: Microbiology | Bacteria | Viruses | Fungi | Parasites
Classification: LCC QR41.2 | NLM QW 4 | DDC 579--dc23 LC record available at https://lccn.loc.gov/2016058724

Executive Content Strategist: James T. Merritt
Content Development Specialist: Kerry Lishon
Publishing Services Manager: Catherine Jackson
Project Manager: Tara Delaney
Design Direction: Maggie Reid

Printed in China

Last digit is the print number: 9 8 7 6 5 4 3 2 1

PREFACE

What is the bigger challenge—for a student or the instructor to understand what is important in medical microbiology? Many years ago when I took my first graduate course in medical microbiology, I read thousands of pages of text, listened to 5 hours of lectures a week, and performed lab exercises 6 hours a week for 1 year. I was given a wonderful foundation in microbiology, but I frequently asked the question—that was voiced by all the students—do I really need to know all this stuff? The answer to that question is certainly no, but the challenge is what information is needed. Years later when I set out to write my first textbook on microbiology, my goal was to only give the students what they need to know, described in a way that is informative, factual, and concise. I think I was successful in that effort, but I also realize that the discipline of microbiology continues to change as do approaches to presenting information to the students. I am still firmly convinced that my efforts in my first textbook, *Medical Microbiology,* and subsequent editions are important, forming the foundation of microbiology knowledge for a student. This cannot be replaced by a quick search of the internet or a published review because much of the subject matter presented in Medical Microbiology—epidemiology, virulence, clinical diseases, diagnostics, treatment—is a distillation of the review of numerous research articles and clinical and technical experience. Having stated that, students frequently turn to review books consisting of abbreviated summaries, illustrations (should I say cartoons), and various mnemonic aids for mastering this subject. As I have watched this evolution of learning microbiology, I am struck by the sacrifice that has been made. I believe microbiology is a beautiful subject, with the balance between health and disease defined by the biology of individual organisms and microbial communities. Without an understanding of the biology, lists of facts are soon forgotten. But I am a realist and know the burden students face, mastering not only microbiology but also a number of other subjects. So the personal question I posed was—is there a better way to present to the student a summary of information that is easy to understand and remember? This book is my approach to solving this question. First, almost by definition, it is not comprehensive. Just as I have carefully selected organisms and diseases to present in this book, I have also intentionally not mentioned others—not because they are unimportant but because they are less common. I have also not presented a detailed discussion of microbial biology and virulence or the immune response of the patient to an infection, but simply presented the association between an organism and disease. Again, I felt those discussions should be reserved for *Medical Microbiology*. Finally, the organization of this book is focused on organisms—bacteria, viruses, fungi, and parasites—rather than diseases. I do this because I think it is easier for a student to remember a limited number of diseases associated with an organism rather than a long list of organisms (or a significantly incomplete list) implicated in a specific disease such as pneumonia. Still, patients present with disease and the observer must develop a list of organisms that could be responsible; so to aid the student, I provide this differential diagnosis in the introductory chapter of each organism section (Chapters 2, 12, 18, and 22). I also provide in these introductory chapters an overview of the classification of the organisms (a structural framework for remembering the organisms) and a listing of antimicrobials that are used to treat infections. The individual chapters in Sections 1–4 are organized in a common theme: brief discussion of the individual organisms, a summary of facts (properties, epidemiology, clinical disease, diagnosis, treatment) provided in a concise table, illustrations provided as a visual learning aid, and clinical cases to reenforce the clinical significance of the organisms. Finally, examination questions are provided to help the student assess their ability to assimilate this material. Again, I will emphasize that this text should not be considered a comprehensive review of microbiology. On the other hand, I believe if the student masters this material, he or she will have a firm foundation in the principles and applications of microbiology. I certainly welcome all comments on how successful my efforts are.

I would like to acknowledge the support and guidance from the Elsevier professionals who help bring this concept to reality, particularly Jim Merritt, Katie DeFrancesco, Nicole DiCicco, and Tara Delaney. Additionally, I want to thank the many students who have challenged me to think about broad world of microbes and distill this into the essential material they must master, and my professional business colleagues who stimulated me to explain complex microbiology information in a factual but coherent story for a novice in this field.

CONTENTS

SECTION IV Fungi

SECTION V Parasites

SECTION VI Review Questions

1

Overview of Medical Microbiology

Microbiology can certainly be overwhelming for the student confronted with the daunting task of learning about hundreds of medically important microbes. I remember well the first day in my introductory graduate course in medical microbiology; the course instructor handed each student a 1000-page syllabus consisting of lecture outlines, notes, and literature references. That became known not so lovingly as *the book of pain*. However, microbiology is not so challenging if the subject matter—the microbes—are subdivided into groups and further subdivided into related units. Let me illustrate this in this introductory chapter.

Microbes are subdivided into one of four groups:

- Viruses
- Bacteria
- Fungi
- Parasites

The structural complexity of these groups increases from viruses (the most simple structure) to parasites (the most complex). There is generally no confusion about which group a microbe should be placed in, although a few fungi were formerly classified with the parasites. Each group of microbes is then further subdivided, generally based on a key feature of the group.

Microbial Classification

Microbes	Primary Classification	Secondary Classification
Viruses	DNA virus	Single- vs. double-stranded nucleic acid Outer envelope or no envelope
	RNA virus	
Bacteria	Gram positive	Cocci vs. rods Aerobic vs. anaerobic Spore-former vs. no spores (only gram-positive bacteria)
	Gram negative	
	Acid-fast	Partial or complete acid-fast staining
	Miscellaneous	Spiral-shaped Obligate intracellular
Fungi	Yeast (single-celled)	
	Mold (multi-celled)	Pigment vs. no pigment Nuclei separated by wall (septum) or nonseptated
	Dimorphic (yeast and mold forms)	

Continued

Microbial Classification—cont'd

Microbes	Primary Classification	Secondary Classification
Parasites	Protozoa	Ameba
		Flagellates
		Sporozoa
	Worms (helminths)	Roundworms (nematodes)
		Flatworms (trematodes)
		Tapeworms (cestodes)
	Bugs (arthropods)	Mosquitos
		Ticks
		Fleas
		Lice
		Mites
		Flies

VIRUSES AND BACTERIA

Viruses

Viruses are very simple microbes, consisting of nucleic acid, a few proteins, and (in some) a lipid envelope. These microbes are completely dependent on the cells they infect for their survival and replication. Medically important viruses are subdivided into 20 families defined by the structural properties of the members. The most important feature is the nucleic acid. Viruses contain either DNA or RNA but not both. The families of DNA viruses and RNA viruses are further subdivided into viruses with either single-stranded or double-stranded nucleic acids. Lastly, these viral families are further subdivided into viruses with an outer envelope, or naked non-enveloped viruses. Now the perceptive student would say that this gives us 8 families of viruses and not 20. Well, the viruses are further subdivided by their shape (spherical or rodlike) and size (big or small ["pico"]). Thus the key to understanding viruses is to place them into their respective families based on their structural features.

Bacteria

Bacteria are a bit more complex, with both RNA and DNA, metabolic machinery for self-replication, and a complex cell wall structure. Bacteria are **prokaryotic** organisms; that is, simple unicellular organisms with no nuclear membrane, mitochondria, Golgi bodies, or endoplasmic reticulum and they reproduce by asexual division. The key feature that is used to separate most bacteria is their staining property, with the Gram stain and acid-fast stain the most important. Most bacteria are either **gram-positive** (retain the blue dye) or **gram-negative** (lose the blue stain and stain with the red dye). These bacteria are then subdivided by their shape (either spherical [cocci] or rod-shaped), whether they grow aerobically or anaerobically (many bacteria grow in both atmospheres and are called **facultative anaerobes**), and whether they form resilient **spores** or not (only gram-positive rods are spore-formers). The other important bacterial stain is the **acid-fast** stain that is retained only by a few bacteria that have a characteristic lipid-rich cell wall. This group is further subdivided by how difficult it is to remove the acid-fast stain (the stain is named because an acid solution removes the stain from most other bacteria). Finally, there are groups of organisms that do not stain with these procedures so they are separated by other features, such as shape (spiral-shaped bacteria) or their need to grow inside a host cell (e.g., leukocyte) or cell cultures in the laboratory.

FUNGI AND PARASITES

Fungi and parasites are more complex **eukaryotic** organisms that contain a well-defined nucleus, mitochondria, Golgi bodies, and endoplasmic reticulum. Single-celled and multi-celled organisms are members of both groups. As can be seen, the line separating these two groups is not as well defined as that separating these organisms from the bacteria or viruses, but the classification is still well recognized.

Fungi

Fungi are subdivided into single-celled organisms **(yeasts)** or multi-celled organisms **(molds)**, with a few medically important members existing in both forms **(dimorphic fungi)**. Molds are complex organisms with the cells organized into threadlike tubular structures **(hyphae)** and specialized asexual reproductive forms **(conidia)**. The molds are then further subdivided by the structure of the hyphae (pigmented or nonpigmented, separated into individual cells [septated molds] or not) and the arrangement of the conidia.

Parasites

Parasites are also subdivided into single-celled organisms **(protozoa)** or multi-celled organisms (**worms** and **bugs**). Members of the family Protozoa are then further divided into amebae, flagellates (think of them as hairy protozoa), and coccidia (some are spherical-shaped but many are not). The worms (technically called **helminthes**) are nicely classified by their shape: roundworms, flatworms, and tapeworms. Pretty simple, although many have very complex lifecycles that unfortunately are important for understanding how they cause disease. The **bugs** are simply "bugs." These include mosquitos, ticks, fleas, lice, mites, and flies. They are important because they are vectors of a number of viruses and bacteria (not fungi) that are responsible for diseases. Other bugs obviously exist (such as spiders), but these generally are not vectors for other pathogenic microbes.

GOOD VERSUS BAD MICROBES

Microbes, particularly the bacteria, have unjustly earned a bad reputation. Most are viewed as bad and recognized only for their ability to cause diseases. We have coined the derogatory term ***germs,*** and great efforts are made to eliminate our exposure to these organisms. The reality is most microbes are not only good but critical for our health. The surfaces of the skin, nose, mouth, gut, and genitourinary tract are covered with bacteria, as well as some fungi and parasites. These organisms are critical for the maturation of our immune system, important metabolic functions such as the digestion of food products, and protection from infection with unwanted pathogens. These organisms are referred to as our **normal flora** or **microbiome**. If these organisms are maintained in their proper balance, then health can be maintained. If they are disrupted either naturally or through man-made interventions (e.g., antibiotics, skin peels, enemas) then we risk disease. Infectious diseases are also initiated when the members of the microbiome are introduced into normally sterile sites (e.g., abdominal cavity, tissues, lungs, urinary tract) through trauma or disease. This is referred to as an **endogenous** infection or an infection caused by the normal microbial population. Finally, infections can be caused by **exogenous** organisms; that is, those introduced from outside. Only a few of the microbes that we encounter from our environment are pathogens, but some of the most serious infections are caused by these exogenous pathogens. So the important lesson is that most microbes are good and not associated with disease. A subset of our endogenous organisms can cause disease when introduced into normally sterile areas, but most endogenous organisms do not have the virulent properties to cause disease. Likewise, most of the exogenous organisms we are exposed to cause no problems at all, but some can cause quite significant disease. It is important to understand which organisms have the necessary properties (**virulence**) to cause disease and under what circumstances this will occur. It is also important to understand which organisms to ignore because they are not associated with disease.

CONCLUSION

The perceived complexity of microbiology is simplified if we understand the relationships between members of each of the four groups of microbes. This is further simplified if we separate the pathogens from nonpathogens and then understand the conditions under which the pathogens produce disease. The following chapters are designed to develop these themes for the individual groups of organisms.

2

Introduction to Bacteria

A WORD OF CAUTION

Alright, there is way too much information in the next few pages. I certainly do not expect the student to master these details before he or she moves on to the rest of the bacteriology chapters. Rather, a quick scan of the information should be done first. Then, as each subsequent chapter is digested, this chapter can provide a framework for linking each of the bacteriology chapters.

OVERVIEW

Bacteria are prokaryotic (*pro*, before; *karyon*, kernel) organisms that are relatively simple in structure. They are unicellular and have no nuclear membrane, mitochondria, Golgi bodies, or endoplasmic reticulum, and they reproduce by asexual division. The bacterial cell wall is complex, consisting of one of two basic forms defined by their staining ability with the **Gram stain**: a gram-positive cell wall with a thick peptidoglycan layer, and a gram-negative cell wall with a thin peptidoglycan layer and an overlying **outer membrane**. Some bacteria lack this cell wall structure and compensate by surviving only inside host cells in a hypertonic environment. The human body is inhabited by thousands of different bacterial species (called the "**microbiome**"), some living transiently, others in a permanent synergistic relationship. Likewise, the environment that surrounds us, including the air we breathe, water we drink, and food we eat is populated with bacteria, many of which are relatively harmless and some of which are capable of causing life-threatening disease. Disease can result from the toxic effects of bacterial products (e.g., toxins) or when bacteria invade normally sterile body tissues and fluids.

CLASSIFICATION

The size (1 to 20 μm or larger), shape (spheres [cocci], rods, or spirals), and spatial arrangement (single cells, pairs, chains, or clusters) of the cells, as well as specific growth properties (e.g., **aerobic** [require oxygen], **anaerobic** [cannot grow in presence of oxygen], or **facultative anaerobes** [grow in presence or absence of oxygen]) are used for the preliminary classification of bacteria. This is a useful exercise that can provide some order to an otherwise confusing list of organisms. The following tables are not comprehensive; rather, these are a listing of the most commonly isolated or clinically important bacteria.

Gram-Positive Bacteria

Aerobic Gram-Positive Cocci: • *Staphylococcus* • *Streptococcus* • *Enterococcus* **Aerobic Gram-Positive Rods:** • *Bacillus* • *Listeria* • *Corynebacterium*	**Anaerobic Gram-Positive Cocci:** • Many genera **Anaerobic Gram-Positive Rods:** • *Clostridium* • *Actinomyces* • *Lactobacillus* • *Propionibacterium*	**Aerobic Acid-Fast Rods:** • *Mycobacterium* • *Nocardia* • *Rhodococcus*

Gram-Negative Bacteria

Aerobic Gram-Negative Cocci and Coccobacilli:
- *Neisseria*
- *Moraxella*
- *Eikenella*
- *Kingella*
- *Haemophilus*
- *Acinetobacter*
- *Bordetella*
- *Brucella*
- *Francisella*

Aerobic Gram-Negative Rods:
- Enterobacteriaceae (many genera)
- *Vibrio*
- *Pseudomonas*
- *Burkholderia*
- *Stenotrophomonas*

Anaerobic Gram-Negative Cocci:
- *Veillonella*

Anaerobic Gram-Negative Rods:
- *Bacteroides*
- *Fusobacterium*

Other Bacteria

Spiral-Shaped Bacteria:
- *Campylobacter*
- *Helicobacter*
- *Treponema*
- *Borrelia*
- *Leptospira*

Obligate Intracellular Organisms:
- *Rickettsia*
- *Orientia*
- *Ehrlichia*
- *Anaplasma*
- *Coxiella*
- *Chlamydia*
- *Chlamydophila*

ROLE IN DISEASE

Occasionally, some diseases have a characteristic presentation and are associated with a single organism. Unfortunately, multiple organisms can produce a similar clinical picture (e.g., sepsis, pneumonia, gastroenteritis, meningitis, urinary tract infection, or genital infection). The clinical management of infections is predicted by the ability to develop an accurate **differential diagnosis** defined by the most common organisms associated with the clinical picture, selection of the appropriate diagnostic tests, and initiation of effective empirical therapy. Once the diagnosis is confirmed, empirical therapy can be modified to provide narrow-spectrum, directed therapy. The following is a list of the most common organisms associated with specific clinical syndromes.

Common Organisms and Their Associated Clinical Syndromes

Disease	Most Common Pathogens
Sepsis	
General sepsis	*Staphylococcus aureus*, coagulase-negative *Staphylococcus*, *Escherichia coli*, *Klebsiella pneumoniae*
Catheter-related sepsis	Coagulase-negative *Staphylococcus*
Septic thrombophlebitis	*S. aureus*, *Bacteroides fragilis*
Cardiovascular Infections	
Endocarditis	Viridans *Streptococcus*, coagulase-negative *Staphylococcus*
Myocarditis	*S. aureus*
Pericarditis	*S. aureus*
Upper Respiratory Infections	
Pharyngitis	*Streptococcus pyogenes* (group A)
Sinusitis	*Streptococcus pneumoniae*, *Haemophilus influenzae*, *Moraxella catarrhalis*, mixed aerobic and anaerobic
Ear Infections	
Otitis externa	*Pseudomonas aeruginosa*, *S. aureus*
Otitis media	*S. pneumoniae*, *H. influenzae*, *M. catarrhalis*
Eye Infections	
Conjunctivitis	*S. aureus*, *S. pneumoniae*, *Haemophilus aegyptius*
Keratitis	*S. aureus*, *S. pneumoniae*, *P. aeruginosa*
Endophthalmitis	*Bacillus cereus*, *S. aureus*, *P. aeruginosa*

Continued

Common Organisms and Their Associated Clinical Syndromes—cont'd	
Disease	**Most Common Pathogens**
Pleuropulmonary and Bronchial Infections	
Bronchitis	*M. catarrhalis, H. influenzae, S. pneumoniae*
Empyema	*S. aureus, S. pneumoniae, S. pyogenes* (group A)
Pneumonia	*S. pneumoniae, S. aureus, K. pneumoniae,* other Enterobacteriaceae
Central Nervous System Infections	
Meningitis	*Streptococcus agalactiae* (group B), *E. coli, H. influenzae, S. pneumoniae, Neisseria meningitidis, Listeria monocytogenes*
Encephalitis	Rarely bacterial
Brain abscess	*S. aureus, Fusobacterium* species, anaerobic cocci
Subdural empyema	*S. aureus, S. pneumoniae*
Intraabdominal Infections	
Peritonitis	*E. coli, B. fragilis, Enterococcus* species
Dialysis-associated peritonitis	Coagulase-negative *Staphylococcus*
Gastrointestinal Infections	
Gastritis	*Helicobacter pylori*
Gastroenteritis	*Salmonella* species, *Shigella* species, *Campylobacter jejuni, Campylobacter coli, E. coli, Vibrio cholera, Vibrio parahaemolyticus, B. cereus, P. aeruginosa*
Antibiotic-associated diarrhea	*Clostridium difficile*
Food intoxication	*S. aureus, B. cereus*
Proctitis	*Neisseria gonorrhoeae*
Genital Infections	
Genital ulcers	*Treponema pallidum, Haemophilus ducreyi*
Urethritis	*N. gonorrhoeae, Chlamydia trachomatis, Mycoplasma genitalium*
Vaginitis	*Mycoplasma hominis, Mobiluncus* species, other anaerobic species
Cervicitis	*N. gonorrhoeae, C. trachomatis, M. genitalium*
Urinary Tract Infections	
Cystitis and pyelonephritis	*E. coli, Proteus mirabilis,* other Enterobacteriaceae, *Staphylococcus saprophyticus*
Renal calculi	*P. mirabilis, S. saprophyticus*
Renal abscess	*S. aureus*
Prostatitis	*E. coli*
Skin and Soft-Tissue Infections	
Impetigo	*S. pyogenes* (group A), *S. aureus*
Folliculitis	*S. aureus, P. aeruginosa*
Furuncles and carbuncles	*S. aureus*
Paronychia	*S. aureus, S. pyogenes* (group A), *P. aeruginosa*
Erysipelas	*S. pyogenes* (group A)
Cellulitis	*S. pyogenes* (group A), *S. aureus*
Necrotizing cellulitis and fasciitis	*S. pyogenes* (group A), *Clostridium perfringens, B. fragilis*
Bacillary angiomatosis	*Bartonella henselae, Bartonella quintana*
Infections of burns	*P. aeruginosa, Enterococcus* species
Surgical wounds	*S. aureus,* coagulase-negative *Staphylococcus*
Bite wounds	*Eikenella corrodens, Pasteurella multocida,* mixed aerobes and anaerobes
Traumatic wounds	*Bacillus* species, *S. aureus*

Common Organisms and Their Associated Clinical Syndromes—cont'd

Disease	Most Common Pathogens
Bone and Joint Infections	
Osteomyelitis	*S. aureus, Salmonella* species
Arthritis	*S. aureus, N. gonorrhoeae*
Prosthetic-associated infection	*S. aureus*, coagulase-negative *Staphylococcus*
Granulomatous Infections	
General	*Mycoplasma tuberculosis, Nocardia* species, *T. pallidum*

ANTIBACTERIAL AGENTS

This section presents an overview of the most commonly used antibacterial agents, their mode of action, and spectrum of activity. By its nature, this is not a comprehensive summary of antibacterial therapy. Additionally, in the following chapters, the recommended therapies for individual organisms are listed.

Commonly Used Antibacterial Agents, Their Mode of Action, and Spectrum of Activity

Mode of Action	Antibiotic	Spectrum of Activity
	DISRUPTION OF CELL WALL	
Binds proteins (penicillin binding proteins) and enzymes responsible for peptidoglycan synthesis	Natural penicillins (penicillin G, penicillin V)	Active against all β-hemolytic streptococci and most other streptococci; limited activity against staphylococci; active against meningococci and most gram-positive anaerobes; poor activity against gram-negative rods
	Penicillinase-resistant penicillins (methicillin, nafcillin, oxacillin, cloxacillin, dicloxacillin)	Similar to the natural penicillins except enhanced activity against staphylococci
	Broad-spectrum penicillins (ampicillin, amoxicillin)	Active against gram-positive cocci equivalent to the natural penicillins; active against some gram-negative rods
	Narrow-spectrum cephalosporins and cephamycins (cephalexin, cephalothin, cefazolin, cephapirin, cephradine)	Activity equivalent to oxacillin against gram-positive bacteria; some gram-negative activity (e.g., *E. coli, Klebsiella, P. mirabilis*)
	Expanded-spectrum cephalosporins and cephamycins (cefaclor, cefuroxime, cefotetan, cefoxitin)	Activity equivalent to oxacillin against gram-positive bacteria; improved gram-negative activity to include *Enterobacter, Citrobacter*, and additional *Proteus* species
	Broad-spectrum cephalosporins (cefixime, cefotaxime, ceftriaxone, ceftazidime, cefepime, cefpirome)	Activity equivalent to oxacillin against gram-positive bacteria; improved gram-negative activity to include *Pseudomonas*
	Carbapenems (imipenem, meropenem, ertapenem, doripenem)	Broad-spectrum antibiotics active against most aerobic and anaerobic gram-positive and gram-negative bacteria except oxacillin-resistant staphylococci, most *Enterococcus faecium*, and selected gram-negative rods (*Pseudomonas, Stenotrophomonas, Burkholderia*)

Continued

Commonly Used Antibacterial Agents, Their Mode of Action, and Spectrum of Activity—cont'd

Mode of Action	Antibiotic	Spectrum of Activity
DISRUPTION OF CELL WALL—cont'd		
	Narrow-spectrum monobactam (aztreonam)	Active against selected aerobic gram-negative rods but inactive against anaerobes and gram-positive cocci
Binds β-lactamases and prevents enzymatic inactivation of β-lactam	Penicillins with β-lactamase inhibitor (ampicillin-sulbactam, amoxicillin-clavulanate, ticarcillin-clavulanate, piperacillin-tazobactam)	Activity similar to natural penicillins plus improved activity against β-lactamase producing staphylococci and selected gram-negative rods
Inhibits cross-linkage of peptidoglycan layers	Glycopeptides (vancomycin)	Active against all staphylococci and streptococci; inactive against many enterococci, gram-positive rods, and all gram-negative bacteria
Inhibits bacterial cytoplasmic membrane and movement of peptidoglycan precursors	Polypeptide (bacitracin)	Active against staphylococci and streptococci; inactive against gram-negative bacteria
Disrupts bacterial outer membrane permeability	Polypeptide (colistin)	Active against most gram-negative bacteria but not gram-positive bacteria (no outer membrane)
Inhibits mycolic acid synthesis	Isoniazid, ethionamide	Active against mycobacteria
Inhibits synthesis of arabinogalactan	Ethambutol	
Inhibits cross-linkage of peptidoglycan precursors	Cycloserine	
INHIBITION OF PROTEIN SYNTHESIS		
Produces premature release of peptide chains from 30S ribosome	Aminoglycosides (streptomycin, kanamycin, gentamicin, tobramycin, amikacin)	Primarily used to treat infections with gram-negative rods; kanamycin with limited activity; tobramycin slightly more active than gentamicin vs *Pseudomonas*; amikacin most active
Prevents polypeptide elongation at 30S ribosome	Tetracyclines (tetracycline, doxycycline, minocycline)	Broad-spectrum antibiotics active against gram-positive and some gram-negative bacteria (*Neisseria*, some Enterobacteriaceae), mycoplasmas, chlamydiae, and rickettsiae
Binds to 30S ribosome and prevents initiation of protein synthesis	Glycylcyclines (tigecycline)	Spectrum similar to tetracyclines but more active against gram-negative bacteria and rapidly growing mycobacteria
Prevents initiation of protein synthesis at 50S ribosome	Oxazolidinone (linezolid)	Active against *Staphylococcus*, *Enterococcus*, *Streptococcus*, gram-positive rods, *Clostridium*, and anaerobic cocci; not active against gram-negative bacteria

Commonly Used Antibacterial Agents, Their Mode of Action, and Spectrum of Activity—cont'd

Mode of Action	Antibiotic	Spectrum of Activity
	INHIBITION OF PROTEIN SYNTHESIS—cont'd	
Prevents polypeptide elongation at 50S ribosome	Macrolides (erythromycin, azithromycin, clarithromycin, roxithromycin)	Broad-spectrum antibiotics active against gram-positive and some gram-negative bacteria, *Neisseria*, *Legionella*, *Mycoplasma*, *Chlamydia*, *Chlamydophila*, *Treponema*, and *Rickettsia*; clarithromycin and azithromycin active against some mycobacteria
	Lincosamide (clindamycin)	Broad-spectrum of activity against aerobic gram-positive cocci and anaerobes
	Streptogramins (quinupristin-dalfopristin)	Primarily active against gram-positive bacteria; good activity against methicillin-susceptible and resistant staphylococci, streptococci, *E. faecium* (no activity against *Enterococcus faecalis*), *Haemophilus*, *Moraxella*, and anaerobes; not active against Enterobacteriaceae or other gram-negative rods
	INHIBITION OF NUCLEIC ACID SYNTHESIS	
Binds α-subunit of DNA gyrase	Narrow-spectrum quinolone (nalidixic acid)	Active against selected gram-negative rods; no useful gram-positive activity
	Broad-spectrum quinolone (ciprofloxacin, levofloxacin)	Broad-spectrum antibiotics with activity against gram-positive and gram-negative bacteria
	Extended-spectrum quinolones (moxifloxacin)	Broad-spectrum antibiotic with enhanced activity against gram-positive bacteria; activity against gram-negative rods similar to that of ciprofloxacin
Prevents transcription by binding DNA-dependent RNA polymerase	Rifampin, rifabutin	Active against aerobic gram-positive bacteria including mycobacteria; no gram-negative activity
Disrupts bacteria DNA	Metronidazole	Active against anaerobic bacteria but not against aerobic or facultative anaerobes
	ANTIMETABOLITE	
Inhibits dihydropteroate synthase and disrupts folic acid synthesis	Sulfonamides	Effective against a broad range of gram-positive and gram-negative organisms and a drug of choice for urinary tract infections
Inhibits dihydropteroate reductase and disrupts folic acid synthesis	Trimethoprim	
Inhibits dihydropteroate synthase	Dapsone	Active against mycobacteria

3

Aerobic Gram-Positive Cocci

INTERESTING FACTS

- The Centers for Disease Control and Prevention (CDC) estimates there are 80,000 methicillin-resistant *Staphylococcus aureus* (MRSA) infections in the United States annually and more than 11,000 related deaths
- *Streptococcus pyogenes* (group A strep) is the most common cause of bacterial pharyngitis
- *Streptococcus agalactiae* (group B strep) is the most common cause of septicemia and meningitis in newborns
- *Streptococcus pneumoniae* is responsible for 3000 to 6000 cases of meningitis, 50,000 cases of septicemia, 400,000 hospitalizations for pneumonia, and 7 million cases of otitis media in the United States annually, despite the availability of effective vaccines
- Vancomycin resistance in enterococci was first described in 1986, spread globally, and now approximately 10% of *Enterococcus faecalis* and >90% of *Enterococcus faecium* are vancomycin resistant

The aerobic gram-positive cocci are a heterogeneous collection of spherical bacteria that are common residents in the mouth, gastrointestinal tract, genitourinary tract, and skin surface. The most important genera are *Staphylococcus*, *Streptococcus*, and *Enterococcus*.

Staphylococcus, Streptococcus, and *Enterococcus*

Genus	Historical Derivation
Staphylococcus	*Staphyle*, bunch of grapes; *coccus*, grain or berry; round, berrylike bacterial cells arranged in grapelike clusters
Streptococcus	*Streptus*, pliant; *coccus*, grain or berry; refers to the appearance of long, flexible chains of cocci
Enterococcus	*Enteron*, intestine; *coccus*, berry; intestinal coccus

The staphylococci, streptococci, and enterococci are gram-positive cocci, typically arranged in clusters (*Staphylococcus*), chains (*Streptococcus*), or pairs (*S. pneumoniae, Enterococcus*), and generally grow well aerobically and anaerobically. The structure of the thick, cross-linked cell wall allows these bacteria to survive on dry surfaces, such as hospital linens, tables, and door knobs. Virulence is determined by the ability to avoid the host immune system, adhere to and invade host cells, and produce toxins and hydrolytic enzymes. The species with the greatest potential for disease are *S. aureus*, *S. pyogenes*, and *S. pneumoniae*, illustrated by the wide variety of virulence factors expressed by each. Particularly noteworthy are a group of toxins: staphylococcal enterotoxins, exfoliative toxins, and toxic shock syndrome toxin, as well as *S. pyogenes* pyrogenic exotoxins. These toxins are termed **"superantigens"** because they stimulate a massive release of cytokines by the patient with resulting pathology.

Although staphylococci, streptococci, and enterococci are among the most common bacteria implicated in disease, it is important to remember that these are also common residents on the human body. Simply recovering these bacteria in a clinical specimen does not define disease. Disease is found in specific populations of patients and under well-defined conditions, so it is important to understand this epidemiology.

Diagnosis of *S. aureus* infections is generally not difficult because the organism grows readily in culture and nucleic acid amplification tests are widely used for the rapid detection of both methicillin-susceptible *S. aureus* (MSSA) and MRSA in clinical specimens. Likewise, diagnosis of infections caused by streptococci and enterococci is not difficult; however, because many of these bacteria are part of the normal microbial population in the body, care must be used to collect uncontaminated specimens.

Treatment of staphylococcal infections is difficult because the majority are MRSA strains. MRSA strains are not only resistant to methicillin but also all of the β-lactam antibiotics (including penicillins, cephalosporins, and carbapenems). Most streptococcal infections can be treated with penicillins, cephalosporins, or macrolides, although resistance is observed with *S. pneumoniae* and some other species of streptococci. Serious enterococcal infections are difficult to manage because antibiotic resistance is common.

Prevention of infections with all of these bacteria is difficult because most infections originate from the patient's own microbial population or through routine daily interactions. The one exception to this is neonatal disease caused by *S. agalactiae* because the infant acquires the infection from the mother. Pregnant women are screened for vaginal carriage with this organism shortly before delivery, and colonized women are treated with antibiotic prophylaxis. Polyvalent vaccines are currently only available for *S. pneumoniae* infections.

The most common species of *Staphylococcus* associated with disease is *S. aureus*, which will be the primary focus in the discussion of this genus. Other species, commonly referred to as **coagulase-negative staphylococci**, are primarily opportunistic pathogens, but three species are noteworthy: *Staphylococcus epidermidis*, *Staphylococcus saprophyticus*, and *Staphylococcus lugdunensis*.

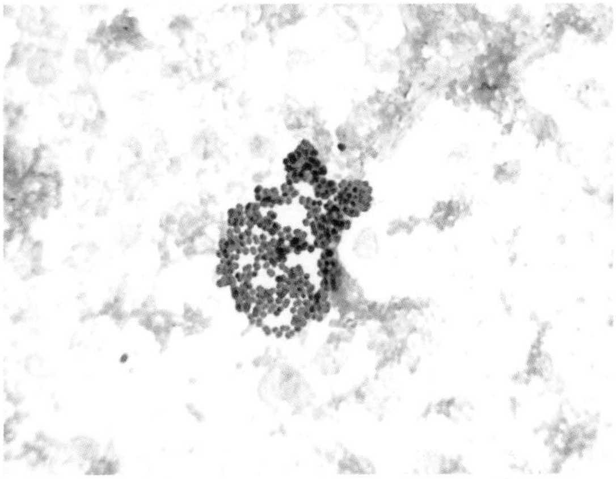

Staphylococcus aureus in a positive blood culture. Note the arrangement of gram-positive cocci in grapelike clusters.

Important Staphylococci

Species	Historical Derivation	Diseases
S. aureus	*Aureus*, golden or yellow; *S. aureus* colonies can turn yellow with age	Pyogenic infections; toxin-mediated infections
S. epidermidis	*Epidermidis*, epidermidis (outer skin)	Opportunistic infections (e.g., catheter-associated infections, surgical site infection where a foreign body is present, such as artificial heart valve [subacute endocarditis])
S. saprophyticus	*Saprophyticus*: *sapros*, putrid; *phyton*, plant (saprophytic or growing on dead tissue)	Urinary tract infections, particularly in sexually active young women
S. lugdunensis	*Lugdunensis*: *Lugdunun*, Latin name for Lyon where the organism was first isolated	Acute endocarditis in patients with native heart valves

The classification of the streptococci is confusing because three different schemes have been used: hemolytic patterns, serologic properties, and biochemical properties. This is an oversimplification but may help sort through the confusion. The streptococci can be divided into two groups: (1) **β-hemolytic** (complete hemolysis on blood agar) species that are subclassified by serologic properties (grouped from A to W); and (2) the **viridans streptococci** group that consists of α-hemolytic (cause partial hemolysis of blood) and γ-hemolytic (no hemolysis) species. Some species of viridans streptococci such as members of the *Streptococcus anginosus* group (with three species) are classified in both the β-hemolytic group and the viridans group because they are biochemically the same but have different hemolytic patterns. Disease caused by the *S. anginosus* group is the same regardless of their hemolytic properties. The following are the most important representatives of the β-hemolytic and viridans group streptococci.

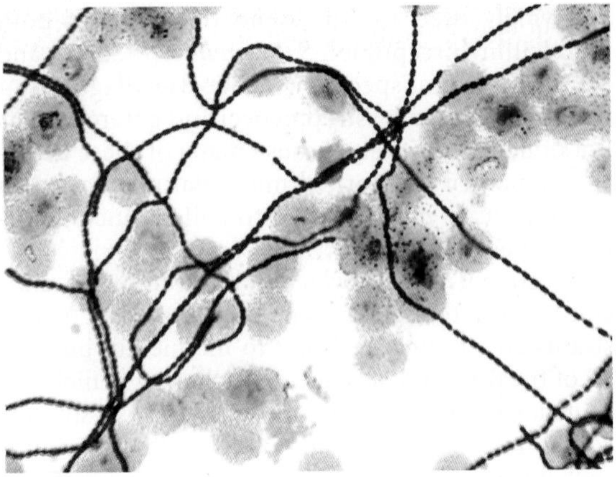

Streptococcus mitis (viridans group) in positive blood culture. Note the long chain of gram-positive cocci.

Important β-Hemolytic Streptococci

Group	Representative Species	Historical Derivation	Diseases
A	*S. pyogenes*	*Pyus*, pus; *gennaio*, producing (producing pus)	Pharyngitis, skin and soft-tissue infections, rheumatic fever, acute glomerulonephritis
	S. anginosus group	*Anginosus*, pertaining to angina	Abscesses
B	*S. agalactiae*	*Agalactia*, want of milk (original isolate associated with bovine mastitis)	Neonatal disease, endometritis, wound infections, urinary tract infections, pneumonia, skin and soft-tissue infections
C	*S. dysgalactiae*	*Dys*, ill; *galactia*, pertaining to milk (associated with bovine mastitis and loss of milk)	Pharyngitis, acute glomerulonephritis

Important Viridans Streptococci

Group	Representative Species	Historical Derivation	Diseases
Anginosus	*S. anginosus* group	*Anginosus*, pertaining to angina	Abscesses
Mitis	*Streptococcus mitis*	*Mitis*, mild (incorrectly thought to cause mild disease)	Subacute endocarditis, sepsis in neutropenic patients
	S. pneumoniae	*Pneumon*, the lungs (causes pneumonia)	Pneumonia, meningitis, sinusitis, otitis media, fulminant septicemia

Important Viridans Streptococci–cont'd

Group	Representative Species	Historical Derivation	Diseases
Mutans	*S. mutans*	*Mutans*, changing (cocci that may appear rodlike)	Dental caries, subacute endocarditis
Salivarius	*Streptococcus salivarius*	*Salivarius*, salivary (found in the mouth in saliva)	Subacute endocarditis
Bovis	*Streptococcus gallolyticus*	*Gallatum*, gallate; *lyticus*, to loosen (able to digest or hydrolyze methyl gallate)	Bacteremia associated with gastrointestinal cancer, meningitis

Enterococcus was classified as a *Streptococcus* but was reclassified in 1984. Two species of enterococci are particularly important because they cause similar diseases and are frequently resistant to most antibiotics.

Important Enterococci

Representative Species	Historical Derivation	Diseases
E. faecalis	*Faecalis*, relating to feces	Urinary tract infections, peritonitis, wound infections, endocarditis
E. faecium	*Faecium*, of feces	

The following are summaries for the major groups of gram-positive cocci.

STAPHYLOCOCCUS AUREUS

Diseases caused by *S. aureus* are divided into two groups: (1) localized pyogenic or "pus-producing" diseases that are characterized by tissue destruction mediated by hydrolytic enzymes and cytotoxins; and (2) diseases mediated by toxins that function as superantigens producing systemic diseases.

STAPHYLOCOCCUS AUREUS

Properties	• Ability to grow aerobically and anaerobically, over a wide range of temperatures, and in the presence of a high concentration of salt; the latter is important because these bacteria are a common cause of food poisoning
	• Polysaccharide **capsule** that protects the bacteria from phagocytosis
	• Cell surface proteins (**protein A**, clumping factor proteins) that mediate adherence of the bacteria to host tissues
	• **Catalase** that protects staphylococci from peroxides produced by neutrophils and macrophages
	• **Coagulase** converts fibrinogen to insoluble fibrin that forms clots and can protect *S. aureus* from phagocytosis
	• **Hydrolytic enzymes and cytotoxins**:
	  • Lipases, nucleases, and hyaluronidase that causes tissue destruction
	  • Cytotoxins (alpha, beta, delta, gamma, leukocidin) that lyse erythrocytes, neutrophils, macrophages, and other host cells
	• Toxins:
	  • **Enterotoxins** (many antigenically distinct) are the heat-stable and acid-resistant toxins responsible for food poisoning
	  • **Exfoliative toxins** A and B cause the superficial layers of skin to peel off (scalded skin syndrome)
	  • **Toxic shock syndrome toxin** is a heat- and protease-resistant toxin that mediates multiorgan pathology

Epidemiology	• Common cause of infections both in the community and in the hospital because the bacteria are easily spread person-to-person and through direct contact or exposure to contaminated bed linens, clothing, and other surfaces • Antibiotic-resistant strains (e.g., MRSA) are widely distributed in both the hospital and community

Continued

STAPHYLOCOCCUS AUREUS—cont'd	
Clinical Disease	*S. aureus* Pyogenic Diseases • **Impetigo**: localized skin infection characterized by pus-filled vesicles on a reddened or erythematous base; seen mostly in children on their face and limbs • **Folliculitis**: impetigo involving hair follicles, such as the beard area • **Furuncles (boils) and carbuncles**: large, pus-filled skin nodules; can progress to deeper layers of the skin and spread into the blood and other areas of the body • **Wound infections**: characterized by erythema and pus at the site of trauma or surgery; more difficult to treat if a foreign body is present (e.g., splinter, surgical suture); majority of infections both in the community and hospital are caused by MRSA; recurrent bouts of infections are common • **Pneumonia**: abscess formation in the lungs; observed primarily in the very young and old and frequently following viral infections of the respiratory tract • **Endocarditis**: infection of the endothelial lining of the heart; disease can progress rapidly and is associated with high mortality rate • **Osteomyelitis**: destruction of bones, particularly the highly vascularized areas of long bones in children • **Septic arthritis**—infection of joint spaces characterized by a swollen, reddened joint with accumulation of pus; the most common cause of septic arthritis in children *S. aureus* Toxin–Mediated Diseases • **Food poisoning**: after consumption of food contaminated with the **heat-stable enterotoxin**, the onset of severe vomiting, diarrhea, and stomach cramps is rapid (2 to 4 hours) but resolves within 24 hours. This is because the intoxication is caused by the preformed toxin present in the food rather than an infection where the bacteria would have to grow and produce toxin in the intestine • **Scalded skin syndrome**: bacteria in a localized infection produce the toxin that spreads through the blood and causes the outermost layer of the skin to blister and peel off; almost exclusively seen in very young children • **Toxic shock syndrome**: bacteria in a localized infection produce the toxin that affects multiple organs; characterized initially by fever, hypotension, and a diffuse, macular, erythematous rash. There is a very high mortality rate associated with this disease unless antibiotics are promptly administered and the local infection managed.

Diagnosis	• **Microscopy**: useful for pyogenic infections but not for bacteremia (too few organisms present), food poisoning (intoxication), or scalded skin syndrome and toxic shock syndrome (toxin production at localized site of infection and bacteria typically not in affected organ tissues)
	• **Culture**: organisms recovered on most laboratory media
	• **Nucleic acid amplification tests**: sensitive method for rapid detection of MSSA and MRSA in clinical specimens
	• **Identification tests**:
	  • **Catalase**: separates *Staphylococcus* (+) from *Streptococcus* and *Enterococcus* (–)
	  • **Coagulase**: separates *S. aureus* (+) from other species of *Staphylococcus* (–)
	  • **Protein A**: separates *S. aureus* (+) from other species of *Staphylococcus* (–)

Treatment, Control, Prevention	• Localized infections managed by incision and drainage
	• Antibiotic therapy indicated for systemic infections; empiric therapy should include antibiotics active against MRSA
	  • Oral therapy can include trimethoprim-sulfamethoxazole, clindamycin, or doxycycline
	  • Vancomycin is the drug of choice for intravenous therapy
	• Treatment is symptomatic for patients with food poisoning although the source of infection should be identified so other individuals will not be exposed
	• Proper cleansing of wounds and use of disinfectant help prevent infections
	• Thorough hand washing and covering exposed skin helps medical personnel prevent infection or spread to other patients
	• No vaccine is currently available

CLINICAL CASE

Staphylococcus aureus Endocarditis

Chen and Li[1] *described a 21-year-old woman with a history of intravenous drug abuse, HIV, and a CD4 count of 400 cells/mm*^{3} *who developed endocarditis caused by* S. aureus. *The patient had a 1-week history of fever, chest pain, and hemoptysis. Physical exam revealed a 3/6 pansystolic murmur and rhonchi in both lung fields. Multiple bilateral, cavitary lesions were observed by chest radiography and cultures of blood and sputum were positive for MSSA. The patient was treated with oxacillin for 6 weeks with resolution of the endocarditis and the pulmonary abscesses. This case illustrated the acute onset of* S. aureus *endocarditis and the frequency of complications caused by septic emboli.*

CLINICAL CASE

Staphylococcal Septic Shock After Treatment of a Furuncle

Moellering and colleagues[2] *described a 30-year-old woman who presented to their hospital with hypotension and respiratory failure. One month earlier the patient, who had previously been in good health, was seen at an urgent care clinic because of a red, hard, painful lump that had developed on her right lower leg 3 days earlier. The lesion was excised and drained, and she was treated with a 10-day course of cephalexin and trimethoprim-sulfamethoxazole. Culture of the lesion grew* S. aureus *that was resistant to oxacillin, penicillins, cephalosporins, levofloxacin, and erythromycin; it was also susceptible to vancomycin, clindamycin, tetracycline, and trimethoprim-sulfamethoxazole. Upon arrival in the emergency department, the patient was agitated, had a temperature of 39.6°C, blood pressure 113/53 mmHg, pulse 156 beats/minute, and respiratory rate 46 breaths/minute. Small cutaneous vesicles were noted on her forehead and abdomen. She rapidly deteriorated and was transferred to the intensive care unit where she was managed for septic shock. Despite clinical efforts, her hypoxemia, hypercardia, acidosis, and hypotension worsened and she died less than 12 hours after arrival at the hospital. Chest radiographs that were obtained upon admission to the hospital showed diffuse pulmonary infiltrates with small areas of cavitation in both lungs; a computed tomography (CT) scan of the abdomen and pelvis showed ascites and lymph node enlargement; and a CT scan of the brain showed multiple foci of hyperintensity in the frontal, temporal, parietal, and occipital lobes.* S. aureus, *with the same antibiotic susceptibility profile as the isolate from the leg furuncle, was cultured from blood and multiple tissue specimens. The clinical diagnosis was that this woman died of sepsis due to infection with community-acquired MRSA that progressed from a localized furuncle to necrotizing pneumonia and then overwhelming sepsis with multiple disseminated septic emboli. This infection illustrates the potential pathogenesis of drug-resistant* S. aureus *in an otherwise healthy individual.*

CLINICAL CASE

Staphylococcal Toxic Shock Syndrome

Todd and colleagues[3] *were the first investigators to describe a pediatric disease they called "toxic shock syndrome". This patient illustrates the clinical course of this disease. A 15-year-old girl was admitted to the hospital with a 2-day history of pharyngitis and vaginitis associated with vomiting and watery diarrhea. She was febrile and hypotensive on admission, with a diffuse erythematous rash over her entire body. Laboratory tests were consistent with acidosis, oliguria, and disseminated intravascular coagulation with severe thrombocytopenia. Her chest radiograph showed bilateral infiltrates suggestive of "shock lung". She was admitted to the hospital intensive care unit where she was stabilized and she improved gradually over a 17-day period. On the 3rd day fine desquamation started on her face, trunk, and extremities and progressed to peeling of the palms and soles by the 14th day. All cultures were negative except from the throat and vagina, from which* S. aureus *was isolated. This case illustrates the initial presentation of toxic shock syndrome, the multiorgan toxicity, and the protracted period of recovery.*

CLINICAL CASE

Staphylococcal Food Poisoning

A report published in the CDC Morbidity and Mortality Weekly Report[4] illustrates many important features of staphylococcal food poisoning. A total of 18 persons attending a retirement party became ill approximately 3 to 4 hours after eating. The most common symptoms were nausea (94%), vomiting (89%), and diarrhea (72%). Relatively few individuals had fever or headache (11%). The symptoms lasted a median of 24 hours. The illness was associated with eating ham at the party. A sample of the cooked ham tested positive for staphylococcal enterotoxin type A. A food preparer had cooked the ham at home, transported it to her workplace, sliced it while it was still hot, and then refrigerated the ham in a large plastic container covered with foil. The ham was served cold the next day. Cooking the ham would kill any contaminating S. aureus, *so it is likely the ham was contaminated after it was cooked. The delays involved in refrigerating the ham and the fact it was stored in a single container allowed the organism to proliferate and produce enterotoxin. Type A toxin is the most common toxin associated with human disease. The rapid onset and short duration of nausea, vomiting, and diarrhea is typical of this disease. Care must be used to avoid contamination of salted meats such as ham because reheating the food at a later time will not inactivate the heat-stable toxin.*

β-HEMOLYTIC STREPTOCOCCI

Two species of β-hemolytic streptococci will be discussed here: *S. pyogenes* and *S. agalactiae*. Other important species should be mentioned here briefly. *S. anginosus* and related bacteria are classified with both the β-hemolytic streptococci and the viridans streptococci and are discussed below; however, it should be recognized that these are important causes of deep tissue abscesses. *Streptococcus dysgalactiae* is an uncommon cause of pharyngitis. This is mentioned because the disease resembles pharyngitis caused by *S. pyogenes* and can be complicated with acute glomerulonephritis but not rheumatic fever (two complications seen with *S. pyogenes*).

Diseases caused by *S. pyogenes* are subdivided into suppurative (characterized by formation of pus) and nonsuppurative. **Suppurative diseases** range from pharyngitis to localized skin and soft-tissue infections to necrotizing fasciitis ("flesh eating" bacterial infection) and streptococcal toxic shock syndrome. **Nonsuppurative diseases** are an autoimmune complication following streptococcal pharyngitis (rheumatic fever, acute glomerulonephritis) and pyodermal infections (only acute glomerulonephritis). Antibodies directed against specific M proteins cross-react with host tissues in nonsuppurative diseases.

STREPTOCOCCUS PYOGENES

Properties

- Outer hyaluronic acid **capsule** (single serotype) protects *S. pyogenes* from phagocytic clearance (nonimmunogenic)
- **M proteins**, M-like proteins, and C5a peptidase in the cell wall blocks complement-mediated phagocytosis
- M proteins and F protein facilitate adherence and invasion into epithelial cells
- **Hydrolytic enzymes**:
  - Streptolysin S and streptolysin O lyse erythrocytes, leukocytes, platelets, and cultured cells
  - Streptokinase lyse blood clots and fibrin deposits, facilitating the rapid spread
  - DNases lyse free DNA in abscesses, facilitating rapid spread
- Toxins:
  - Four distinct heat-labile **streptococcal pyrogenic exotoxins** enhance release of proinflammatory cytokines responsible for clinical manifestations of severe streptococcal diseases

STREPTOCOCCUS PYOGENES—cont'd	
Epidemiology	• Person-to-person spread by respiratory droplets (pharyngitis) or through breaks in skin after direct contact with infected person, fomite, or arthropod vector • Pharyngitis and soft-tissue infections typically caused by strains with different M proteins • Transient colonization in upper respiratory tract and skin surface with disease caused by recently acquired strains (before protective antibodies are produced) • Most common cause of bacterial pharyngitis • Individuals at higher risk for disease include children from 5 to 15 years old (pharyngitis); children from 2 to 5 years old with poor personal hygiene (pyoderma); patients with soft-tissue infection (streptococcal toxic shock syndrome); patients with prior streptococcal pharyngitis (rheumatic fever, glomerulonephritis) or soft-tissue infection (glomerulonephritis) • Pharyngitis is most common in the cold months; no seasonal incidence for soft-tissue infections
Clinical Disease	• **Pharyngitis**: reddened pharynx with exudates generally present; cervical lymphadenopathy can be prominent • **Scarlet fever**: complication of streptococcal pharyngitis; diffuse erythematous rash beginning on the chest and spreading to the extremities • **Pyoderma**: localized skin infection with vesicles progressing to pustules; no evidence of systemic disease • **Erysipelas**: localized skin infection with pain, inflammation, lymph node enlargement, and systemic symptoms • **Cellulitis**: infection of the skin that involves the subcutaneous tissues • **Necrotizing fasciitis**: deep infection of the skin that involves destruction of muscle and fat layers • **Streptococcal toxic shock syndrome**: multiorgan systemic infection resembling staphylococcal toxic shock syndrome; however, most patients are bacteremic and with evidence of fasciitis
	• **Rheumatic fever**: nonsuppurative complication of streptococcal pharyngitis characterized by inflammatory changes of the heart (pancarditis), joints (arthralgias to arthritis), blood vessels, and subcutaneous tissues • **Acute glomerulonephritis**: nonsuppurative complication of streptococcal pharyngitis or soft-tissue infections characterized by acute inflammation of the renal glomeruli with edema, hypertension, hematuria, and proteinuria
Diagnosis	• Microscopy is useful in soft-tissue infections but not pharyngitis or nonsuppurative complications • Direct tests for the group A antigen are useful for the diagnosis of streptococcal pharyngitis • Isolates identified by catalase (negative), positive L-pyrrolidonyl arylamidase reaction, susceptibility to bacitracin, and presence of group-specific antigen (group A antigen) • Antistreptolysin O (ASO) test is useful for confirming rheumatic fever or glomerulonephritis associated with streptococcal pharyngitis; anti-DNase B test (not antistreptolysin O) should be performed for glomerulonephritis associated with pharyngitis or soft-tissue infections
Treatment, Control, Prevention	• Penicillin V or amoxicillin used to treat pharyngitis; oral cephalosporin or macrolide for penicillin-allergic patients; intravenous penicillin plus clindamycin used for systemic infections • Oropharyngeal carriage occurring after treatment can be retreated; treatment is not indicated for prolonged asymptomatic carriage because antibiotics disrupt normal protective flora • Starting antibiotic therapy within 10 days in patients with pharyngitis prevents rheumatic fever • For patients with a history of rheumatic fever, antibiotic prophylaxis is required before procedures (e.g., dental) that can induce bacteremias leading to endocarditis • For glomerulonephritis, no specific antibiotic treatment or prophylaxis is indicated

CLINICAL CASE

Streptococcal Necrotizing Fasciitis and Toxic Shock Syndrome

Filbin and colleagues[5] describe the dramatic clinical course of disease caused by group A Streptococcus *in a previously healthy 25-year-old man. Two days before admission to the hospital he noticed a lesion on the dorsum of his right hand and thought it was an insect bite. The next day the hand became swollen and painful and he felt ill. The next morning he had chills and a temperature of 38.6°C. That evening his mother found him obtunded, vomiting, and incontinent and he was rushed to the emergency department. At the time of admission his blood pressure was 73/25 mmHg, temperature 37.9°C, pulse 145 beats/minute, and respiratory rate 30 breaths/minute. The right hand was mottled and swollen, with a 1-cm black eschar on the dorsum, and swelling up his forearm. Manipulations of the fingers resulted in extreme pain. A radiograph of the hand revealed prominent soft-tissue swelling and chest radiograph showed findings consistent with interstitial edema. A diagnosis of severe sepsis was made and intravenous vancomycin and clindamycin were administered. The patient was taken to surgery 4 hours after arrival in the hospital and complete debridement of the skin and fascia up to the elbow of the right arm was required. Pathologic examination of the tissues revealed liquefactive necrosis involving the fascial planes and superficial fat. Small blood vessel intraluminal thrombi and infiltration of mononuclear cells and neutrophils was also observed in the tissues, as well as abundant gram-positive cocci subsequently identified as group A streptococci. Over the course of this patient's hospitalization he developed severe systemic manifestations of hypotension, coagulopathy, renal failure, and respiratory insufficiency, consistent with the diagnosis of streptococcal toxic shock syndrome. The patient was aggressively treated with penicillin G, clindamycin, vancomycin, and cefepime, and slowly improved until his discharge 16 days after hospitalization. This case illustrates the rapid progression of disease from a relatively innocuous superficial skin lesion to necrotizing fasciitis, septic shock, and multiorgan involvement. Mortality with necrotizing fasciitis and toxic shock syndrome approaches 50%, and is only successfully managed with aggressive surgical debridement and antibiotic therapy.*

CLINICAL CASE

Acute Rheumatic Fever Associated with *Streptococcus pyogenes* Infection

Acute rheumatic fever is relatively rare in the United States, which can complicate the diagnosis. Casey and colleagues[6] described a 28-year-old woman who presented with a history of joint pain and swelling, initially in her right foot and ankle that resolved after a few days and then pain and swelling in other joints. Upon physical examination, diffuse tenderness of the joints was noted on palpation but no swelling or erythema. Cardiovascular examination was notable for tachycardia, but no murmurs were detected. The diagnosis of a "viral infection" was made and she was discharged with a course of nonsteroidal antiinflammatory drugs. After 5 days, the patient returned with progressive shortness of breath and persistent pain in her knee. Physical examination revealed a low-grade temperature, tachycardia, and a new heart murmur with mitral valve regurgitation. The left knee was warm to the touch, the range of motion was limited, and it was painful on flexion. The diagnosis of bacterial endocarditis was considered but all blood cultures were negative. Medical history revealed that as a child she became short of breath easily and was unable to play with other children. The patient's history of dyspnea is consistent with rheumatic heart disease, as is the combination of fever, mitral regurgitation, and migratory arthritis. Recent evidence of infection with group A Streptococcus *is required to confirm the diagnosis, but throat culture is insensitive because symptoms of acute rheumatic fever appear 2 to 3 weeks after the infection. The diagnosis was confirmed by demonstrating elevated antistreptolysin and anti-DNase B antibodies.*

S. agalactiae infections are most common in newborns, acquired either *in utero* or during the first week of life, and are associated with a high mortality or significant neurologic sequelae.

STREPTOCOCCUS AGALACTIAE	
Properties	• Outer polysaccharide **capsule** (multiple serotypes) protects from phagocytic clearance • **Sialic acid** blocks complement mediated phagocytosis
Epidemiology	• Asymptomatic colonization of the upper respiratory tract and genitourinary tract • Early-onset disease acquired by neonates from mother during pregnancy or at time of birth • Women with genital colonization are at risk for postpartum disease • Neonates are at higher risk for infection if: (1) there is premature rupture of membranes, prolonged labor, preterm birth, or disseminated maternal group B streptococcal disease; and (2) mother is without type-specific antibodies and has low complement levels • Men and nonpregnant women with diabetes mellitus, cancer, or alcoholism are at increased risk for disease • No seasonal incidence
Clinical Disease	• **Early-onset neonatal disease**: within 7 days of birth, infected newborns develop signs and symptoms of pneumonia, meningitis, and sepsis • **Late-onset neonatal disease**: more than 1 week after birth, neonates develop signs and symptoms of bacteremia with meningitis • **Infections in pregnant women**: most often present as postpartum endometritis, wound infections, and urinary tract infections; disseminated complications may occur • **Infections in other adult patients**: most common diseases include pneumonia, bone and joint infections, and skin and soft-tissue infections
Diagnosis	• Microscopy useful for meningitis (cerebrospinal fluid), pneumonia (lower respiratory secretions), and wound infections (exudates) • Antigen tests are less sensitive than microscopy and should not be used
	• Culture is a sensitive test for detection of vaginal carriage in pregnant women if a selective broth (i.e., LIM) is used • Nucleic acid amplification tests are commercially available and are as sensitive as culture and more rapid • Isolates are identified by demonstration of group-specific cell wall carbohydrate or positive nucleic acid amplification test
Treatment, Control, Prevention	• Penicillin G is the drug of choice; combination of penicillin and aminoglycoside is used in patients with serious infections; a cephalosporin or vancomycin is used for patients allergic to penicillin • For high-risk babies, penicillin is given at least 4 hours before delivery • No vaccine is currently available

CLINICAL CASE

Group B Streptococcal Disease in a Neonate

The following is a description of late-onset group B streptococcal disease in a neonate.[7] An infant male weighing 3400 g was delivered spontaneously at term. Physical examinations of the infant were normal during the first week of life; however, the child started feeding irregularly during the second week. On day 13, the baby was admitted to the hospital with generalized seizures. A small amount of cloudy cerebrospinal fluid was collected by lumbar puncture, and S. agalactiae *serotype III was isolated from culture. Despite the prompt initiation of therapy, the baby developed hydrocephalus, necessitating implantation of an atrioventricular shunt. The infant was discharged at age 3.5 months with retardation of psychomotor development. This patient illustrates neonatal meningitis caused by the most commonly implicated serotype of group B streptococci in late-onset disease and the complications associated with this infection.*

STREPTOCOCCUS PNEUMONIAE

S. pneumoniae is the most important member of the viridans streptococci and is typically considered separately because it is one of the most common causes of a spectrum of diseases: pneumonia, meningitis, otitis, and sinusitis. Recurrent infections with this bacterium are common because immunity to infection is mediated by the presence of antibodies to the polysaccharide capsule, and nearly 100 unique serotypes have been described.

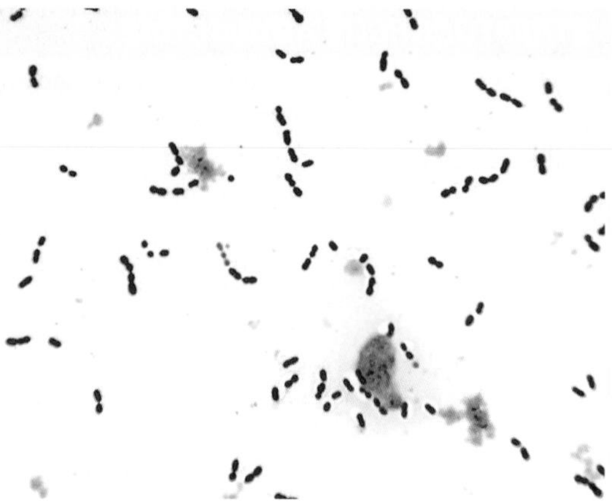

Streptococcus pneumoniae in positive blood culture. Note the arrangement of cocci in pairs and short chains.

STREPTOCOCCUS PNEUMONIAE	
Properties	• Outer **polysaccharide capsule** (multiple serotypes) protects from phagocytic clearance • Surface protein adhesins bind bacteria to epithelial cells • Phosphorylcholine binds to receptors on the surface of endothelial cells, leukocytes, and platelets; upon entering the cells, the bacteria are protected from opsonization and phagocytosis • Immunoglobulin (Ig)A protease prevents inactivation of bacteria trapped in mucus by secretory IgA • Pneumolysis is a cytotoxin similar to streptolysin O; binds to cholesterol in host cell wall and creates pores, destroying epithelial and phagocytic cells
Epidemiology	• The most virulent member of the viridans streptococci • Most infections are caused by endogenous spread from the colonized nasopharynx or oropharynx to distal site (e.g., lungs, sinuses, ears, meninges) • Person-to-person spread through infectious droplets is rare • Colonization is highest in young children and their contacts • Individuals with antecedent viral respiratory tract disease or other conditions that interfere with bacterial clearance from respiratory tract are at increased risk for pneumonia, otitis media (young children), and sinusitis (all ages) • Children and the elderly are at greatest risk for meningitis • People with hematologic disorder (e.g., malignancy, sickle cell disease) or functional asplenia are at risk for fulminant sepsis • Although the organism is ubiquitous, disease is more common in cool months
Clinical Disease	• **Pneumonia**: acute onset of chills and sustained fever; productive cough with blood-tinged sputum; lobar consolidation • **Meningitis**: severe infection involving the meninges, with headache, fever, and sepsis; high mortality and severe neurologic deficits in survivors • **Sinusitis and otitis media**: common cause of acute infections of the paranasal sinuses and ear; typically preceded by a viral infection of the upper respiratory tract with leukocytes infiltration and obstruction of the sinuses and ear canal • **Fulminant sepsis**: bacteremia is more common in patients with pneumonia and meningitis than with sinusitis or otitis media; fulminant sepsis in asplenic patients

***STREPTOCOCCUS PNEUMONIAE*—cont'd**	
Diagnosis	• Microscopy is highly sensitive, as is culture, unless the patient has been treated with antibiotics • Specific antigen tests for pneumococcal C polysaccharide are sensitive with cerebrospinal fluid for the diagnosis of meningitis but should not be used with other specimen types or infections • Nucleic acid amplification tests are not commonly used for diagnosis except for meningitis • Culture requires use of enriched-nutrient media (e.g., sheep blood agar); organism is susceptible to many antibiotics, so culture can be negative in partially treated patients • Isolates identified by catalase (negative), susceptibility to optochin, and solubility in bile
Treatment, Control, Prevention	• Penicillin is the drug of choice for susceptible strains, although resistance is increasingly common • Vancomycin combined with ceftriaxone is used for empiric therapy; monotherapy with a cephalosporin, fluoroquinolone, or vancomycin can be used in patients with susceptible isolates • Immunization with 13-valent **conjugated vaccine** is recommended for all children younger than 2 years of age; a 23-valent **polysaccharide vaccine** is recommended for adults at risk for disease

CLINICAL CASE

Pneumonia Caused by *Streptococcus pneumoniae*

Costa and associates[8] described a 68-year-old woman who was in good health until 3 days before hospitalization. She developed fever, chills, increased weakness, and a productive cough with pleuritic chest pain. On admission, she was febrile, had an elevated pulse and respiration rate, and was in moderate respiratory distress. Initial laboratory values showed leucopenia, anemia, and acute renal failure. Chest radiograph demonstrated infiltrates in the right and left lower lobes with pleural effusions. Therapy with a fluoroquinolone was initiated, and blood and respiratory cultures were positive for S. pneumoniae. *Additional tests (serum and urine protein electrophoresis) revealed the patient had multiple myeloma. The patient's infection resolved with a 14-day course of antibiotics. This patient illustrates the typical picture of pneumococcal lobar pneumonia and the increased susceptibility to infection in patients with defects in their ability to clear encapsulated organisms.*

VIRIDANS STREPTOCOCCI

The viridans streptococci are commonly thought of as a homogeneous collection of streptococci, but in reality the individual species of bacteria are associated with distinct infections (e.g., abscess formation, dental caries, subacute endocarditis, septicemia, and meningitis) so it is important to know the specific disease associations.

VIRIDANS STREPTOCOCCI	
Properties	• Although relatively avirulent, individual species have a predilection of producing disease in specific anatomic sites (abscess formation, endocarditis, meningitis)
Epidemiology	• Ubiquitous colonizers of mucosal surfaces (mouth, gastrointestinal tract, genitourinary tract); not commonly found on skin surface • Opportunistic pathogen • No seasonal incidence of disease
Clinical Disease	• Abscess formation in deep tissues: associated with the *S. anginosus* group • Septicemia in neutropenic patients: associated with *S. mitis* • Subacute endocarditis: associated with *S. mitis*, *S. mutans*, and *S. salivarius* • Dental caries: associated with *S. mutans* • Malignancies of gastrointestinal tract: associated with *S. gallolyticus* subsp. *gallolyticus* • Meningitis: associated with *S. gallolyticus* subsp. *pasteurianus* and *S. mitis*

Continued

VIRIDANS STREPTOCOCCI—cont'd	
Diagnosis	• Diagnosis of most viridans group infections is based on clinical presentation and isolation of the organism in blood or surgically collected specimens • Biochemical identification of most species is not accurate so either sequencing or mass spectrometry must be done
Treatment, Control, Prevention	• With the exception of the *S. mitis* group, most viridans streptococci are highly susceptible to penicillins and cephalosporins • Vancomycin should be used for resistant bacteria or in penicillin-allergic patients

CLINICAL CASE

Endocarditis Caused by *Streptococcus mutans*

Greka and colleagues[9] described a 50-year-old man who was admitted to their hospital complaining of acute left flank pain that developed while bicycling. The patient's medical history included the diagnosis of Hodgkin disease 15 years previously, which was treated with chemotherapy, radiation therapy, and splenectomy. On examination the patient had a temperature of 37.3°C, blood pressure 158/72 mmHg, pulse 76 beats/minute, and respiratory rate 20 breaths/minute. A holosystolic soft murmur, grade 2/6 was heard at the apex, with radiation to the axilla (consistent with mitral regurgitation), and a crescendo–decrescendo systolic murmur, grade 2/6 also was heard at the border (consistent with aortic stenosis). Seven hours after the presentation, the patient's temperature rose to 37.8°C and he was admitted to the hospital. Urinalysis was performed and blood and urine cultures were collected. The urinalysis was negative, which is inconsistent with flank pain related to pyelonephritis. Renal ischemia is consistent with the acute onset and severe pain and imaging studies revealed a hypodense renal area. The presence of fever, new heart murmurs, and renal infarction are strongly suggestive of an infectious process, specifically endocarditis. This was confirmed by the isolation of S. mutans *from multiple blood cultures collected during the first week of the patient's hospitalization.* S. mutans*, a well-recognized cause of bacterial endocarditis, is able to spread from the mouth to the heart valve, adhere to the valve and grow, leading to vegetations that can shed microcolonies resulting in emboli. This patient was at particular risk for this because he was asplenic and unable to effectively clear the organisms when they were initially introduced into the blood. The patient was treated successfully with a 4-week course of ceftriaxone.*

ENTEROCOCCUS

Enterococci are one of the most common causes of nosocomial (hospital-acquired) infections, particularly in patients treated with broad-spectrum cephalosporins (antibiotics that are inherently inactive against enterococci).

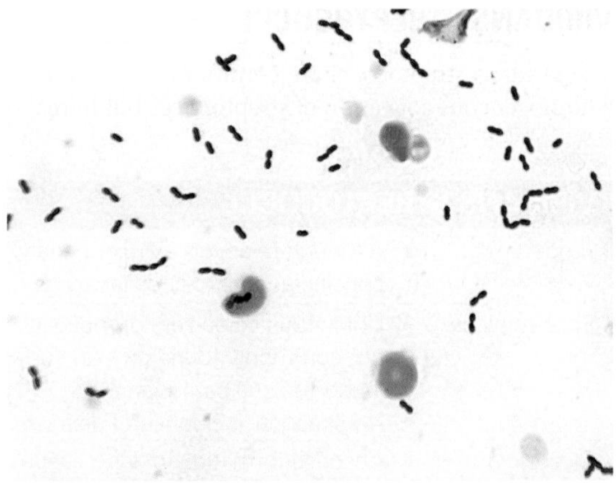

Enterococcus faecium in positive blood culture. Note the arrangement of pairs of cocci resemble *Streptococcus pneumoniae.*

ENTEROCOCCUS FAECALIS AND *ENTEROCOCCUS FAECIUM*	
Properties	• **Antibiotic resistance** limits effective antibiotic therapy
Epidemiology	• Colonizes the gastrointestinal tracts of humans and animals; spreads to other mucosal surfaces if broad-spectrum antibiotics eliminate the normal bacterial population • Cell wall structure typical of gram-positive bacteria, which allows survival on environmental surfaces for prolonged periods • Most infections endogenous (from patient's bacterial flora); some caused by patient-to-patient spread • Patients at increased risk include those hospitalized for prolonged periods and treated with broad-spectrum antibiotics (particularly cephalosporins, to which enterococci are naturally resistant)
Clinical Disease	• **Urinary tract infection**: dysuria and pyuria, cost commonly in hospitalized patients with an indwelling urinary catheter and receiving broad-spectrum cephalosporin antibiotics • **Peritonitis**: abdominal swelling and tenderness after abdominal trauma or surgery; patients are typically acutely ill and febrile; most infections are polymicrobial • **Bacteremia and endocarditis**: bacteremia associated with localized infection or endocarditis; endocarditis can be acute or chronic, involving the heart endothelium or valves
Diagnosis	• Grows readily on common, nonselective media • Differentiated from related organisms by simple tests (catalase negative, L-pyrrolidonyl arylamidase–positive, resistant to bile and optochin)
Treatment, Control, Prevention	• Therapy for serious infections requires combination of an aminoglycoside with a cell wall–active antibiotic (penicillin, ampicillin, or vancomycin); newer agents used for antibiotic-resistant bacteria include linezolid, daptomycin, tigecycline, and quinupristin/dalfopristin • Antibiotic resistance to each of these drugs is becoming increasingly common, and infections with many isolates (particularly *E. faecium*) are not treatable with any antibiotics • Prevention and control of infections require careful restriction of antibiotic use and implementation of appropriate infection-control practices

CLINICAL CASE

Enterococcal Endocarditis

Zimmer and associates[10] described the epidemiology of enterococcal infections and the difficulties in treating a patient with endocarditis. The patient was a 40-year-old man with hepatitis C, hypertension, and end-stage renal disease who developed fevers and chills during hemodialysis. In the 2 months before this episode, he was treated with ampicillin, levofloxacin, and gentamicin for group B streptococcal endocarditis. Cultures performed during the hemodialysis grew E. faecalis *resistant to levofloxacin and gentamicin. Because the patient had an allergic reaction to ampicillin, he was treated with linezolid. Echocardiography showed vegetation on the mitral and tricuspid valves. Over a 3-week period, the patient's cardiac output deteriorated so that the patient was desensitized to ampicillin, and therapy was switched to ampicillin and streptomycin. After 25 days of hospitalization, the patient's damaged heart valves were replaced, and therapy was extended for an additional 6 weeks. Thus use of broad-spectrum antibiotics predisposed this patient with previously damaged heart valves to endocarditis caused by* Enterococcus, *and treatment was complicated by resistance of the isolate to many commonly used antibiotics.*

REFERENCES

1. Chen JY, Li YH. Images in clinical medicine. Multiple pulmonary bacterial abscesses. *N Engl J Med.* 2006;355:e27.
2. Moellering Jr RC, Abbott GF, Ferraro MJ. Case records of the Massachusetts General Hospital. Case 2-2011. A 30-year-old woman with shock after treatment of a furuncle. *N Engl J Med.* 2011;364:266–275.
3. Todd J, Fishaut M, Kapral F, Welch T. Toxic-shock syndrome associated with phage-group-I staphylococci. *Lancet.* 1978;2:1116–1118.
4. Centers for Disease Control and Prevention. Outbreak of staphylococcal food poisoning associated with precooked ham—Florida. *MMWR Morb Mortal Wkly Rep.* 1997;1997(46):1189–1191.
5. Filbin MR, Ring DC, Wessels MR, Avery LL, Kradin RL. Case records of the Massachusetts General Hospital. Case 2-2009. A 25-year-old man with pain and swelling of the right hand and hypotension. *N Engl J Med.* 2009;360:281–290.
6. Casey JD, Solomon DH, Gaziano TA, Miller AL, Loscalzo J. Clinical problem-solving. A patient with migrating polyarthralgias. *N Engl J Med.* 2013;369:75–80.
7. Hammersen G, Bartholomé K, Oppermann HC, Wille L, Lutz P. Group B streptococci: a new threat to the newborn. *Eur J Pediatr.* 1977;126:189–197.
8. Costa DB, Shin B, Cooper DL. Pneumococcemia as the presenting feature of multiple myeloma. *Am J Hematol.* 2004;77:277–281.
9. Greka A, Bhatia RS, Sabir SH, Dekker JP. Case records of the Massachusetts General Hospital. Case 4-2013. A 50-year-old man with acute flank pain. *N Engl J Med.* 2013;368:466–472.
10. Zimmer SM, Caliendo AM, Thigpen MC, Somani J. Failure of linezolid treatment for enterococcal endocarditis. *Clin Infect Dis.* 2003;37:e29–30.

4

Aerobic Gram-Positive Rods

INTERESTING FACTS

- Anthrax is primarily a disease of herbivores (e.g., cattle, sheep) acquired by ingestion or inhalation of the spores of *Bacillus anthracis.* Humans are accidental victims with infections most commonly acquired by contact with contaminated animal products
- It is estimated that *Bacillus cereus* is responsible for almost 65,000 episodes of acute food poisoning, characterized by nausea and vomiting and indistinguishable from *Staphylococcus aureus* food poisoning
- The most common food products associated with *Listeria monocytogenes* infections are processed meats, including hot dogs and turkey franks, soft cheeses, unpasteurized milk, and uncooked vegetables. The bacteria tolerates salt and grows in refrigerator temperatures down to freezing
- Before vaccination, between 100,000 and 200,000 people in the United States were infected with *Corynebacterium diphtheriae*; today, only one case has been reported since 2002

The aerobic gram-positive rods can be subdivided into spore-forming rods (*Bacillus* is the most common) and non–spore-forming rods (*Listeria* and *Corynebacterium* are the most common). For this chapter, I will focus on four clinically important species, recognizing that there are many other species that may be isolated in clinical specimens.

Clinically Important Species

Species	Derivation	Diseases
B. anthracis	*Bacillum*, a small rod; *anthrax*, charcoal (refers to the black, necrotic wound associated with cutaneous anthrax)	Anthrax (cutaneous, gastrointestinal, inhalation)
B. cereus	*Cereus*, waxen (refers to typical dull surface of colonies)	Gastroenteritis; ocular infections; anthrax-like pulmonary disease
L. monocytogenes	*Listeria*, named after the English surgeon, Lord Joseph Lister; *monocytum*, monocyte; *gennaio*, produce (stimulates monocyte production in rabbits although not seen in human infections)	Neonatal disease with abscesses, granulomas, and meningitis; influenza-like illness in healthy adults; primary septicemia and meningitis in pregnant women and immunocompromised adults
C. diphtheriae	*Coryne*, a club (club-shaped rods); *diphthera*, leather or skin (reference to leathery membrane that forms over the pharynx)	Diphtheria (respiratory, cutaneous)

BACILLUS ANTHRACIS AND BACILLUS CEREUS

Due to their nature of producing endospores (heat-resistant, dormant bacterial forms), *Bacillus* can survive for years in the most harsh environments, so many species can be isolated in nature. Of this diverse collection, two are clinically important for very different reasons: *B. anthracis* because it causes anthrax and *B. cereus* because it is an opportunistic pathogen. In order for *B. anthracis* to produce disease, it must carry genes for capsule production, and three individual proteins (protective antigen, edema factor, and lethal factor) that combine to form two toxins (edema toxin and lethal toxin). *B. cereus* carries genes for heat-stable and heat-labile enterotoxins, which are responsible for gastrointestinal infections, and cytotoxic enzymes that cause tissue destruction in opportunistic infections.

Anthrax is primarily an animal disease, so we should call this a **zoonotic disease** and acknowledge that humans are accidental victims. Animal herds in industrial countries are vaccinated for anthrax; therefore this is primarily a disease of resource-limited countries. That is, until it was recognized that this is an ideal biological weapon. For that reason, we can never consider this a disease of exclusive historical interest. *B. cereus* food poisoning is all too common because the organism is ubiquitous in the environment. So it is important to recognize the symptoms of disease and the public health implications of improperly prepared and stored foods.

Diagnosis of *B. anthracis* and *B. cereus* is challenging, but for different reasons. *B. anthracis* is rarely seen, so it may not be initially suspected and the microbiologist would generally have little or no experience identifying this organism. Obviously this would change if there was a recognized bioterrorism outbreak. In contrast, *B. cereus* is commonly isolated in the lab and is easy to identify; however, because most isolates are clinically insignificant contaminants, the importance of the organism may not be initially recognized.

BACILLUS ANTHRACIS	
Properties	• **Polypeptide capsule** consisting of poly-D-glutamic acid; inhibits phagocytosis • **Edema toxin** (protective antigen + edema factor) with adenylate cyclase activity that is responsible for fluid accumulation • **Lethal toxin** (protective antigen + lethal factor) stimulates macrophages to release TNF-α, IL-1β, and other proinflammatory cytokines
Epidemiology	• *B. anthracis* primarily infects herbivores, with humans as accidental hosts • Rarely isolated in industrial countries but is prevalent in impoverished areas where vaccination of animals is not practiced • The greatest danger of anthrax in industrial countries is the use of *B. anthracis* as an agent of bioterrorism
Clinical Disease	• **Cutaneous anthrax** (most common in humans): painless papule progresses to ulceration with surrounding vesicles and then to eschar formation; painful lymphadenopathy, edema, and systemic signs may develop • **Gastrointestinal anthrax** (most common in herbivores): ulcers form at site of invasion (e.g., mouth, esophagus, intestine) leading to regional lymphadenopathy, edema, and sepsis • **Inhalation anthrax (bioterrorism)**: initial nonspecific signs followed by the rapid onset of sepsis with fever, edema, and lymphadenopathy (mediastinal lymph nodes); meningeal symptoms in half of the patients, and most patients will die unless treatment is initiated immediately
Diagnosis	• Microscopy of wound specimens and blood typically positive; grows readily in culture • Preliminary identification is based on microscopic (gram-positive, nonmotile rods) and colonial (nonhemolytic, adherent colonies) morphology; confirmed by demonstrating capsule and either a positive direct fluorescent antibody test for the specific cell wall polysaccharide or positive nucleic acid amplification test for the toxin genes

BACILLUS ANTHRACIS—cont'd	
Treatment, Control, Prevention	• Inhalation or gastrointestinal anthrax should be treated with ciprofloxacin or doxycycline, combined with one or two additional antibiotics (e.g., rifampin, vancomycin, penicillin, imipenem, clindamycin, clarithromycin) • Naturally acquired cutaneous anthrax can be treated with amoxicillin • Vaccination of animal herds and people in endemic areas can control disease, but spores are difficult to eliminate from contaminated soils • Vaccination of animal herds and at-risk humans is effective, although the development of a less toxic vaccine is desired

CLINICAL CASE

Inhalation Anthrax

Bush and associates[1] reported the first case of inhalation anthrax in the 2001 bioterrorism attack in the United States. The patient was a 63-year-old man living in Florida who had a 4-day history of fever, myalgias, and malaise without localizing symptoms. His wife brought him to the regional hospital because he awoke from sleep with fever, emesis, and confusion. On physical examination he had a temperature of 39°C, blood pressure of 150/80 mmHg, pulse of 110 beats/minute, and respiration of 18 breaths/minute. No respiratory distress was noted. Treatment was initiated for presumed bacterial meningitis. Basilar infiltrates and a widened mediastinum were noted on the initial chest radiograph. Gram stain of cerebrospinal fluid (CSF) revealed many neutrophils and large gram-positive rods. Anthrax was suspected and penicillin treatment was initiated. Within 24 hours of admission, CSF and blood cultures were positive for B. anthracis. *During the 1st day of hospitalization, the patient had a* grand mal *seizure and was intubated. On the 2nd hospital day, hypotension and azotemia developed, with subsequent renal failure. On the 3rd hospital day, refractory hypotension developed and the patient had a fatal cardiac arrest. This patient illustrates the rapidity with which patients with inhalation anthrax can deteriorate, despite a rapid diagnosis and appropriate antimicrobial therapy. Although the route of exposure is via the respiratory tract, patients do not develop pneumonia; rather, the abnormal chest radiograph is caused by hemorrhagic mediastinitis.*

CLINICAL CASE

Intestinal *Bacillus anthracis* Disease with Sepsis

Klempner and colleagues[2] described an unusual presentation of anthrax. The patient was a 24-year-old woman who was transferred to their hospital because of severe abdominal pain, vomiting, ascites, and shock. The patient had been healthy until 9 days before admission, when she developed fatigue, fevers, headache, and diffuse body aches. She subsequently developed a progressive cough, and 3 days before admission, nausea and vomiting. Upon admission, blood cultures were collected and intravenous fluids and ertapenem were administered. Exploratory laparotomy revealed ascites, hemorrhagic lesions in the mesentery, and necrotic small bowel. Although cultures of the ascites were negative, gram-positive rods were recovered in multiple blood cultures. These were initially dismissed as contaminants but subsequently identified as B. anthracis. *Treatment was adjusted to include ciprofloxacin. Her clinical course was stormy, requiring hospitalization for nearly 2 months, followed by 3 weeks in a rehabilitation facility. She continued to have ascites, nausea, vomiting, and abdominal pain that resolved very slowly. This patient was a resident of Massachusetts and had not traveled outside the area, so the discovery of* B. anthracis *infection was alarming. Exposure was traced to imported drums made of animal hides. The most common forms of anthrax in this setting would either be cutaneous exposure (development of wound anthrax) or inhalation anthrax (aerosolization of anthrax spores). The patient's disease is attributed to ingestion of spores, presumably when the aerosolized spores contaminated either her food or drink. It should be noted that* Bacillus *species are an uncommon contaminant in blood cultures, so any isolate should be carefully examined. In my experience, if the isolate is not associated with a patient's disease, commercial contamination of the blood culture bottles should be considered.*

BACILLUS CEREUS	
Properties	• **Heat-stable enterotoxin** produces emetic form of disease (vomiting) and **heat-labile enterotoxin** produces diarrheal form of disease • **Cereolysin** and **phospholipase C** with hemolysin and lecithinase activity, respectively; responsible for pathology associated with eye infections and tissue destruction
Epidemiology	• Ubiquitous in soils throughout the world • People at risk include those who consume food contaminated with the bacterium (e.g., rice, meat, vegetables, sauces), those with penetrating injuries (e.g., to the eye), those who receive intravenous injections, and immunocompromised patients exposed to *B. cereus*
Clinical Disease	• **Gastroenteritis**: emetic form characterized by a rapid onset (a few hours) of vomiting and abdominal pain and a short duration (generally <24 hours); diarrheal form characterized by a longer onset (8 to 12 hours) and duration (1 to 2 days) of diarrhea and abdominal cramps • **Traumatic eye infection**: rapid, progressive destruction of the eye after traumatic introduction of the bacteria into the eye • **Opportunistic infections**: sepsis associated with contaminated intravenous catheter • **Anthrax-like pulmonary disease**: severe pulmonary disease in immunocompetent patients infected with strains that have acquired genes for capsule formation and edema and lethal toxins (rare but important for biosafety concerns)
Diagnosis	• Isolation of the organism in implicated food product or nonfecal specimens (e.g., eye, wound)
Treatment, Control, Prevention	• Gastrointestinal infections are treated symptomatically • Ocular infectious or other invasive diseases require removal of foreign bodies and treatment with vancomycin, clindamycin, ciprofloxacin, or gentamicin • Gastrointestinal disease is prevented by proper preparation of food (e.g., foods should be consumed immediately after preparation or refrigerated)

CLINICAL CASE

Bacillus cereus Traumatic Endophthalmitis

Endophthalmitis caused by the traumatic introduction of B. cereus *into the eye is unfortunately not uncommon. This is a typical presentation. A 44-year-old man suffered a traumatic eye injury while working in a vegetable garden, when a piece of metal was deflected into his left eye, damaging the cornea and anterior and posterior lens capsule. Over the next 12 hours he developed increasing pain and purulence in his eye. He underwent surgery to relieve the ocular pressure, drain the purulence, and introduce intravitreal antibiotics (vancomycin, ceftazidime) and dexamethasone. Culture of the aspirated fluid was positive for* B. cereus. *Ciprofloxacin was added to his therapeutic regimen postoperatively. Despite the prompt surgical and medical intervention, and subsequent intravitreal antibiotic injections, the intraocular inflammation persisted and evisceration was required. This patient illustrates the risks involved with penetrating eye injuries and the need to intervene aggressively if the eye is to be saved.*

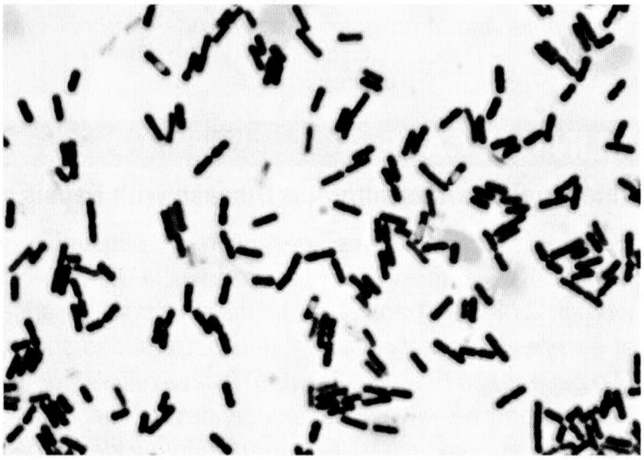

Bacillus cereus. The spores typically do not take up the Gram stain and appear as clear areas in the rods.

LISTERIA MONOCYTOGENES

L. monocytogenes is a short gram-positive rod that grows aerobically and anaerobically over a broad temperature range (including refrigerator temperatures) and in high salt concentrations. Human exposure is primarily through ingestion of contaminated food products, so survival when exposed to gastric pH, digestive enzymes, and bile salts is important for this pathogen. It is a facultative intracellular pathogen, so it must also penetrate into cells, survive intracellular killing, replicate, and migrate from cell to cell while avoiding the host's immune response.

Listeria is of public health concern because most infections are in fact outbreaks, involving many individuals over a potentially wide geographic distribution (e.g., multistate outbreaks involving improperly prepared commercial food products).

Diagnosis of *Listeria* is challenging because the bacteria are slow-growing organisms that may initially resemble either streptococci or nonpathogenic *Corynebacterium* species. These other organisms are commonly isolated and considered part of the normal bacterial population on the skin; therefore the significance of this isolate may also not be recognized.

LISTERIA MONOCYTOGENES	
Properties	• Bacterial **surface proteins** (internalins A, B) interact with host surface receptor • **Hemolysins** (listeriolysin O, two phospholipase C enzymes) allow intracellular survival and growth of bacteria
Epidemiology	• Isolated in soil, water, and vegetation and from a variety of animals, including humans (transient gastrointestinal carriage) • Disease associated with consumption of contaminated food products (e.g., milk and cheese, processed meats such as turkey franks, raw vegetables [especially cabbage]) or transplacental spread from mother to neonate; sporadic cases and epidemics occur throughout the year • Neonates, elderly, pregnant women, and patients with defects in cellular immunity are at increased risk for disease
Clinical Disease	• **Early-onset neonatal disease**—acquired transplacentally *in utero* and is characterized by disseminated abscesses and granulomas in multiple organs • **Late-onset neonatal disease**—acquired at or shortly after birth and presents as meningitis or meningoencephalitis with septicemia • Disease in pregnant women or adults with cell-mediated immune defects—can present as a primary febrile bacteremia or as disseminated disease with hypotension and meningitis • Disease in healthy adults—typically an influenza-like illness with or without gastroenteritis
Diagnosis	• Microscopy is insensitive; culture may require incubation for 2 to 3 days or enrichment at 4°C (refrigerate specimen so *Listeria* grows slowly while other insignificant organisms die) • Characteristic properties include motility at room temperature, weak β-hemolysis, and growth at 4°C and in high salt concentrations
Treatment, Control, Prevention	• The treatment of choice for severe disease is penicillin or ampicillin, alone or in combination with gentamicin • People at high risk should avoid eating raw or partially cooked foods of animal origin, soft cheese, and unwashed raw vegetables

CLINICAL CASE

Listeria Meningitis in Immunocompromised Man

The following patient, described by Bowie and associates,[3] illustrates the clinical presentation of Listeria *meningitis. A 73-year-old man with refractory rheumatoid arthritis was brought to the local hospital by his family because he had a decreased level of consciousness and a 3-day history of headache, nausea, and vomiting. His current medications were infliximab, methotrexate, and prednisone for his rheumatoid arthritis. On physical examination, the patient had a stiff neck and was febrile, with a pulse of 92 beats/minute, and blood pressure of*

CLINICAL CASE—cont'd

Listeria Meningitis in Immunocompromised Man

179/72 mmHg. Meningitis was suspected; therefore blood and CSF was collected for culture. The Gram stain of the CSF was negative, but Listeria *grew from both blood and CSF. The patient was treated with vancomycin, the infliximab was discontinued, and he made an uneventful recovery despite using less-than-optimal antimicrobial therapy. Infliximab has been associated with a dose-dependent monocytopenia. Monocytes are key effectors for clearance of* Listeria, *which meant this immunocompromised patient was specifically at risk for infection with this organism. Failure to detect* Listeria *in CSF by Gram stain is typical of this disease, because the bacteria fail to multiply to detectable levels.*

CLINICAL CASE

Listeria Gastroenteritis and Bacteremia

A 53-year-old man who was receiving immunosuppressive therapy for Crohn disease presented to the hospital with diarrhea and fever.[4] *He had been in his usual state of health until 2 days before admission, when he woke with severe malaise and headache. Over the next 2 days his symptoms included sharp, fluctuating abdominal pain, and episodes of urgent, uncontrollable nonbloody diarrhea. When his symptoms did not improve and he developed a temperature of 39.8°C, he went to the hospital. Blood cultures that were collected in the Emergency Department were positive within 24 hours for small gram-positive rods. Although a variety of bacteria and viruses can produce clinical symptoms such as this patient's, the positive blood culture was highly suggestive of* L. monocytogenes, *which was confirmed by biochemical tests and mass spectrometry. Other gram-positive bacteria associated with gastrointestinal disease include* B. cereus *(much larger than this organism) and* Clostridium difficile, *both of which are much larger than this isolate and neither cause bacteremia. The patient reported a recent history of eating cantaloupe, which was provocative because cantaloupes were implicated in a multistate outbreak of* Listeria *gastroenteritis at the time of this patient's disease; however, the patient's strain was a different serotype from that implicated in the outbreak. This case illustrates the syndrome of fever and nonbloody diarrhea that is typical of* Listeria *infections, and the increased risk of bacteremia (as well as meningitis) for specific risk groups: immunocompromised patients such as in this case, as well as very young children, pregnant women, and the elderly. A careful food history (such as consumption of raw vegetables, unpasteurized mild soft cheeses, and delicatessen foods) is important because the individual case may be part of a broader outbreak of disease.*

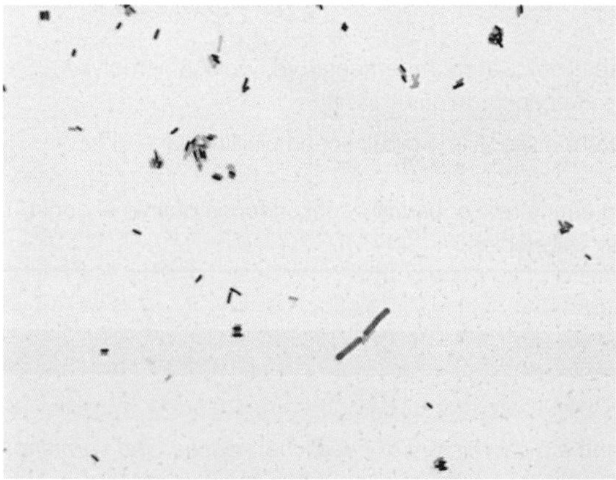

Listeria monocytogenes. Note the gram-positive rods are very small compared with the much larger pair of gram-negative rods.

CORYNEBACTERIUM DIPHTHERIAE

There are many corynebacteria species on the human skin and mucosal membranes, most of which only cause opportunistic infections (e.g., catheter-related bacteremia). The exception is *C. diphtheriae*, a strictly human pathogen that is not commonly isolated but causes a significant disease, **diphtheria**. This disease is mediated by diphtheria toxin, an **A-B exotoxin** that is introduced into strains of *C. diphtheriae* by a lysogenic bacteriophage, β-phage (so not all species have the toxin). A-B toxins consist of: (1) a catalytic region (active toxin molecule) on the A subunit; and (2) a receptor-binding region (binds to the target) and a translocation region (moves the active toxin into the cell) on the B subunit. We will see A-B toxins with other bacteria, but this was one of the first described.

CORYNEBACTERIUM DIPHTHERIAE	
Properties	• **Diphtheria exotoxin** is an A-B toxin that inhibits protein synthesis by inactivating protein chain elongation factor-2
Epidemiology	• Worldwide distribution maintained in asymptomatic carriers and infected patients • Humans are the only known reservoir, with carriage in oropharynx or on skin • Spread person-to-person by exposure to respiratory droplets or skin contact • Disease observed in unvaccinated or partially immune children or adults traveling to countries with endemic disease • Diphtheria is very uncommon in the United States and other countries with active vaccination programs
Clinical Disease	• **Respiratory diphtheria**: sudden onset with exudative pharyngitis, sore throat, low-grade fever, and malaise; a thick pseudomembrane develops over the pharynx; in critically ill patients, cardiac and neurologic complications are most significant • **Cutaneous diphtheria**: a papule can develop on the skin, which progresses to a nonhealing ulcer; systemic signs can develop
Diagnosis	• Microscopy is nonspecific • Culture should be performed on nonselective (blood agar) and selective media developed for recovery of *C. diphtheria* • Definitive identification is by biochemical tests or species-specific gene sequencing • Demonstration of exotoxin is performed by Elek test or nucleic acid amplification test for the encoding gene
Treatment, Control, Prevention	• Infections are treated with combination of: (1) diphtheria antitoxin to neutralize exotoxin; (2) penicillin or erythromycin to eliminate *C. diphtheriae* and terminate toxin production; and (3) immunization of convalescing patients with diphtheria toxoid to stimulate protective antibodies • Diphtheria vaccine and booster shots should be administered to susceptible population

CLINICAL CASE

Respiratory Diphtheria

Lurie and associates[5] reported the last patient with respiratory diphtheria seen in the United States. An unvaccinated 63-year-old man developed a sore throat while on a week-long trip in rural Haiti. Two days after he returned home to Pennsylvania, he visited a local hospital with complaints of a sore throat and difficulties in swallowing. He was treated with oral antibiotics but returned 2 days later with chills, sweating, difficulty swallowing and breathing, nausea, and vomiting. He had diminished breath sounds in the left lung, and radiographs confirmed pulmonary infiltrates as well as enlargement of the epiglottis. Laryngoscopy revealed yellow exudates on the tonsils, posterior pharynx, and soft palate. He was admitted to the intensive care unit and treated with azithromycin, ceftriaxone, nafcillin, and steroids, but over the next 4 days became hypotensive with a low-grade fever. Cultures were negative for C. diphtheriae. *By the 8th day of illness, a chest radiograph showed infiltrates in the right and left lung bases, and a white exudate consistent with* C. diphtheriae *pseudomembrane was observed over the supraglottic structures. At this time, cultures remained negative for* C. diphtheriae, *but polymerase chain reaction testing for the exotoxin gene was positive. Despite aggressive therapy the patient continued to deteriorate, and on the 17th day of hospitalization the patient developed cardiac complications and died. This patient illustrates: (1) the risk factor of unimmunized patients traveling to an endemic area; (2) the classic presentation of severe respiratory diphtheria; (3) delays associated with diagnosis of an uncommon disease; and (4) the difficulties that most laboratories would now have isolating the organism in culture.*

Diphtheria has fortunately been eliminated in most industrial countries through the use of vaccination, but it is still an important disease in resource-limited countries where vaccination use is not widespread. Diagnosis of these infections is also a challenge. *C. diphtheriae* is a well-known pathogen, but many other species of corynebacteria colonize the mouth, so the pathogen may not be initially recognized unless infection was suspected.

REFERENCES

1. Bush LM, Abrams BH, Beall A, Johnson CC. Index case of fatal inhalational anthrax due to bioterrorism in the United States. *N Engl J Med.* 2001;345:1607–1610.
2. Klempner MS, Talbot EA, Lee SI, Zaki S, Ferraro MJ. Case records of the Massachusetts General Hospital. Case 25-2010. A 24-year-old woman with abdominal pain and shock. *N Engl J Med.* 2010;363:766–777.
3. Bowie VL, Snella KA, Gopalachar AS, Bharadwaj P. Listeria meningitis associated with infliximab. *Ann Pharmacother.* 2004;38:58–61.
4. Hohmann EL, Kim J. Case records of the Massachusetts General Hospital. Case 8-2012. A 53-year-old man with Crohn's disease, diarrhea, fever, and bacteremia. *N Engl J Med.* 2012;366:1039–1045.
5. Centers for Disease Control and Prevention. Fatal respiratory diphtheria in a U.S. traveler to Haiti—Pennsylvania. *MMWR Morb Mortal Wkly Rep.* 2003;2004(52):1285–1286.

5

Acid-Fast Bacteria

INTERESTING FACTS

- In the last 25 years, the number of new cases of tuberculosis increased from 7.5 million to 9.6 million, and deaths decreased from 2.5 million to 1.5 million despite the appearance of multidrug-resistant strains, accounting for 480,000 new infections in 2014
- Leprosy has been eliminated from 119 of 122 countries where the disease was considered a public health problem in 1985, with antileprosy treatment (a combination of dapsone, rifampicin, and clofazimine) available globally at no charge through the World Health Organization
- The risk of *Mycobacterium avium* infections in HIV patients is inversely related to CD4 lymphocyte counts; this was the most common opportunistic infection in AIDS patients before the widespread use of clarithromycin or azithromycin prophylaxis
- *Nocardia* is present in organically rich soils, causing opportunistic infections in immunocompromised patients, most commonly presenting initially as pneumonia and then with dissemination to the brain (abscess) or skin

The bacteria discussed in this chapter are nonmotile, non–spore-forming, aerobic gram-positive rods that stain acid-fast. That is, these bacteria are resistant to decolorization with weak to strong acid solutions due to the presence of medium to long chains of **mycolic acids** in their cell wall. This staining property is important because only five genera of acid-fast bacteria are medically important: *Mycobacterium*, *Nocardia*, *Rhodococcus*, *Gordonia*, and *Tsukamurella*. Mycobacteria and *Nocardia* will be the focus of this chapter. *Rhodococcus* is a pathogen of immunocompromised patients, primarily causing invasive pulmonary disease, and *Gordonia* and *Tsukamurella* are uncommon opportunistic pathogens, responsible for pulmonary infections in immunocompromised patients and intravenous catheter infections. The latter three genera will not be discussed further.

All acid-fast organisms are relative slow-growing, requiring incubation for 3 to 7 days (*Nocardia* and some mycobacterial species), to as long as 4 weeks or more (*Mycobacterium* species such as *Mycobacterium tuberculosis*). *Mycobacterium leprae*, the etiologic agent of leprosy, has not been grown in culture. Acid-fast organisms are resistant to many disinfectants, survive in relatively harsh environmental conditions, and are resistant to many of the antibiotics that are used to treat other bacterial infections. Although more than 350 species of acid-fast bacteria have been described, only a few will be discussed in this chapter. A few species of mycobacteria are closely related to *M. avium* and produce similar human diseases, so they will be referred to as the *M. avium* complex. Likewise, I am not distinguishing between the many species of *Nocardia*.

ACID-FAST ORGANISMS

Some "rapid-growing" mycobacteria (e.g., *Mycobacterium fortuitum*, *Mycobacterium chelonae*, *Mycobacterium abscessus*, and *Mycobacterium mucogenicum*) are common opportunistic pathogens, and some "slow-growing" mycobacteria (e.g., *Mycobacterium kansasii* and *Mycobacterium marinum*) are relatively common pathogens. I will not discuss them in this chapter but the following clinical case illustrates disease caused by rapidly growing mycobacteria.

CLINICAL CASE

Mycobacterial Infections Associated with Nail Salons

In September 2000[1] a physician reported to the California Department of Health four females who developed lower extremity furunculosis. Each patient presented with small erythematous papules that became large, tender, fluctuant, violaceous boils over several weeks. Bacterial cultures of the lesions were negative, and the patients failed empiric antibacterial therapy. All of the patients had visited the same nail salon before the furuncles developed. As a result of an investigation of the nail salon, a total of 110 patients with furunculosis were identified. M. fortuitum *was cultured from the lesions of 32 patients, as well as from the footbaths used by the patients before their pedicures. Shaving the legs was identified as a risk factor for disease. Similar outbreaks have been reported in the literature, which illustrates the risks associated with contamination of waters with rapidly growing mycobacteria; the difficulties of confirming these infections by routine bacterial cultures, which are typically incubated for only 1 to 2 days; and the need for effective antibiotic therapy.*

It is difficult to list virulence properties for acid-fast bacteria, because much of the pathology results from the infected host's response to the organism. *M. tuberculosis* is an intracellular pathogen that is able to establish a lifelong infection. Maintenance of persistent infections, without progression to disease, involves a delicate host–parasite relationship: balance between growth of the bacteria and immunologic control by the host. When the host regulation is disrupted, progressive disease develops. At the time of exposure, *M. tuberculosis* enters the respiratory airways and penetrates the alveoli, where the bacteria are phagocytized by alveolar macrophages. The bacteria prevent fusion of the phagosome with lysosomes and evade macrophage killing. However, in response to infection with *M. tuberculosis,* macrophages secrete the cytokines IL-12 and TNF-α that in turn recruit T-cells and natural killer cells into the area of the infected macrophages, activate the macrophages, and stimulate intracellular killing. The subsequent mass of necrotic cells (termed **granuloma**) will contain the infection, but also permits some surviving bacteria. These are the bacteria that will subsequently cause disease when the immune process is disrupted.

The ability of *M. leprae* to produce disease is also a manifestation of the slow growth properties of the organism and the host immunologic response. This organism is acquired through inhalation of infectious aerosols or through skin contact with respiratory secretions or wound exudates. The bacteria replicate very slowly and disease may take years before it is clinically apparent. Two forms of disease develop in direct response to the host immune response: (1) **tuberculoid**

Acid-Fast Organisms

Species	Derivation	Diseases
M. tuberculosis	*Myces*, a fungus; *bakterion*, a small rod (fungus-like rod); *tuberculum* a small swelling or tubercle (characterized by tubercles in lungs of infected patients)	Tuberculosis (pulmonary, disseminated)
M. leprae	*Lepra*, of leprosy	Leprosy, also called Hansen disease (tuberculoid, lepromatous)
M. avium complex	*Avis*, of birds (original isolate from birds with tuberculosis-like illness)	Pulmonary disease in immunocompetent patients; cervical adenitis in children; disseminated disease in immunocompromised patients
Nocardia species	*Nocard*, named after the French veterinarian Edmond Nocard	Pulmonary disease; primary or secondary cutaneous infections; meningitis; brain abscesses

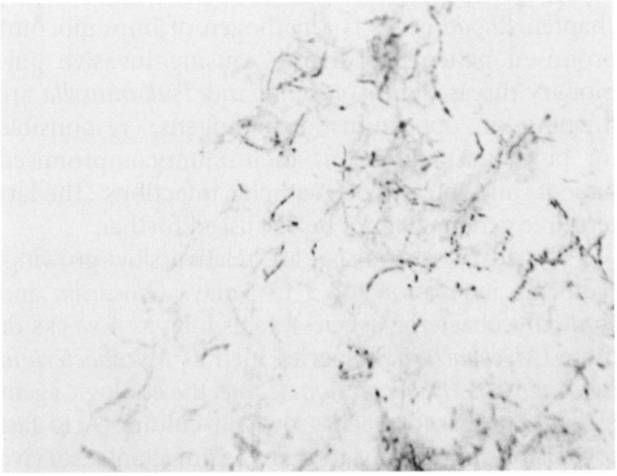

Acid-fast stain of *Mycobacterium tuberculosis* in sputum specimen. Note the "beaded" appearance of the individual rods.

leprosy, where there is a strong cellular immune reaction with the induction of cytokine production that mediates macrophage activation, phagocytosis, and bacillary clearance; and (2) **lepromatous leprosy**, where a strong antibody response is observed, but the cellular response is defective. Mycobacterial diseases are primarily controlled by cellular immunity; as a result, the lepromatous form is characterized by the presence of abundant acid-fast bacteria and extensive tissue destruction, the most familiar form of leprosy.

M. avium is an intracellular pathogen that produces either a slowly progressive disease in patients with compromised pulmonary function, or a rapidly progressive, disseminated disease in patients with severe depression of cellular immunity.

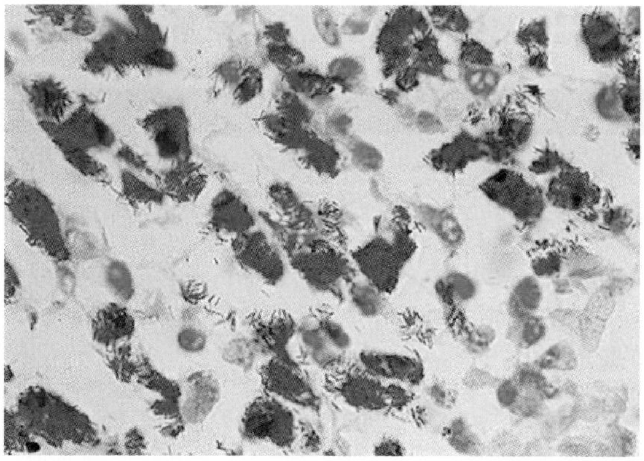

Mycobacterium avium complex in tissue from an AIDS patient. The abundant bacilli in the tissue of immunocompromised patients is typical.

Nocardia, like its mycobacterial relatives, is an intracellular pathogen that effectively produces disease by avoiding the host immune response.

Mycobacterial and nocardial infections are exogenous—caused by organisms that are not normally part of the normal human microbial population. *M. tuberculosis* and *M. leprae* are transmitted person-to-person, while all other members of these genera are acquired directly from the environment. Isolation of acid-fast bacteria in a clinical specimen is always noteworthy, but the significance of an isolate, with the exception of *M. tuberculosis* and *M. leprae*, must be proven; that is, the isolate could represent transient colonization with an environmental contaminant.

Diseases with these pathogens are well-characterized, so demonstration of the significance of an isolate should not be difficult. The possible exception to this rule would be with *M. avium*. It may be necessary to isolate the organism from multiple sputum specimens in elderly patients with chronic pulmonary disease.

Diagnosis of these infections is by a combination of microscopy (observation of acid-fast bacteria in clinical specimens), culture, and molecular tests such as nucleic acid amplification tests. Detection of a cellular immune response to infection is useful for *M. tuberculosis* and the tuberculoid form of *M. leprae* disease, but this does not distinguish between active disease and past exposure.

MYCOBACTERIUM TUBERCULOSIS

MYCOBACTERIUM TUBERCULOSIS	
Properties	• Acid-fast rods frequently observed in clump • Growth in culture is slow, typically 2 to 6 weeks incubation is required
Epidemiology	• Worldwide; one-third of the world's population is infected with this organism • A total of 9.6 million new cases in 2014 and 1.5 million deaths • Disease most common in China, India, Eastern Europe, Pakistan, sub-Saharan Africa, and South Africa • Fewer than 10,000 new cases in United States annually; most infections observed in immigrants from countries with endemic disease • Populations at greatest risk for disease are immunocompromised patients (particularly those with HIV infection), drug or alcohol abusers, homeless persons, and individuals exposed to diseased patients • Humans are the only natural reservoir • Person-to-person spread by infectious aerosols
Clinical Disease	• **Tuberculosis**: infections in immunocompetent patients primarily restricted to the lungs; typically present with nonspecific symptoms (malaise, weight loss, cough, night sweats) with sputum production (bloody and purulent with cavitary disease) • **Extrapulmonary tuberculosis**: disseminated disease following hematogenous spread; kidneys, bones, spleen, and meninges most common foci of disseminated disease

Continued

MYCOBACTERIUM TUBERCULOSIS—cont'd	
Diagnosis	• **Tuberculin skin test** and **interferon-γ release assay (IGRA)** are sensitive markers for exposure to organism • Microscopy and culture are sensitive and specific • Direct detection of *M. tuberculosis* in clinical specimens commonly performed by nucleic acid amplification tests • Identification of clinical isolates most commonly made using species-specific molecular probes
Treatment, Control, Prevention	• Prolonged treatment with multiple drugs is required to prevent development of drug-resistant strains • Isoniazid, ethambutol, pyrazinamide, and rifampin for 2 months, followed by 4 to 6 months of isoniazid and rifampin or alternative combination drugs • Drug-resistant strains are common, so treatment for patients who fail initial therapy must be guided by drug susceptibility tests • Prophylaxis for exposure to tuberculosis can include isoniazid for 6 to 9 months or rifampin for 4 months; pyrazinamide and ethambutol or levofloxacin are used for 6 to 12 months after exposure to drug-resistant *M. tuberculosis* • Immunoprophylaxis with **Bacille Calmette-Guérin (BCG)** vaccination is used in countries with endemic disease, but the effectiveness of this is limited • Control of disease is through active surveillance, prophylactic and therapeutic intervention, and careful case monitoring

CLINICAL CASE

Drug-Resistant *Mycobacterium tuberculosis*

The risk of active tuberculosis is significantly increased in HIV-infected individuals. Unfortunately, this problem is complicated by the development of drug-resistant M. tuberculosis *strains in this population. This was illustrated in the report by Gandhi and associates,*[2] *who studied the prevalence of tuberculosis in South Africa from January 2005 to March 2006. They identified 475 patients with culture-confirmed tuberculosis, of whom 39% had multidrug-resistant strains (MDR TB) and 6% with extensively drug-resistant strains (XDR TB). All patients with XDR TB were co-infected with HIV, and 98% of these patients died. The high prevalence of MDR TB and the evolution of XDR TB pose a serious challenge for tuberculosis treatment programs, and emphasize the need for rapid diagnostic tests.*

MYCOBACTERIUM LEPRAE

MYCOBACTERIUM LEPRAE	
Properties	• Acid-fast rods
Epidemiology	• Fewer than 300,000 new cases were reported in 2005, with most cases in India, Nepal, and Brazil • 64 new cases reported in United States in 2013 • Lepromatous form of the disease, but not the tuberculoid form, is highly infectious • Person-to-person spread by direct contact or inhalation of infectious aerosols
Clinical Disease	• **Tuberculoid leprosy**: skin lesions characterized by scant erythematous or hypopigmented plaques with flat centers and raised, demarcated borders; peripheral nerve damage with complete sensory loss; visible enlargement of nerves • **Lepromatous leprosy**: skin lesions with many erythematous macules, papules, or nodules; extensive tissue destruction (e.g., nasal cartilage, bones, ears); diffuse nerve involvement with patchy sensory loss; lack of nerve enlargement
Diagnosis	• Microscopy is sensitive for the lepromatous form but not for the tuberculoid form • *M. leprae* does **not grow in culture; skin test** • Skin testing is required to confirm tuberculoid leprosy; poorly reactive in lepromatous leprosy
Treatment, Control, Prevention	• Tuberculoid form is treated with rifampicin and dapsone for 6 months; clofazimine is added to this regimen for treatment of the lepromatous form, and therapy is extended to a minimum of 12 months • Disease is controlled through the prompt recognition and treatment of infected people

MYCOBACTERIUM AVIUM COMPLEX

MYCOBACTERIUM AVIUM COMPLEX	
Properties	• Small acid-fast rods
Epidemiology	• Worldwide distribution, but disease is seen most commonly in countries where tuberculosis is less prevalent • Acquired primarily through ingestion of contaminated water or food; inhalation of infectious aerosols is believed to play a minor role in transmission • Patients at greatest risk for disease are those who are immunocompromised (particularly patients with AIDS) or those with long-standing pulmonary disease
Clinical Disease	• **Pulmonary disease** in immunocompetent patients: slowly progressive chronic pulmonary disease that resembles tuberculosis, or may present as chronic bronchiectasis • **Cervical adenitis** in children: development of a solitary enlarged lymph node • **Disseminated disease** in immunocompromised patients: overwhelming disseminated infection in AIDS patients with CD4 T-lymphocytes less than 10 cells/mm^3.
Diagnosis	• Microscopy and culture are sensitive and specific • Identification of clinical isolates most commonly made using species-specific molecular probes
Treatment, Control, Prevention	• Infections treated for prolonged period with clarithromycin or azithromycin, combined with ethambutol and rifabutin • Prophylaxis in AIDS patients who have a low CD4 cell count consists of clarithromycin, azithromycin or rifabutin, and such treatment has greatly reduced the incidence of disease

CLINICAL CASE

Mycobacterium avium Infections in an AIDS Patient

Woods and Goldsmith[3] described a patient with advanced AIDS who died of disseminated M. avium *infection. The patient was a 27-year-old man, who initially presented in October 1985 with a 2-week history of progressive dyspnea and a nonproductive cough. Pneumocystis was detected in a bronchoalveolar lavage, and serology confirmed the patient had an HIV infection. The patient was successfully treated with trimethoprim-sulfamethoxazole and discharged. The patient remained stable until May 1987, when he presented with persistent fever and dyspnea. Over the next week he developed severe substernal chest pain, and a pericardial friction rub. Echocardiogram revealed a small effusion. The patient left the hospital against medical advice but returned 1 week later with a persistent cough, fever, and pain in the chest and left arm. A diagnostic pericardiocentesis was performed, and 220 mL of fluid was aspirated. Tuberculous pericarditis was suspected, and appropriate antimycobacterial therapy was initiated. However, over the next 3 weeks the patient developed progressive cardiac failure and died.* M. avium *was recovered from the pericardial fluid, as well as autopsy cultures of the pericardium, spleen, liver, adrenal glands, kidneys, small intestine, lymph nodes, and pituitary gland. Although* M. avium *pericarditis was unusual, the extensive dissemination of the mycobacteria in patients with advanced AIDS was common before azithromycin prophylaxis became widely used.*

NOCARDIA SPECIES

NOCARDIA SPECIES	
Properties	• **Partially acid-fast** bacteria typically arranged in long branching filaments
Epidemiology	• Worldwide distribution in soil rich with organic matter • Exogenous infections acquired by inhalation (pulmonary) or traumatic introduction (cutaneous) • Opportunistic pathogen causing disease most commonly in immunocompromised patients with T-cell deficiencies (transplant recipients, patients with malignancies, HIV patients, patients receiving corticosteroids) or in healthy individuals with traumatic infections

Continued

NOCARDIA SPECIES—cont'd	
Clinical Disease	• **Bronchopulmonary disease**: indolent pulmonary disease with necrosis and abscess formation; dissemination to central nervous system or skin is common • **Mycetoma**: chronic progressive, destructive disease, generally of extremities, characterized by suppurative granulomas, progressive fibrosis and necrosis, and sinus tract formation • **Lymphocutaneous disease**: primary infection or secondary spread to cutaneous site characterized by chronic granuloma formation and erythematous subcutaneous nodules, with eventual ulcer formation • **Cellulitis and subcutaneous abscesses**: granulomatous ulcer formation with surrounding erythema, but minimal or no involvement of the draining lymph nodes • **Brain abscess**—chronic infection with fever, headache, and focal deficits related to the location of the slowly developing abscesses
Diagnosis	• Microscopy is sensitive and relatively specific when branching, partially acid-fast organisms are seen • Culture is slow, requiring incubation for up to 1 week; selective media (e.g., buffered charcoal yeast extract agar) may be required for isolating *Nocardia* in mixed cultures • Identification at the genus level can be made by the microscopic and macroscopic appearances (branching, weakly acid-fast rods, forming colonies with fuzzy aerial hyphae) • Identification at the species level requires genomic analysis for most isolates; the species cannot be reliably identified by biochemical tests
Treatment, Control, Prevention	• Infections are treated with antibiotics and proper wound care • Trimethoprim-sulfamethoxazole used as initial empiric therapy for cutaneous infections in immunocompetent patients; therapy for severe infections and cutaneous infections in immunocompromised patients should include trimethoprim-sulfamethoxazole plus amikacin for pulmonary or cutaneous infections and trimethoprim-sulfamethoxazole plus imipenem or a cephalosporin for central nervous system infections; prolonged treatment (up to 12 months) is recommended • Exposure cannot be avoided because nocardiae are ubiquitous

CLINICAL CASE

Disseminated Nocardiosis

Shin and associates[4] described a 63-year-old man who received a liver transplant for liver cirrhosis caused by hepatitis C. The patient was treated with immunosuppressive drugs, including tacrolimus and prednisone for 4 months, at which time he returned to the hospital with fever and lower leg pain. Although the chest radiograph was normal, ultrasound revealed an abscess in the soleus muscle. Poorly staining gram-positive rods were observed in the Gram stain of the pus aspirated from the abscess, and Nocardia *grew after 3 days of incubation. Treatment with imipenem was started; however, the patient developed convulsions 10 days later and partial left-sided paralysis. Brain imaging studies revealed three lesions. Treatment was switched to ceftriaxone and amikacin. The subcutaneous abscess and brain lesions gradually improved, and the patient was discharged after 55 days of hospitalization. This patient illustrates the propensity of* Nocardia *to infect immunocompromised patients, disseminate to the brain, and the slow rate of growth of the organism in culture and related need for prolonged treatment.*

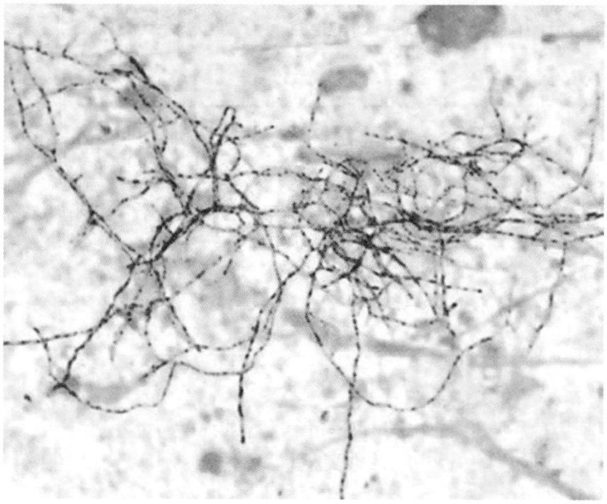

Gram stain of *Nocardia* in expectorated sputum. The long, delicate filaments and irregular staining is characteristic of *Nocardia.*

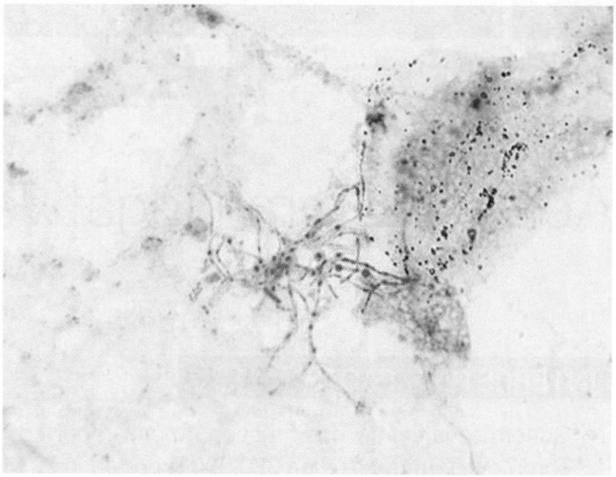

Acid-fast stain of *Nocardia* in expectorated sputum. Note the branching filaments that partially retain the acid-fast stain.

REFERENCES

1. Winthrop KL, Abrams M, Yakrus M, et al. An outbreak of mycobacterial furunculosis associated with footbaths at a nail salon. *N Engl J Med.* 2002;346:1366–1371.
2. Gandhi NR, Moll A, Sturm AW, et al. Extensively drug-resistant tuberculosis as a cause of death in patients co-infected with tuberculosis and HIV in a rural area of South Africa. *Lancet.* 2006;368:1575–1580.
3. Woods GL, Goldsmith JC. Fatal pericarditis due to *Mycobacterium avium-intracellulare* in acquired immunodeficiency syndrome. *Chest.* 1989;95:1355–1357.
4. Shin N, Sugawara Y, Tsukada K, et al. Successful treatment of disseminated *Nocardia farcinica* infection in a living-donor liver transplantation recipient. *Transplant Infect Dis.* 2006;8:222–225.

6

Aerobic Gram-Negative Cocci and Coccobacilli

INTERESTING FACTS

- Gonorrhea is the second most commonly reported notifiable disease in the United States (chlamydia is the most common), with more than 350,000 reported in 2014, and the incidence is increasing, particularly in men aged 20 to 24 years
- In contrast with viral meningitis, bacterial meningitis caused by *Neisseria meningitidis* and *Haemophilus influenzae* is contagious, so person-to-person spread with development of meningitis can occur
- Although pediatric disease with *Haemophilus influenzae* has been virtually eliminated with the HIB vaccine, this is a significant pathogen in countries where vaccination is not widely used
- *Acinetobacter baumannii* was largely ignored until multidrug-resistant strains were observed in military hospitals during the Iraq and Afghanistan conflicts. Now these bacteria are widely disseminated worldwide, and treatment is increasingly challenging
- Although the highest incidence of pertussis and complications is in children <1 year of age, disease in older children and adults is frequently not appreciated, and these patients serve as an unrecognized reservoir for *Bordetella pertussis*

The focus of this chapter is on a broad collection of bacteria that are gram-negative cocci or coccobacilli (short rods). There are many species of *Neisseria*, but the two most important are *Neisseria gonorrhoeae* and *Neisseria meningitidis*. Two genera, *Eikenella* and *Kingella*, are members of the same family of bacteria as *Neisseria*, with a single important species in each genus, *Eikenella corrodens* and *Kingella kingae*. Both bacteria are normal residents of the human mouth, as are two other genera, *Moraxella* and *Haemophilus*. I will discuss *Moraxella catarrhalis* and *H. influenzae* as representatives of their genera, and I should point out that *M. catarrhalis* was formerly classified as *Neisseria*, because both genera are typically arranged in pairs (diplococci) with the adjacent sides flattened together (resembling coffee beans). Four additional genera are considered in this chapter. The genus *Acinetobacter* contains many species but *A. baumannii* is the most important, because many strains that cause opportunistic infections in hospitalized patients are multidrug-resistant and virtually untreatable. *Bordetella*, *Francisella*, and *Brucella* all cause specific diseases (pertussis, tularemia, and brucellosis, respectively) that are of significant public health interest. These bacteria and their diseases are distinct; therefore each will be considered individually.

Aerobic Gram-Negative Cocci and Coccobacilli

Bacteria	Historical Derivation
N. gonorrhoeae	Named after the German physician Albert Neisser, who originally described the organism responsible for gonorrhea; *gone*, seed; *rhoia*, a flow (a flow of seeds in reference to the purulent exudate produced in the disease gonorrhea)
N. meningitidis	*meningis*, the covering of the brain; *itis*, inflammation (inflammation of the meninges as in meningitis)
E. corrodens	Named after M. Eiken who first described the organism and observed the ability of the organism to pit or "corrode" agar
K. kingae	Named after Elizabeth King who described the organism
M. catarrhalis	Named after Morax who first described the organism; *catarrhus*, catarrh (refers to inflammation of respiratory membranes)

Aerobic Gram-Negative Cocci and Coccobacilli—cont'd	
Bacteria	**Historical Derivation**
H. influenzae	*Haemo*, blood; *hilos*, lover (blood lover, requires blood for growth in culture); originally thought to cause influenza
A. baumannii	*Akinetos*, unable to move; *bactrum*, rod (nonmotile rods); *baumannii*, named after the microbiologist Baumann
B. pertussis	Named after Bordet who first isolated the organism; *per*, severe; *tussis*, cough (a severe cough)
F. tularensis	Named after Francis who first described the disease; tularensis, pertaining to Tulare County, California, where the disease was first described
B. melitensis	Named after Bruce who first recognized the organism as a cause of "undulant fever"

NEISSERIA GONORRHOEAE

Despite the fact *N. gonorrhoeae* survives poorly when exposed to cold temperatures, and requires humidity and carbon dioxide when grown in laboratory cultures, it has managed to become the most common cause of sexually transmitted diseases worldwide. In fact, it is interesting that the three most common bacteria responsible for sexually transmitted diseases—*N.gonorrhoeae*, *Treponema pallidum* (syphilis), and *Chlamydia trachomatis*—all survive poorly outside their human hosts. This illustrates how important close physical contact is for the maintenance of these diseases.

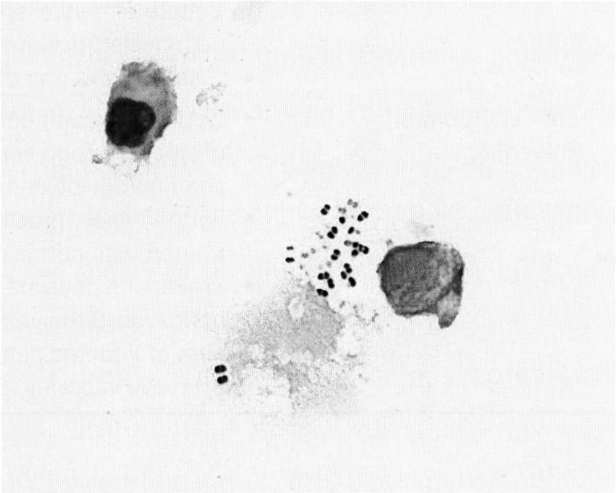

Neisseria gonorrhoeae in urethral exudate. Note the gram-negative cocci are arranged in pairs with flattened sides (gram-negative diplococci).

NEISSERIA GONORRHOEAE	
Properties	• Pilin protein mediates initial attachment to nonciliated epithelial cells in the vagina, fallopian tube, and buccal cavity; interferes with neutrophil killing • Porin proteins promote intracellular survival by preventing phagolysosome fusion and subsequent bacterial death in neutrophils • Opacity proteins mediate firm attachment to host cells • Transferrin, lactoferrin, and other hemoglobin binding proteins mediate acquisition of iron for bacterial metabolism and growth • Cell wall lipooligosaccharide (LOS) has endotoxin activity • β-Lactamase mediates resistance to penicillin
Epidemiology	• Humans are the only natural hosts • Carriage can be asymptomatic, particularly in women, facilitating transmission • Transmission is primarily by sexual contact • Most common cause of septic arthritis in sexually active adults • Almost 335,000 cases reported in United States in 2012 (true incidence of disease believed to be at least twice that); estimated 100 million new cases worldwide annually • Incidence of disease highest in people aged 15 to 24 years, blacks, residents of southeastern United States, and people who have multiple sexual encounters • Higher risk of disseminated disease in patients with deficiencies in late components of complement

Continued

NEISSERIA GONORRHOEAE—cont'd	
Clinical Disease	• **Gonorrhea**: characterized by purulent discharge from involved site (e.g., urethra, cervix, epididymis, prostate, rectum) after a 2- to 5-day incubation period • **Disseminated infections**: spread of infection from genitourinary tract through blood to skin or joints; characterized by pustular rash with erythematous base and suppurative arthritis in involved joints • **Ophthalmia neonatorum**: purulent ocular infection acquired by neonate at birth
Diagnosis	• Gram stain of urethral specimens (presence of gram-negative diplococci) is accurate only for symptomatic males • Gram stain of synovial fluid is diagnostic for septic arthritis • Culture of genital specimens is sensitive and specific but has been replaced with nucleic acid amplification tests (NAATs) in most laboratories • Culture is the test of choice for all other specimens
Treatment, Control, Prevention	• Ceftriaxone with either azithromycin or doxycycline is currently the treatment of choice, although high-level resistance to cephalosporins, as well as to penicillins and fluoroquinolones, has been observed • For neonates, prophylaxis with 1% silver nitrate; ophthalmia neonatorum is treated with ceftriaxone • Prevention consists of patient education, use of condoms or spermicides with nonoxynol-9 (only partially effective), and aggressive follow-up of sexual partners of infected patients • Effective vaccines are not available

CLINICAL CASE

Gonococcal Arthritis

Gonococcal arthritis is a common presentation of disseminated Neisseria gonorrhoeae *infection. Fam and associates*[1] *described six patients with this disease, including the following patient, who has a typical presentation. A 17-year-old girl was admitted to the hospital with a 4-day history of fever, chills, malaise, sore throat, skin rash, and polyarthralgia. She reported being sexually active and having a 5-week history of a profuse yellowish vaginal discharge that was untreated. Upon presentation, she had erythematous maculopapular skin lesions over her forearm, thigh, and ankle, and her metacarpophalangeal joint, wrist, knee, ankle, and midtarsal joints were acutely inflamed. She had an elevated leukocyte count and sedimentation rate. Cultures of her cervix were positive for* N. gonorrhoeae, *but blood specimens, exudates from the skin lesions, and synovial fluid were all sterile. The diagnosis of disseminated gonorrhea with polyarthritis was made, and she was successfully treated with penicillin G for 2 weeks. This case illustrates the limitations of culture in disseminated infections and the value of a careful history.*

NEISSERIA MENINGITIDIS

Rarely does a bacterial pathogen strike such fear in a community as *N. meningitidis*, for it is able to produce meningitis and overwhelming sepsis in healthy children and adults, and rapidly spreads through contact with the initial victims.

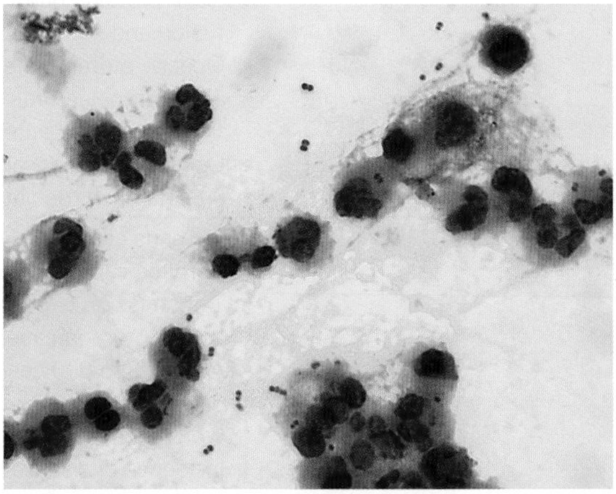

Neisseria meningitidis in cerebrospinal fluid of a child with meningitis. Note the morphology is identical to *Neisseria gonorrhoeae*.

NEISSERIA MENINGITIDIS	
Properties	• Pilin protein mediates initial attachment to host cells; interferes with neutrophil killing • Polysaccharide capsule protects bacteria from antibody-mediated phagocytosis; a number of immunologic distinct serogroups have been described • Cell wall LOS has endotoxin activity
Epidemiology	• Humans are the only natural hosts • Person-to-person spread occurs via aerosolization of respiratory tract secretions • Highest incidence of disease is in children younger than 5 years (particularly infants <6 months of age), young adults in college or military settings, institutionalized people, and patients with late complement deficiencies • Endemic and epidemic disease most commonly caused by serogroups A, B, C, W135, and Y (meningitis by serogroups A, B, C; pneumonia by serogroups W135 and Y); serogroups A and W135 infections are most common in resource-limited countries, while serogroup B infections are most common in industrial countries • Disease occurs worldwide, most commonly in the dry, cold months of the year
Clinical Disease	• **Meningitis**: purulent inflammation of meninges associated with headache, meningeal signs, and fever; high mortality rate unless promptly treated with effective antibiotics • **Meningococcemia**: disseminated infection characterized by thrombosis of small blood vessels and multiorgan involvement; small, petechial skin lesions coalesce into larger hemorrhagic lesions • **Pneumonia**: milder form of meningococcal disease characterized by bronchopneumonia in patients with underlying pulmonary disease
Diagnosis	• Gram stain of CSF (gram-negative diplococci) is sensitive and specific but is of limited value for blood specimens (too few organisms are generally present, except in overwhelming sepsis) • Culture is definitive, but organism is fastidious and dies rapidly when exposed to cold or dry conditions • Tests to detect meningococcal antigens are insensitive and nonspecific • NAATs are not yet widely used
Treatment, Control, Prevention	• Empiric treatment of patients with suspected meningitis or bacteremia should be initiated with ceftriaxone; if the isolate is penicillin susceptible, treatment can be changed to penicillin G • Chemoprophylaxis for contact with persons with the disease is with rifampin, ciprofloxacin, or ceftriaxone • Breast-feeding infants have passive immunity (first 6 months). For immunoprophylaxis, vaccination is an adjunct to chemoprophylaxis; it is used only for serogroups A, C, Y, and W135; no effective vaccine is available for serogroup B; vaccination for serogroup A has been introduced in Africa, which is important.

CLINICAL CASE

Meningococcal Disease

Gardner[2] described a previously healthy 18-year-old man who presented to a local emergency department with the acute onset of fever and headache. His temperature was elevated (40°C), and he was tachycardic (pulse of 140 beats/minute) and hypotensive (blood pressure at 70/40 mmHg). Petechiae were noted over his chest. Although the result of a cerebrospinal fluid (CSF) culture was not reported, N. meningitidis *was recovered in the patient's blood cultures. Despite the prompt administration of antibiotics and other support measures, the patient's condition rapidly deteriorated, and he died 12 hours after arrival in the hospital. This patient illustrates the rapid progression of meningococcal disease, even in healthy young adults.*

EIKENELLA CORRODENS

In contrast with *N. gonorrhoeae* and *N. meningitidis*, *E. corrodens* is a relatively unknown pathogen to the medical community, although disease caused by this organism, particularly bite-related infections, is well-documented. A basic knowledge of this organism is important, because antibiotic treatment of these infections is very different from traditional gram-negative infections.

EIKENELLA CORRODENS	
Properties	• Opportunistic pathogen
Epidemiology	• Normal resident of human mouth
Clinical Disease	• **Human bite wound** or fist fight injury • **Subacute endocarditis** in patients with preexisting heart disease • **Opportunistic infections** (pneumonia, lung or brain abscesses, sinusitis) in immunocompromised patients or patients with trauma of the oral cavity
Diagnosis	• Slow-growing facultative anaerobe that requires 2 or more days of incubation • Preliminary identification of the cultured organism is possible based on the Gram stain morphology and whether the colonies pit the agar ("corrodes" agar; about half the isolates will do this) and produce a bleachlike odor (very common) • Definitive identification by biochemical tests or mass spectrometry
Treatment, Control, Prevention	• Susceptible to **penicillin** (unusual for gram-negative bacteria), ampicillin, extended spectrum cephalosporins, tetracycline, fluoroquinolones • Resistant to oxacillin, first generation cephalosporins, clindamycin, erythromycin

KINGELLA KINGAE

This organism also remains in the shadows, unknown to many medical practitioners. This fact is emphasized because the organism most commonly produces disease with a nonspecific but insidious presentation, and is frequently difficult to recover in culture unless extended incubation is used.

KINGELLA KINGAE	
Properties	• Opportunistic pathogen
Epidemiology	• Normal resident of the human mouth, particularly in children
Clinical Disease	• **Septic arthritis** in children • **Subacute endocarditis** in patients with preexisting heart disease
Diagnosis	• Slow-growing facultative anaerobe that requires 3 or more days of incubation • Definitive identification by biochemical tests or mass spectrometry
Treatment, Control, Prevention	• Susceptible to **penicillin**, erythromycin, tetracycline, fluoroquinolones

MORAXELLA CATARRHALIS

For many years, *M. catarrhalis* was considered a relatively insignificant member of the genus *Neisseria*. This changed when it was realized that the only thing the two genera had in common was their gram-negative diplococci morphology. Additionally, you only have to look at a Gram stain of sputum collected from a patient with *M. catarrhalis* pneumonia to recognize the presence of abundant organisms, surrounded by equally numerous inflammatory cells. Any organism capable of triggering such a vigorous immune response has to be significant.

MORAXELLA CATARRHALIS	
Properties	• Opportunistic pathogen
Epidemiology	• Normal resident of the human mouth
Clinical Disease	• **Bronchitis** or **bronchopneumonia** in patients with chronic pulmonary disease • **Sinusitis** and **otitis** in previously healthy individuals
Diagnosis	• Gram stain (gram-negative diplococci) is suggestive of *Moraxella* but cannot be differentiated from *Neisseria* • Strict aerobic growth in 1 to 2 days on most nonselective laboratory media • Identification by biochemical tests or mass spectrometry
Treatment, Control, Prevention	• Most isolates product β-lactamase and are resistant to all penicillins • Susceptible to most other antibiotics including cephalosporins, erythromycin, tetracyclines, trimethoprim-sulfamethoxazole

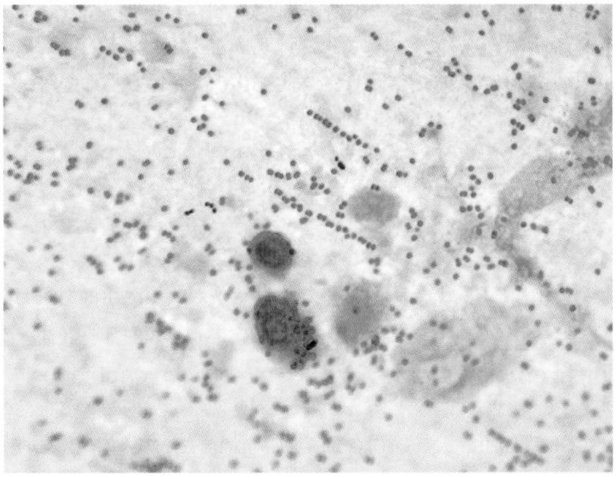

Typical appearance of *Moraxella catarrhalis* in sputum with large numbers of gram-negative diplococci and host inflammatory cells. *M. catarrhalis* resembles and is frequently mistaken for *Neisseria*.

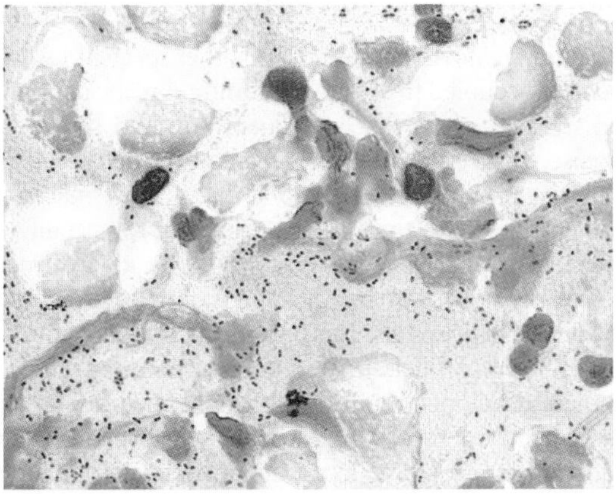

Haemophilus influenzae in sputum. Bacteria typically appear as very small coccobacilli, arranged as single cells or occasionally in pairs.

HAEMOPHILUS INFLUENZAE

H. influenzae is a bacterium almost relegated to historical value. I say "almost" because despite the fact that the disease has been virtually eliminated in vaccinated populations of children, vaccination has not been universally adopted worldwide. That remains the challenge—and promise—for the future. A few other species of *Haemophilus* should be mentioned here:

- *Haemophilus aegyptius,* an important cause of acute purulent **conjunctivitis** ("pinkeye"); associated with epidemics during the warm months of the year
- *Haemophilus ducreyi,* the etiologic agent of the sexually transmitted disease soft chancre, or **chancroid**; characterized by a tender papule with an erythematous base that progresses to painful ulceration with associated lymphadenopathy
- Other species of *Haemophilus* are opportunistic pathogens primarily responsible for **sinusitis, otitis,** or **bronchitis**

HAEMOPHILUS INFLUENZAE	
Properties	• *H. influenzae* subdivided serologically based on capsular antigens (types a to f); **serotype b** is clinically the most virulent • The major virulence factor in ***H. influenzae* type b (HIB)** is the antiphagocytic **polysaccharide capsule**, which contains ribose, ribitol, and phosphate; commonly referred to as polyribitol phosphate or PRP; antigen used for preparation of the vaccine • Antibodies developed against PRP are protective • Bacterial cell wall lipopolysaccharide lipid A induces meningeal inflammation
Epidemiology	• *Haemophilus* species are normal residents of the human mouth although *H. influenzae* type b is relatively uncommon • Disease caused by *H. influenzae* type b is primarily a pediatric problem (<5 years of age) although vaccination has eliminated this pathogen in many populations • Patients at greatest risk for disease are those with inadequate levels of protective antibodies, those with depleted complement, and those who have undergone splenectomy
Clinical Disease	• **Meningitis**: the most common cause of pediatric meningitis in unvaccinated populations; starts with mild upper respiratory symptoms and then progresses to meningeal signs • **Epiglottitis**: cellulitis and swelling of the supraglottic tissues; represents a life-threatening emergency in young children with naturally narrow airways • **Cellulitis**: development of reddish-blue patches on the cheeks or periorbital areas; accompanied by fever • **Arthritis**: prior to vaccination, this was the most common cause of arthritis in children younger than 2 years of age
Diagnosis	• Gram stain and culture of CSF or synovial fluid is diagnostic • Blood cultures typically positive for most diseases • Immunoassays for PRP are antigen sensitive with CSF or urine (antigen concentrated in urine) specimens, but rarely used today following the introduction of the vaccine in the community
Treatment, Control, Prevention	• Broad-spectrum cephalosporins used for initial empiric therapy; use of alternative antibiotics should be guided by *in vitro* susceptibility tests • Primary approach to prevent *H. influenzae* type b disease is through immunization with a **conjugated PRP vaccine** (combined with protein to stimulate immune response in very young children); vaccine administered before 6 months of age, followed by booster vaccination between age 12 to 15 months; vaccine only effective against type b strains of *H. influenzae*

CLINICAL CASE

Pneumonia Caused by *Haemophilus Influenzae*

Holmes and Kozinn[3] described a 61-year-old woman with pneumonia caused by H. influenzae *serotype d. The patient had a long history of smoking, chronic obstructive lung disease, diabetes mellitus, and congestive heart failure. She presented with left upper lobe pneumonia, producing purulent sputum with many gram-negative coccobacilli. Both sputum and blood cultures were positive for* H. influenzae *serotype d. The organism was susceptible to ampicillin, to which the patient responded. This case illustrates the susceptibility of patients with chronic underlying pulmonary disease to infections with nonserotype b strains of* H. influenzae.

ACINETOBACTER BAUMANNII

For many years *A. baumannii* and other species of *Acinetobacter* occupied the relatively common niche of opportunistic pathogens that infrequently caused significant disease. This has changed in recent years, because these bacteria, particularly *A. baumannii*, added one additional property to their assets: resistance to virtually all antimicrobials. This ability has not only made treatment a challenge, it has also handicapped control of the spread of bacteria in hospitals. This became most evident during the military conflicts in Iraq and Afghanistan. Injured soldiers developed wound infections, pneumonia, and overwhelming sepsis in the military hospitals where infection control practices were inadequate, and then became reservoirs for infections when the soldiers were transferred back to their home countries. The organisms now persist in many hospitals worldwide, and certainly will remain a challenge for many years to come.

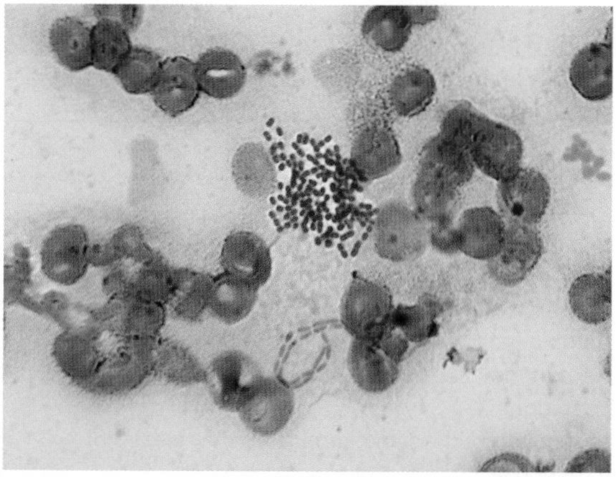

Acinetobacter baumannii in a positive blood culture with *Pseudomonas aeruginosa*. This gram-negative coccobacillus resembles fat gram-positive cocci, arranged as single cells or in pairs. In contrast, *P. aeruginosa* are gram-negative rods arranged in a chain.

ACINETOBACTER BAUMANNII	
Properties	• Opportunistic pathogen • Many strains are **multidrug resistant**
Epidemiology	• *Acinetobacter* species are ubiquitous saprophytes present in the environment inside and outside the hospital; able to survive on both moist surfaces such as mechanical ventilation equipment, and on dry surfaces such as the human skin • Although other *Acinetobacter* species can colonize the human mouth, *A. baumannii* is not considered a normal resident, so isolation from clinical specimens is considered significant • Patients at risk of infection include those receiving broad-spectrum antibiotics, recovering from surgery, or on respiratory ventilation
Clinical Disease	• **Opportunistic pathogen** causing infections in the respiratory tract, urinary tract, wounds, and sepsis
Diagnosis	• Gram stain morphology is characteristic—large, plump coccobacilli that may appear gram-positive and typically in pairs (larger and more round than *Streptococcus pneumoniae* or *Enterococcus* so this will not cause confusion) • Growth on nonselective media is typically seen after 1 day of incubation • Identification of *A. baumannii* can be made using biochemical tests, but these are generally unreliable for other *Acinetobacter* species; gene sequencing used for identification of these organisms
Treatment, Control, Prevention	• Treatment must be guided by *in vitro* susceptibility tests because multidrug resistance is common • Colistin may be the only active antibiotic • Proper infection control practices are required to prevent the spread of this organism in critically ill hospitalized patients, particularly for wound care and use of mechanical respiratory devices

BORDETELLA PERTUSSIS

One should question why we are seeing a resurgence of infections with an organism whose biology, epidemiology, and pathogenesis are so well known, and where vaccines to control the disease are readily available. The reality is we know so much about this organism because it is such an important pathogen. The use of effective, nontoxic vaccines has only recently been introduced, and disease in adult patients persists because the initial vaccines did not provide lasting immunity. Elimination of pertussis will only be achieved by an aggressive vaccine program and vigilance in monitoring for subclinical disease. Until that is accomplished, understanding the importance of this organism will remain paramount.

BORDETELLA PERTUSSIS	
Properties	• **Filamentous hemagglutinin** and **pertactin** bind to the membranes of ciliated cells in trachea; these proteins are highly immunogenic and are used in the current vaccines • **Pertussis toxin** binds to ciliated epithelial cells of the oropharynx as well as to the surface of phagocytic cells • Pertussis toxin (A-B toxin) inactivates G1α, a protein that controls adenylate cyclase activity, resulting in increased levels of cyclic adenosine monophosphate (AMP) with subsequent increase in respiratory secretions and mucus production; also inhibits phagocytic killing and monocyte migration • **Adenylate cyclase/hemolysin toxin** increases cyclic AMP levels; also inhibits phagocytic killing and monocyte migration • **Tracheal cytotoxin** kills ciliated respiratory cells and stimulates the release of interleukin-1 resulting in febrile response
Epidemiology	• Strict human pathogen • Worldwide distribution • Unvaccinated individuals are at greatest risk for disease • Disease was traditionally restricted primarily to children younger than 1 year; however, disease is now commonly observed in older children and adults, most likely due to waning immunity • Disease spreads person-to-person by infectious aerosols
Clinical Disease	• **Pertussis**: develops after a 7- to 10-day incubation period; characterized by: (1) **catarrhal** stage (resembles a common cold); progressing to the (2) **paroxysmal** stage (repetitive coughs followed by inspiratory whoops); and then the (3) **convalescence** stage (diminishing paroxysms and secondary complications) • Paroxysmal stage may be less prominent in older children and adults because their airways may not be obstructed as in infants
Diagnosis	• Microscopy is insensitive and nonspecific • Culture on selective media is specific but insensitive • NAATs are the most sensitive and specific tests and have generally replaced microscopy and culture • Serology can be used as a confirmatory test but is not widely used
Treatment, Control, Prevention	• Treatment with a macrolide (i.e., azithromycin, clarithromycin) is effective • Azithromycin is used for prophylaxis • Vaccines containing inactivated pertussin toxin, filamentous hemagglutinin, and pertactin are highly effective • Pediatric vaccine is administered in five doses (ages 2, 4, 6, 15 to 18 months, and 4 to 6 years); adult vaccine is administered at ages 11 to 12 years and 19 to 65 years)

CLINICAL CASE

Pertussis Outbreak in Health Care Workers

Pascual and associates[4] reported an outbreak of pertussis among hospital workers. The index case, a nurse anesthetist, presented acutely with cough, paroxysms followed by vomiting, and apneic episodes that led to loss of consciousness. Surgical service personnel, exposed patients, and family members were surveyed, and cultures, polymerase chain reaction tests, and serology were obtained from patients with respiratory symptoms. Twelve (23%) health care workers and 0 of 146 patients had clinical pertussis. The lack of disease in patients was attributed to mask use, cough etiquette, and limited face-to-face contact. This outbreak emphasizes the susceptibility of adults to infection, and the highly infectious nature of B. pertussis.

FRANCISELLA TULARENSIS

F. tularensis has reached the "lofty" status of **Select Agent**, an organism of potential bioterrorism. The importance of this organism and the high degree of infectivity was not wasted on me as a young microbiologist when I started my career in St. Louis, and recovered this organism in culture every summer (it is well established in the area's rabbit population). My staff quickly realized how dangerous this organism was, and exercised extreme caution when the almost submicroscopic gram-negative coccobacilli were observed in a positive blood culture. The ease with which this can be transmitted to a technologist in the laboratory is similar to the ease of transmission from infected animal tissues or a tick bite.

FRANCISELLA TULARENSIS	
Properties	• Polysaccharide capsule protects bacteria for antibody-mediated phagocytosis • Intracellular pathogen resistant to killing in serum and by phagocytes
Epidemiology	• Humans are accidental hosts • Wild mammals, domestic animals, and blood sucking arthropods are reservoirs; **rabbits**, cats, **hard ticks**, and biting flies are most commonly associated with human disease • Worldwide distribution, with disease in the United States most common in Oklahoma, Missouri, and Arkansas • Infectious dose is small when exposure is by arthropod, through skin penetration, or by inhalation; larger numbers of organisms must be ingested for disease by this route • Ticks must feed for a prolonged time before transmission of the bacteria in their feces
Clinical Disease	• **Ulceroglandular tularemia**: characterized by the development of a painful papule that is initially observed at the site of inoculation, and then progresses to ulceration with localized lymphadenopathy • **Oculoglandular tularemia**: after inoculation into the eye (e.g., rubbing the eye with a contaminated finger), infection is characterized by the development of conjunctivitis with regional lymphadenopathy • **Pneumonic tularemia**: pneumonitis with signs of sepsis develops rapidly after exposure to contaminated aerosols; high mortality unless disease is promptly diagnosed and treated
Diagnosis	• Microscopy is insensitive because the organism is very small (this morphology is similar to *Brucella* and is quite characteristic for both organisms) • Growth of the organism must be on cysteine-supplemented media (e.g., chocolate agar, buffered charcoal yeast extract agar) and prolonged incubation (3 or more days) is required; culture is insensitive unless the organism is suspected and culture plates incubated longer than what is typical • *Francisella* is highly contagious so care must be used if the organism is isolated in culture • Serology can be used to confirm the diagnosis, but antibodies persist for years and cross-react with *Brucella* infections
Treatment, Control, Prevention	• Gentamicin is the antibiotic of choice; fluoroquinolones and doxycycline have good activity; penicillins and some cephalosporins are ineffective • Disease prevented by avoiding reservoirs and vectors of infections • Prompt removal of infected ticks is usually effective • Live attenuated vaccine is available but rarely used for preventing human disease

CLINICAL CASE

Cat-Associated Tularemia

Capellan and Fong[5] described a 63-year-old man who developed ulceroglandular tularemia complicated by pneumonia after a cat bite. He initially presented with pain and localized swelling of his thumb 5 days after the bite. Oral penicillins were prescribed, but the patient's condition worsened, with increased local pain, swelling, and erythema at the wound site, and systemic signs (fever, malaise, and vomiting). Incision of the wound was performed, but no abscess was found; culture of the wound was positive for a light growth of coagulase-negative staphylococci. Intravenous penicillins were prescribed, but the patient continued to deteriorate, with the development of tender axillary lymphadenopathy and pulmonary symptoms. A chest radiograph revealed pneumonic infiltrates in the right middle and lower lobes of the lung. The patient's therapy was changed to clindamycin and gentamicin, which was followed by defervescence and improvement of his clinical status. After 3 days of incubation, tiny colonies of faintly staining gram-negative coccobacilli were observed on the original wound culture. The organism was referred to a national reference laboratory, where it was identified as F. tularensis. *A more complete history revealed the patient's cat lived outdoors and fed on wild rodents. This case illustrates the difficulty in making the diagnosis of tularemia, and the lack of responsiveness to penicillins.*

BRUCELLA SPECIES

Much like *Francisella, Brucella* species are extremely small gram-negative coccobacilli that are now classified as **Select Agents**. The most common species responsible for human disease is *Brucella melitensis,* an organism that unfortunately finds its way into the United States primarily via unpasteurized dairy products from Mexico. This is the species that is also responsible for the most acute, severe systemic disease and associated complications.

***BRUCELLA* SPECIES**	
Properties	• Intracellular pathogen of reticuloendothelial system and is able to resist being killed in serum and by phagocytes
Epidemiology	• Animal reservoirs are goats and sheep (*B. melitensis*), cattle and American bison (*Brucella abortus*), swine, reindeer, and caribou (*Brucella suis*) and dogs, foxes, and coyotes (*Brucella canis*) • Humans are accidental hosts that can develop disease from any of the listed species • Infects animal tissues rich in erythritol (e.g., breast, uterus, placenta, epididymis), with shedding of organisms in high numbers in milk, urine, and birth products • Worldwide distribution; vaccination of herds has controlled disease in the United States • Most disease in the United States is reported in California and Texas, and in travelers from Mexico • Individuals at greatest risk for disease are people who consume unpasteurized dairy products such as milk and cheeses, people in direct contact with infected animals, and laboratory workers
Clinical Disease	• **Brucellosis**: initially presents with nonspecific symptoms of malaise, chills, sweats, fatigue, myalgias, weight loss, arthralgias, and fever; typically progresses to systemic symptoms and involvement (gastrointestinal tract, bones or joints, respiratory tract, other organs) • Fever can be intermittent (termed "**undulant fever**")
Diagnosis	• Microscopy is insensitive because the organism is very small, although characteristic when observed • Culture (blood, bone marrow, infected tissue) is sensitive if prolonged incubation is used (3 days to 2 weeks) • Serology can be used to confirm the clinical diagnosis, but high titers can persist for months to years and cross-reactivity is observed with other infections
Treatment, Control, Prevention	• Recommended treatment is with doxycycline combined with rifampin for a minimum of 6 weeks for nonpregnant adults; trimethoprim-sulfamethoxazole for pregnant women and for children younger than 8 years • Human disease is controlled by eradication of the disease in the animal reservoir through vaccination, and serologic monitoring of the animals for evidence of disease; pasteurization of dairy products; and use of proper safety practices in clinical laboratories working with this organism

CLINICAL CASE

Brucellosis

Lee and Fung[6] described a 34-year-old woman who developed brucellosis caused by B. melitensis. *The woman presented with recurrent headaches, fever, and malaise that developed after she had handled goat placenta in China. Blood cultures were positive for* B. melitensis *after extended incubation. She was treated for 6 weeks with doxycycline and rifampicin, and had a successful response. The case was a classical description of exposure to contaminated tissues high in erythritol, a presentation of recurrent fevers and headaches, and response to the combination of doxycycline and rifampicin.*

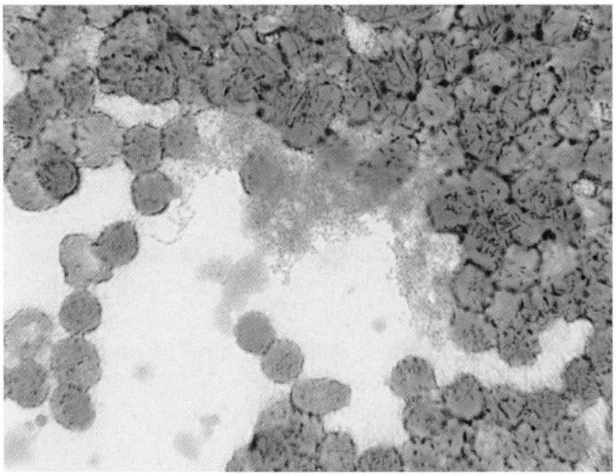

Brucella melitensis in a positive blood culture. The bacteria are extremely small, poorly staining coccobacilli, arranged in clumps around the much larger erythrocytes. Individual cells of the bacteria would be very difficult to detect due to their size and staining properties. *Francisella* has a very similar morphology.

REFERENCES

1. Fam A, McGillivray D, Stein J, Little H. Gonococcal arthritis: a report of six cases. *Can Med Assoc J.* 1973;108:319–325.
2. Gardner P. Clinical practice. Prevention of meningococcal disease. *N Engl J Med.* 2006;355:1466–1473.
3. Holmes RL, Kozinn WP. Pneumonia and bacteremia associated with *Haemophilus influenzae* serotype d. *J Clin Microbiol.* 1983;18:730–732.
4. Pascual FB, McCall CL, McMurtray A, Payton T, Smith F, Bisgard KM. Outbreak of pertussis among healthcare workers in a hospital surgical unit. *Infect Control Hosp Epidemiol.* 2006;27:546–552.
5. Capellan J, Fong IW. Tularemia from a cat bite: case report and review of feline-associated tularemia. *Clin Infect Dis.* 1993;16:472–475.
6. Lee MK, Fung KS. A case of human brucellosis in Hong Kong. *Hong Kong Med J.* 2005;11:403–406.

7

Aerobic Fermentative Gram-Negative Rods

INTERESTING FACTS

- The Centers for Disease Control and Prevention (CDC) estimates that there are more than 250,000 infections with Shiga toxin–producing *Escherichia coli* (STEC) annually in the United States and only about one-third are caused by *E. coli* O157
- The CDC estimates that there are approximately 1.2 million illnesses and 450 deaths annually in the United States due to nontyphoidal *Salmonella.* Children less than 5 years of age are most likely to be infected and the very young and elderly are most likely to have adverse complications
- There are approximately 500,000 cases of shigellosis in the United States annually, with young children and gay males at greatest risk for infection. In contrast to the United States, *Shigella* is the most common cause of diarrheal disease in young children in resource-limited countries
- Although cholera is rare in the United States and other industrialized countries, outbreaks are still reported in Africa, Southeast Asia, and Haiti

Two large and important families of bacteria are discussed in this chapter: **Enterobacteriaceae** and **Vibrionaceae**. Members of the Enterobacteriaceae family are the most common gram-negative bacteria responsible for human disease. Although somewhat less common, one member of the Vibrionaceae, ***Vibrio cholerae***, is responsible for one of the most feared and deadly diseases in developing countries: cholera. These two families share the common property of fermenting glucose, as well as having several diseases in common, such as gastroenteritis and wound infections. It is not practical to discuss individual members of these families without first understanding the common properties found in all family members that contribute to their virulence, epidemiology, and diseases they produce.

The family Enterobacteriaceae is the largest, most heterogeneous collection of medically important gram-negative rods, home to more than 50 genera and hundreds of species and subspecies. Members of this family are **ubiquitous**, found worldwide in soil, water, and vegetation, and are part of the normal intestinal flora of most animals, including humans. All members can grow rapidly, aerobically and anaerobically, on a variety of nonselective (e.g., blood agar) and selective (e.g., MacConkey agar) media. The Enterobacteriaceae have simple nutritional requirements, they ferment glucose, and are oxidase negative. The absence of cytochrome oxidase activity is an important characteristic because it can be measured rapidly with a simple test and is used to distinguish the Enterobacteriaceae from many other fermentative (e.g., *Vibrio*) and nonfermentative (e.g., *Pseudomonas*) gram-negative rods. The appearance of the bacteria on culture media has been used to differentiate common members of the Enterobacteriaceae. For example, **fermentation of lactose** (detected by color changes in lactose-containing media such as the commonly used MacConkey agar) has been used to differentiate some enteric pathogens that do not ferment lactose (e.g., *Salmonella*, *Shigella*; colorless colonies on MacConkey agar) from lactose-fermenting species (e.g., *Escherichia*, *Klebsiella*; pink-purple colonies on MacConkey agar). **Resistance to bile salts** in some selective media has also been used to separate enteric pathogens (e.g., *Shigella*, *Salmonella*) from commensal organisms that are inhibited by bile salts. In this example, use of culture media that assess lactose fermentation and resistance to bile salts is a rapid screening test for enteric pathogens that would be otherwise difficult to detect in diarrheal stool specimens where many different organisms may be present. Some Enterobacteriaceae, such as *Klebsiella*, are also characteristically mucoid (wet, heaped, viscous colonies with prominent **capsules**), whereas a loose-fitting, diffusible slime layer surrounds other species.

The heat-stable **lipopolysaccharide (LPS)** is a major cell wall antigen in the Enterobacteriaceae, and consists of three components: the outermost somatic **O polysaccharide,** a core polysaccharide common to all Enterobacteriaceae (**enterobacterial common antigen**), and **lipid A**. The lipid A component of LPS is responsible for endotoxin activity, and many of the systemic manifestations of gram-negative bacterial infections are initiated by endotoxin—activation of complement, release of cytokines, leukocytosis, thrombocytopenia, disseminated intravascular coagulation, fever, decreased peripheral circulation, shock, and death.

The epidemiologic (serologic) classification of the Enterobacteriaceae is based on three major groups of antigens: **somatic O polysaccharides, K antigens** in the capsule (type-specific polysaccharides), and the **H proteins** in the bacterial flagella. Detection of these various antigens has important clinical significance beyond epidemiologic investigations, some pathogenic species of bacteria are associated with specific O and H serotypes (e.g., *E. coli* O157:H7 is associated with hemorrhagic colitis).

The family Vibrionaceae is also large, consisting of more than 100 species, with *V. cholerae* the most important. All of the species can grow on a variety of simple media, but require salt for growth (halophilic or "salt loving"). These species can also tolerate a wide range of temperatures and pH, but are susceptible to gastric acid. For this reason, exposure to a large inoculum is required for disease. As with the Enterobacteriaceae, the cell wall of Vibrionaceae contains LPS consisting of the outer O polysaccharide, core polysaccharide, and inner lipid A components. The O polysaccharide is used to subdivide *Vibrio* species into serogroups. There are more than 200 serogroups of *V. cholerae*, with *V. cholerae* O1 the most important. This is the serogroup responsible for worldwide pandemics of cholera.

Although the discussion of *Vibrio* species in this chapter focuses on *V. cholerae*, two other species deserve mention: *Vibrio parahaemolyticus* and *Vibrio vulnificus*. Following ingestion of contaminated seafood, *V. parahaemolyticus* can cause **diarrheal disease**, ranging from self-limited, watery diarrhea to a mild form of cholera. Illness lasts 3 days or more, but results in an uneventful recovery. In contrast, *V. vulnificus* is a particularly virulent species, with the most common presentations as a **primary septicemia** after consumption of contaminated raw oysters, or a rapidly **progressive wound infection** after exposure to contaminated seawater. Mortality can approach 50% in septic patients, and 20% to 30% in patients with wound infections. Immunocompromised patients are at particular risk, or those with preexisting hepatic disease, hematopoietic disease, or chronic renal failure.

CLINICAL CASE

Raw Oysters and *Vibrio parahaemolyticus*

One of the largest known outbreaks of V. parahaemolyticus *in the United States was reported in 2005.*[1] *On July 19, the Nevada Office of Epidemiology reported isolation of* V. parahaemolyticus *from a person who developed gastroenteritis 1 day after eating raw oysters served on an Alaskan cruise ship. Epidemiologic investigations determined that 62 individuals (29% attack rate) developed gastroenteritis following consumption of as few as one raw oyster. In addition to watery diarrhea, the ill individuals reported abdominal cramping (82%), chills (44%), myalgias (36%), headache (32%), and vomiting (29%), with symptoms lasting a median of 5 days. None of the persons required hospitalization. All of the oysters were harvested from a single farm, where the water temperatures in July and August were recorded at 16.6°C and 17.4°C. Water temperatures above 15°C are considered favorable for growth of* V. parahaemolyticus. *Since 1997, the mean water temperatures at the oyster farm have increased by 0.21°C per year, and now remain consistently above 15°C. Thus this seasonal warming has extended the range of* V. parahaemolyticus *and the associated gastrointestinal disease. This outbreak illustrates the role of contaminated shellfish in* V. parahaemolyticus *disease and the clinical symptoms typically observed.*

CLINICAL CASE

Septicemia Caused by *Vibrio vulnificus*

Septicemia and wound infections are well-known complications following exposure to V. vulnificus. *The following clinical case, published in* Morbidity and Mortality Weekly Report,[2] *illustrates typical features of these diseases. A 38-year-old man with a history of alcoholism and insulin-dependent diabetes developed fever, chills, nausea, and myalgia 3 days after eating raw oysters. He was admitted to the local hospital the next day with high fevers and two necrotic lesions on his left leg. The clinical diagnosis of sepsis was made, and the patient was transferred to the intensive care unit. Antibiotic therapy was initiated, and on the second hospital day* V. vulnificus *was isolated from blood specimens collected at the time of admission. Despite aggressive medical management, the patient continued to deteriorate and died on the third day of hospitalization. This case illustrates the rapid, often fatal progression of* V. vulnificus *disease, and the risk factor of eating raw shellfish, particularly for individuals with liver disease. A similar progression of disease could have been observed if this individual had been exposed to* V. vulnificus *through a contaminated, superficial wound.*

Enterobacteriaceae and Vibrionaceae

Bacteria	Historical Derivation
Family Enterobactericeae	
E. coli	*Escherichia*, named after the discoverer Theodor Escherich; *coli*, of the colon
Klebsiella pneumoniae	*Klebsiella*, named after the German microbiologist Edwin Klebs; *pneumoniae*, inflammation of the lungs
Proteus mirabilis	*Proteus*, a god able to change himself into different shapes; *mirabilis*, surprising (refers to pleomorphic colony forms)
Salmonella typhi	*Salmonella*, named after Daniel Salmon, chairman of the department where the discoverer, Theobald Smith, worked; *typhi*, of typhoid (referring to the disease typhoid fever)
Shigella dysenteriae	*Shigella*, named after the discoverer Kiyoshi Shiga; *dysenteriae*, dysentery
Yersinia pestis	*Yersinia*, named after Yersin who identified the first isolate; *pestis*, plague
Family Vibrionaceae	
V. cholerae	*Vibrio*, move rapidly or vibrate (rapid movement caused by the polar flagella); *cholerae*, cholera or an intestinal disease

Discussion of the Enterobacteriaceae and Vibrionaceae cannot be comprehensive due to the large number of species responsible for disease; however, I believe the species I have selected are representative of these families.

ESCHERICHIA COLI

E. coli is the most common and important member of the family Enterobacteriaceae. This organism is associated with a variety of diseases, including gastroenteritis and extraintestinal infections such as cystitis and pyelonephritis, intraabdominal infection, meningitis, and sepsis. A multitude of strains are capable of causing disease, with some serotypes associated with greater virulence (e.g., *E. coli* O157 is the most common cause of hemorrhagic colitis and hemolytic uremic syndrome). Five different clusters of *E. coli* are responsible for intestinal disease, each possessing unique virulence properties.

ESCHERICHIA COLI	
Properties	• **Enterotoxigenic *E. coli* (ETEC)** attach to the small intestine by colonization factor antigens and produce heat-labile and heat-stable toxins • **Enteropathogenic *E. coli* (EPEC)** attach to the small intestine by adhesins (bundle-forming pili, intimin) and disrupt the surface • **Enteroaggregative *E. coli* (EAEC)** attach to the small intestine by aggregative adherence fimbriae (AAF) and also disrupt the surface • **Shiga Toxin Producing *E. coli* (STEC)** initially attach to intestines by bundle-forming pili and intimin, and then produce shiga toxins Stx1 and Stx2 that affect the colonic epithelium • EIEC invade and destroy the colonic epithelium • Uropathogenic strains bind to cells of bladder and upper urinary tract by adhesins (P pili, AAF, others), and produce hemolysin HlyA that lyses cells leading to cytokine release in stimulation of inflammatory response • Majority of strains that cause neonatal meningitis possess the K1 capsular antigen
Epidemiology	• Most common aerobic gram-negative rods in the gastrointestinal tract • Urinary tract infections, intraabdominal infections and sepsis are primarily endogenous (patient's microbial flora); strains causing gastroenteritis are generally acquired exogenously • Meningitis primarily restricted to neonates • Intraabdominal infections related to spillage of intestinal bacteria into abdomen during trauma or surgery; infections typically polymicrobial

Clinical Disease	• **Gastroenteritis**: caused by variety of strains with specific virulence factors; clinical illness reflection of site of infection and pathology
	  • Infections of small intestine (ETEC, EPEC, EAEC): characterized by watery diarrhea, vomiting, and low-grade fever
	  • Infections of large intestine (STEC, EIEC): characterized by bloody diarrhea (hemorrhagic colitis) and abdominal cramps
	• **Hemolytic uremic syndrome**: a complication of STEC and EIEC infections
	• **Urinary tract infections**: may be restricted to inflammation of the bladder or may involve the upper tract, primarily kidneys, with associated flank pain and fever
	• Polymicrobial **intraabdominal infection**: characterized by abscess formation (caused by associated bacteria) and septicemia
	• **Meningitis**: in neonates cannot be differentiated from other causes of meningitis (e.g., group B *Streptococcus*)

Diagnosis	• Gram stains of Enterobacteriaceae isolates stain most intensely at the end, with a characteristic "bipolar" appearance • Organisms grow rapidly on most culture media • Enteric pathogens, with the exception of STEC, are detected primarily by nucleic acid amplification tests (NAATs) which have recently become commercially available • STEC-producing strains detected on selective media or by assays for detection of the toxins or the encoding genes
Treatment, Control, Prevention	• Enteric pathogens are treated symptomatically unless disseminated disease occurs • Antibiotic therapy is guided by *in vitro* susceptibility tests because of increased resistance to penicillins, cephalosporins, and carbapenems, mediated by extended spectrum β-lactamases and carbapenemases • Appropriate infection-control practices are used to reduce the risk of nosocomial infections (e.g., restricting use of antibiotics, avoiding unnecessary use of urinary tract catheters) • Maintenance of high hygienic standards to reduce the risk of exposure to gastroenteritis strains, particularly for travelers to less developed regions • Proper cooking of beef products to reduce risk of STEC infections

CLINICAL CASE

Multistate Outbreak of STEC Infections

In 2006, E. coli *O157 was responsible for a large, multistate outbreak of gastroenteritis. The outbreak was linked to the contamination of spinach, with a total of 173 cases reported in 25 states, primarily over an 18-day period. The outbreak resulted in the hospitalization of more than 50% of the patients with documented disease, a 16% rate of hemolytic uremic syndrome, and one death. Despite the wide distribution of the contaminated spinach, publication of the outbreak and the rapid determination that spinach was responsible resulted in prompt removal of spinach from grocery stores and termination of the outbreak. This outbreak illustrates how contamination of a food product, even with small numbers of organisms, can lead to a widespread outbreak with a particularly virulent organism, such as strains of STEC.*

KLEBSIELLA PNEUMONIAE

The most important member of the genus *Klebsiella* is *K. pneumoniae*, a prominent cause of **pneumonia**. Members of the genus are covered with a prominent mucoid capsule, which makes recognition of the bacteria by Gram stain (large rods surrounded by large capsule) and culture relatively easy. The bacteria in this genus cause both community- and hospital-acquired pneumonia, with destruction of the alveolar spaces, formation of cavities, and production of blood-tinged sputum prominent. Treatment of disease caused by this organism has also become a challenge, because many strains are resistant to all β-lactam antibiotics through the production of carbapenemases. The term "**KPC**" or *K. pneumoniae*–producing carbapenemases has unfortunately become an all too familiar part of our conversation today.

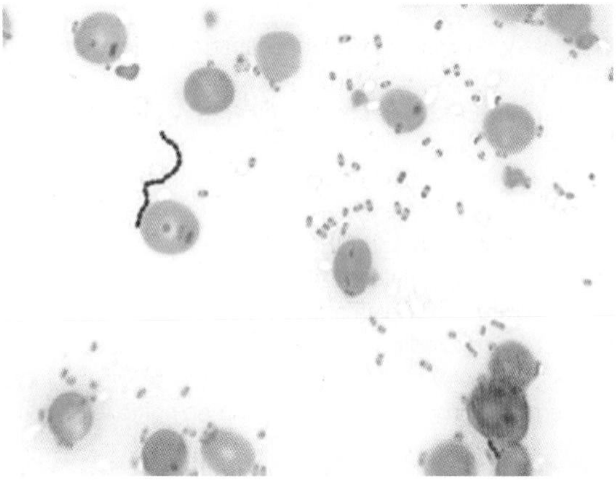

Escherichia coli and *Streptococcus* spp. in a positive blood culture. All members of the Enterobacteriaceae have bipolar staining; that is, the ends of the rods stain more intensely than the center of the cell, giving the initial appearance of diplococci.

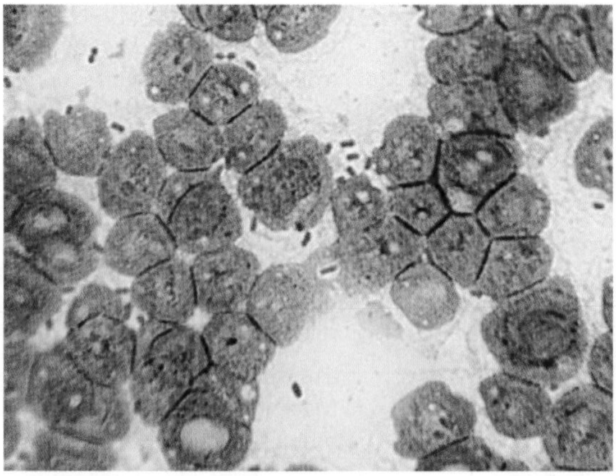

Klebsiella pneumoniae are large rods frequently surrounded by a prominent capsule. Note in this slide many of the rods are surrounded by a clear area (particularly noticeable in the pair of rods in the center of the photo). The clear area is the capsule that excludes the stain.

KLEBSIELLA PNEUMONIAE	
Properties	• Prominent mucoid polysaccharide capsule • Production of carbapenemases and other β-lactamases
Epidemiology	• Widely distributed in nature and low level colonization of healthy individuals • Disease primarily in patients with depressed pulmonary function or control of respiratory secretions (e.g., alcoholics, moribund hospitalized patients)
Clinical Disease	• **Pneumonia**: prominently involving one or more lobes ("lobar pneumonia") with cavity formation and production of bloody sputa
Diagnosis	• Gram stain of sputa with characteristic bacteria associated with a vigorous cellular immune response • Relatively easy to grow in culture

KLEBSIELLA PNEUMONIAE—cont'd	
Treatment, Control, Prevention	• Treatment must be guided by *in vitro* susceptibility tests because multidrug-resistant strains are common, particularly in hospital settings • Appropriate infection-control practices are used to reduce the risk of nosocomial infections, including screening asymptomatic patients for carriage of resistant strains and limited use of antibiotics

PROTEUS MIRABILIS

The most commonly isolated member of the genus *Proteus* is *P. mirabilis*, which is an important cause of **urinary tract infections** in previously healthy adults. *P. mirabilis* produces large quantities of urease, an enzyme that splits urea into carbon dioxide and ammonia. This process raises the urine pH, precipitating magnesium and calcium in the form of struvite and apatite crystals, respectively, and results in the formation of renal stones. Other bacteria that infect the urinary tract and produce urease can produce the same effect (e.g., *Staphylococcus saprophyticus*).

PROTEUS MIRABILIS	
Properties	• Urease production
Epidemiology	• Present in the gastrointestinal tract and can migrate to the urinary tract to produce disease • Patients with a history of infections with this organism are at increased risk of reinfections
Clinical Disease	• **Urinary tract infections** including cystitis (bladder) and pylenephritis (kidney) with stone formation
Diagnosis	• Grows readily in culture and has a characteristic swarming motility on the surface of the agar plates (colony will rapidly spread and cover the entire plate surface with a thin sheet of bacteria) • Definitive identification by biochemical tests or mass spectrometry
Treatment, Control, Prevention	• Generally susceptible to ampicillin and cephalosporins; resistant to tetracycline • Restricted use of urinary tract catheters will reduce risk of hospital-acquired infections

SALMONELLA SPECIES

More than 2500 serotypes of *Salmonella* are described, and are frequently listed as individual species, with the most common being *S. typhi*, *Salmonella enteritidis*, *Salmonella choleraesuis*, and *Salmonella typhimurium*. In reality most of these serotypes are members of a single species, *Salmonella enterica*. I don't believe the student is particularly interested in these taxonomic debates, but there is some confusion in the literature that should be recognized. To simplify this presentation, I will focus on the most important member of this genus, *S. typhi*, and provide general commentary on the other species.

Salmonella species can colonize all animals, particularly poultry, and cause disease in a variety of hosts including humans; however, *S. typhi* is a strictly human pathogen that can cause severe disease, and survive in the gallbladder establishing chronic carriage.

SALMONELLA SPECIES	
Properties	• Virulence of *S. typhi* is regulated by genes on two large pathogenicity islands that facilitate the attachment, engulfment, and replication of bacteria in intestinal cells and macrophages • Bacteria are transported from the intestines to liver, spleen, and bone marrow by macrophages

Continued

SALMONELLA SPECIES—cont'd	
Epidemiology	• In contrast with most *Salmonella* species that are acquired by eating contaminated food products (e.g., poultry, eggs, dairy products), *S. typhi* is a **strict human pathogen** and is acquired by person-to-person contact or ingestion of food or water contaminated by infected individuals • 400 to 500 *S. typhi* infections occur annually in the United States, most of which are acquired during foreign travel; more than 27 million cases worldwide with an estimated 200,000 deaths annually • Infectious dose is low, so person-to-person spread is common • Asymptomatic long-term colonization occurs commonly
Clinical Disease	• **Enteric fever**: 10 to 14 days after ingestion of *S. typhi*, patients experience gradually increasing fever with nonspecific complaints of headache, myalgias, fever, and anorexia; symptoms persist for 1 week or more followed by gastrointestinal symptoms • **Asymptomatic colonization**: chronic low-grade infection with *S. typhi*, localized to the gallbladder
Diagnosis	• *S. typhi* present in the **blood** during the first phase of illness and then recovered in **stool specimens** after infection is localized in the gallbladder • Culture is frequently negative because the bacteremic phase is transient and low numbers of organisms present in the stool specimen may be difficult to detect • Although serologic tests have been used historically to document present or past infections, these tests are considered insensitive and nonspecific
Treatment, Control, Prevention	• Infections with *S. typhi* or disseminated infections with other organisms should be treated with an effective antibiotic (selected by *in vitro* susceptibility tests); fluoroquinolones (e.g., ciprofloxacin), chloramphenicol, trimethoprim-sulfamethoxazole, or a broad-spectrum cephalosporin may be used, but regional antibiotic resistance is common due to unrestricted use of antibiotics in some communities • Carriers of *S. typhi* should be identified and treated • Vaccination against *S. typhi* can reduce the risk of disease for travelers into endemic areas

CLINICAL CASE

Salmonella typhi Infection

Scully and associates[3] described a 25-year-old woman who was admitted to a Boston hospital with a history of persistent fever that did not respond to amoxicillin, acetaminophen, or ibuprofen. She was a resident of the Philippines who had been traveling in the United States for the previous 11 days. On physical examination she was febrile, had an enlarged liver, abdominal pain, and an abnormal urinalysis. Blood cultures were collected upon admission to the hospital and were positive the next day with S. typhi. The organism is susceptible to fluoroquinolones; therefore this therapy was selected. Within 4 days, she had defervesced and was discharged to return home to the Philippines. Although typhoid fever can be a very serious, life-threatening illness, it can initially present with nonspecific symptoms, as was seen in this woman.

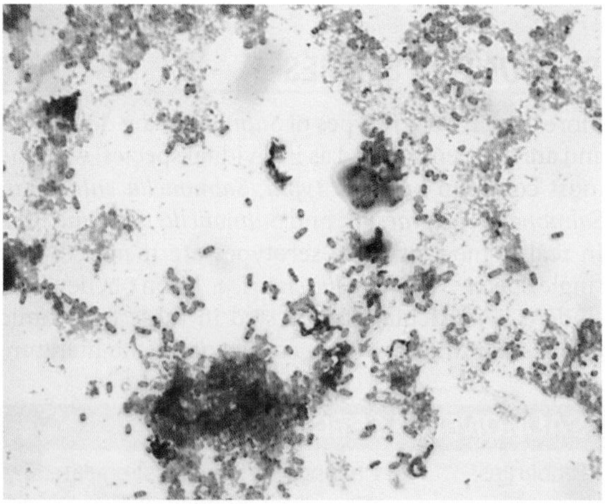

Salmonella typhi in a positive blood culture. Note the prominent bipolar staining.

SHIGELLA SPECIES

Species in the genus *Shigella* are actually biochemical variants (biogroups) of *E. coli*; however, they remain in a separate genus for historical reasons. It is probably easiest to think of *Shigella* as variants of Enteroinvasive *E. coli* (EIEC) and STEC. Four species of *Shigella* are recognized, with *Shigella sonnei* responsible for the vast majority of infections in the United States, and *Shigella flexneri* predominating in developing countries. Although *Shigella dysenteriae* infections are less common, primarily observed in West Africa and Central America, this is the most virulent species of *Shigella* and is associated with mortality rates of 5% to 15%. The fourth species, *Shigella boydii*, is infrequently isolated.

SHIGELLA SPECIES	
Properties	• Attach, invade, and replicate in cells lining the colon • Replicate in the cytoplasm of phagocytic cells and move cell-to-cell without extracellular exposure, thus protected from immune-mediated clearance • Induce programed cell death of macrophages, resulting in the release of interleukin-1β with resulting stimulation of localized inflammatory response • A-B exotoxin (**Shiga toxin** similar to STEC toxin) produced by *S. dysenteriae* disrupts protein synthesis and produces endothelial damage • Shiga toxin can also mediate damage to the glomerular endothelial cells, resulting in renal failure: **hemolytic uremic syndrome**
Epidemiology	• Estimated 500,000 cases of *Shigella* infections occur annually in the United States; 90 million cases worldwide (one of the most common causes of bacterial gastroenteritis) • **Humans are the only reservoir** for these bacteria • Disease spread person-to-person by fecal–oral route • Primarily a pediatric disease with young children in day-care centers, nurseries, and custodial institutions at highest risk for disease; also at risk are siblings and parents of these children; communities with poor hygienic standards; male homosexuals • Relatively few organisms can produce disease (highly infectious) • Disease occurs worldwide with no seasonal incidence (consistent with person-to-person spread involving a low inoculum)
Clinical Disease	• **Shigellosis** presents initially as a watery diarrhea progressing within 1 to 2 days to abdominal cramps and tenesmus (with or without bloody stools) • **Bacterial dysentery** is a severe form of disease, caused by *S. dysenteriae* • **Asymptomatic carriage** develops in a small number of patients (reservoir for future infections)
Diagnosis	• Microscopy is not useful because *Shigella* cannot be differentiated from *E. coli* and other gram-negative rods present in stool specimens from healthy individuals • Culture using selective media designed for the recovery of *Shigella* is useful but care is needed in handling positive cultures because this organism is highly infectious (laboratory-acquired infections are not uncommon) • Multiplex NAATs (simultaneously testing for multiple enteric pathogens) are becoming common and may replace cultures within the next few years in laboratories where resources are available
Treatment, Control, Prevention	• Antibiotic therapy shortens the course of symptomatic disease, fecal shedding, and infectivity for contacts • Treatment should be guided by *in vitro* susceptibility tests • Empirical therapy can be initiated with a fluoroquinolone or trimethoprim-sulfamethoxazole • Appropriate infection-control measures should be instituted to prevent spread of the organism, including hand washing and proper disposal of soiled linens

CLINICAL CASE

Shigella Infections in Day-Care Centers

In 2005, three states reported outbreaks of multidrug-resistant Shigella *infections in day-care centers. A total of 532 infections were reported in the Kansas City area, with the patients' median age of 6 years old.*[4] *The predominant pathogen was a multidrug-resistant strain of S. sonnei, with 89% of the isolates resistant to ampicillin and trimethoprim-sulfamethoxazole. Shigellosis spreads easily in day-care centers because of the increased risk of fecal contamination and the low infectious dose responsible for disease. Parents and teachers, as well as classmates, are at significant risk for disease.*

YERSINIA PESTIS

The best known human pathogens in this genus are *Y. pestis* and *Yersinia enterocolitica*. *Y. pestis* causes the highly fatal systemic disease known as **plague**, and will be the focus of this section. *Y. enterocolitica* is responsible for **gastroenteritis** in cold weather climates in Northern European and North American, as well as two additional diseases: (1) chronic inflammation of the terminal ileum with enlargement of the mesenteric lymph nodes resulting in "**pseudoappendicitis**" (primarily a disease in children); and (2) **blood transfusion-related bacteremia**. *Y. enterocolitica* can grow at 4°C, so this organism can multiply to high concentrations in blood products stored in a refrigerator.

YERSINIA PESTIS	
Properties	• *Y. pestis* is covered with a protein capsule and inhibits phagocytosis • Protease that degrades: (1) complement component C3b preventing opsonization; (2) C5a preventing phagocytic migration; and (3) fibrin clots permitting spread of the bacteria • Induces macrophage killing and suppression of cytokine production, resulting in diminished inflammatory response to infection • *Y. pestis* is resistant to serum killing
Epidemiology	• Plague was one of the most devastating diseases in history, with major epidemics recorded in the Old Testament; worldwide from 540 AD to mid-700 AD, in Europe in the 1320s (30%–40% of the population died), and beginning in China in the 1860s, Epidemics and sporadic cases continue to occur • *Y. pestis* is a zoonotic infection with humans the accidental host • Two epidemiologic forms of disease: (1) **urban plague** with rats as reservoir; (2) **sylvatic plague** with squirrels, rabbits, and domestic animals as reservoirs • Disease is spread by bites from the flea vector (infected reservoir host to humans), direct contact with infected tissues, or person-to-person by inhalation of infectious aerosols from a patient with pulmonary disease (patients with pulmonary disease highly infectious) • Fewer than 10 cases are reported annually in the United States with disease primarily sylvatic plague
Clinical Disease	• Two clinical manifestations: bubonic plague and pneumonic plague • **Bubonic plague**: characterized by incubation period of less than 1 week, followed by development of high fever and painful swelling or bubo of regional lymph nodes (groin or axilla) with bacteremia. High mortality rate unless promptly treated • **Pneumonic plague**: characterized by development of fever and pulmonary symptoms within 1 to 2 days after inhalation of bacteria; high mortality rate
Diagnosis	• Microscopy of bubo or pulmonary secretions suggestive if disease is clinically suspected but not specific (resembles other Enterobacteriaceae) • Organisms grow on most culture media but may require 2 days of incubation • Identification by biochemical testing or mass spectrometry

YERSINIA PESTIS—cont'd	
Treatment, Control, Prevention	• *Y. pestis* infections are treated with streptomycin; tetracyclines, chloramphenicol, or trimethoprim-sulfamethoxazole can be administered as alternative therapy • Enteric infections with other *Yersinia* species are usually self-limited; if antibiotic therapy is indicated, most organisms are susceptible to broad-spectrum cephalosporins, aminoglycosides, chloramphenicol, tetracyclines, and trimethoprim-sulfamethoxazole • Plague is controlled by reduction of the rodent population • Vaccine is no longer available in the United States

CLINICAL CASE

Human Plague in the United States

In 2006, a total of 13 human plague cases were reported in the United States—7 in New Mexico, 3 in Colorado, 2 in California, and 1 in Texas.[5] The following is a description of a 30-year-old man with a classic presentation of bubonic plague. On July 9, the man presented to his local hospital with a 3-day history of fever, nausea, vomiting, and right inguinal lymphadenopathy. He was discharged without treatment. Three days later, he returned to the hospital and was admitted with sepsis and bilateral pulmonary infiltrates. He was placed on respiratory isolation and treated with gentamicin, to which he responded. Cultures of his blood and enlarged lymph node were positive for Y. pestis. *The bacteria were also recovered in fleas collected near the patient's home. Typically, the reservoirs for sylvatic plaque are small mammals, and the vectors are fleas. When the mammals die off, the fleas will seek human hosts.*

VIBRIO CHOLERAE

Much like *Y. pestis*, *V. cholerae* is responsible for one of the most feared diseases in history—**cholera**. We are currently in the midst of the seventh pandemic (worldwide epidemic) of cholera since 1817, with disease reported in most coastal countries with poor hygiene. In contrast with *Y. pestis*, *V. cholerae* is present in most oceans and seas, so most exposures result in no disease or self-limited diarrhea. Significant disease occurs only following ingestion of a large number of organisms, so control of epidemics is simple in principle but difficult to realize.

VIBRIO CHOLERAE	
Properties	• Cholera toxin is an A-B toxin that binds to receptors on intestinal epithelial cells, which results in hypersecretion of electrolytes and water • Toxin-coregulated pilus serves as the receptor site for the bacteriophage that transfers the two toxin genes into the bacteria; also mediates bacterial adherence to intestinal mucosal cells • Accessory cholera enterotoxin increases intestinal fluid secretion • Zonula occludens toxin increases intestinal permeability
Epidemiology	• Seven major pandemics of cholera have occurred since 1817, including the current pandemic that began in Asia and has spread worldwide • Estimated 3 to 5 million cases of cholera annually with 120,000 deaths • **Serotype 01** is responsible for major pandemics, with significant mortality in countries with substandard hygiene • Organisms are found in marine environments worldwide; associated with shellfish • Bacterial levels increase in warm months so infections are seasonal • Infections most commonly acquired by consumption of contaminated water or shellfish • Person-to-person spread is rare because the infectious dose is high
Clinical Disease	• **Cholera**: begins with an abrupt onset of watery diarrhea and vomiting, and can progress rapidly to severe dehydration, metabolic acidosis and hypokalemia, and hypovolemic shock • **Gastroenteritis**: milder forms of diarrheal disease can occur in toxin-negative strains of *V. cholerae* O1 and in non-O1 serotypes

Continued

VIBRIO CHOLERAE—cont'd	
Diagnosis	• Microscopic examination of stool can be useful in acute infections, but rapidly become negative as the disease progresses because organisms are "flushed" out of the intestines with the profuse watery diarrhea • Immunoassays for cholera toxin or O1 antigen are useful although the analytic performance can be quite variable • Culture should be performed early in course of disease with fresh stool specimens; delays in processing the specimen may result in a shift to acidic pH which will result in loss of viable bacteria • Multiplex NAATs (simultaneously testing for multiple enteric pathogens) are becoming common and may replace cultures within the next few years in laboratories where resources are available
Treatment, Control, Prevention	• Fluid and electrolyte replacement are crucial • Antibiotics (e.g., azithromycin) reduce the bacterial burden and exotoxin production, but play a secondary role in patient management • Improved community hygiene is critical for control of disease • Combination inactivated whole cell and cholera toxin B subunit vaccines provide limited protection

CLINICAL CASE

Cholera Caused by *V. cholerae*

Harris and colleagues[6] describe a 4-year-old Haitian boy who was admitted to a Haiti hospital because of vomiting and persistent diarrhea. The boy was healthy until about 10 hours before admission. He was extremely dehydrated, not producing urine, and passed a clear, watery stool during his initial examination. Oral rehydration solution was administered, but little fluid was retained because of vomiting and numerous episodes of diarrhea. Intravenous lines were established and 2 L of isotonic crystalloid solution was infused over a 2-hour period. Approximately 4 hours after admission, episodes of diarrhea were occurring too often to count and no urine output had occurred; however, the patient was able to drink an oral rehydrating solution and his mental status had improved. Azithromycin was administered orally, and fluids continued to be administered orally and intravenously. During the remainder of the day, the frequency of diarrhea decreased and vomiting ceased; however, the patient appeared dehydrated on the morning of the second day. Additional fluids were administered with resolution of the dehydration. The patient remained in the hospital for an additional day before discharge, with instructions to the parents about the need for adequate oral hydration. This patient illustrates the severity of diarrhea caused by cholera and the difficulty in managing the fluid loss. This patient was fortunate to have received treatment in the hospital because it was highly likely that he would not have survived without the medical care. This is illustrated by how rapidly he became dehydrated during the first night of hospitalization.

REFERENCES

1. McLaughlin JB, DePaola A, Bopp CA, et al. Outbreak of *Vibrio parahaemolyticus* gastroenteritis associated with Alaskan oysters. *N Engl J Med.* 2005;353:1463–1470.
2. Centers for Disease Control and Prevention. *Vibrio vulnificus* infections associated with eating raw oysters—Los Angeles, 1996. *MMWR Morb Mortal Wkly Rep.* 1996;45:621–624.
3. Case records of the Massachusetts General Hospital. Weekly clinicopathological exercises. Case 22-2001. A 25-year-old woman with fever and abnormal liver function. *N Engl J Med.* 2007;345:201–205.
4. Centers for Disease Control and Prevention. Outbreaks of multidrug-resistant *Shigella sonnei* gastroenteritis associated with day care centers—Kansas, Kentucky, and Missouri, 2005. *MMWR Morb Mortal Wkly Rep.* 2006;5:1068–1071.
5. Centers for Disease Control and Prevention. Human plague—four states, 2006. *MMWR Morb Mortal Wkly Rep.* 2006;55:940–943.
6. Harris JB, Ivers LC, Ferraro MJ. Case records of the Massachusetts General Hospital. Case 19-2011. A 4-year-old Haitian boy with vomiting and diarrhea. *N Engl J Med.* 2011;364:2452–2461.

8

Aerobic Nonfermentative Gram-Negative Rods

INTERESTING FACTS

- Due to its ability to tolerate high temperatures and many disinfectants, *Pseudomonas aeruginosa* is a common cause of "hot tub rash", a pustular dermatitis associated with immersion in hot tubs
- The "pseudomonads" (as *Pseudomonas*, *Burkholderia*, and *Stenotrophomonas* are commonly known) have been responsible for infections associated with contaminated disinfectants, mouthwash, and hospital equipment such as ventilators
- Although *Stenotrophomonas maltophilia* is listed in the National Institutes of Health Genetic and Rare Diseases Center, it is a common pathogen of immunocompromised patients who are treated with carbapenem antibiotics, to which this bacterium is naturally resistant

The nonfermentative gram-negative rods discussed in this chapter are opportunistic pathogens of plants, animals, and humans. Originally all were classified in the genus *Pseudomonas*, based on their inability to ferment carbohydrates and their morphologic appearance—small rods typically arranged in pairs. *Pseudomonas* was subdivided into a number of new genera, with *Burkholderia* and *Stenotrophomonas* the most common human pathogens. Members of these genera are found in the soil, decaying organic matter, and water, as well as in moist areas of the hospital. These bacteria can use many organic compounds as a source of carbon and nitrogen, so they can survive and replicate in environments where nutrients are minimal. The bacteria, particularly *Pseudomonas*, produce an impressive array of virulence factors, and all are resistant to the most commonly used antibiotics. It is not surprising that these bacteria are particularly important opportunistic pathogens in hospitalized patients. In this chapter I will focus on the most commonly isolated species for each genus: *P. aeruginosa*, *Burkholderia cepacia*, and *S. maltophilia*.

The genus *Pseudomonas* consists of more than 200 species and a number of these will be encountered in the hospital environment. Likewise, there are a number of species closely related to *B. cepacia* (frequently these are referred to as the *B. cepacia* complex), as well as one species, *Burkholderia pseudomallei*, that is a significant cause of **respiratory infections** ranging from asymptomatic colonization to cavitary disease resembling tuberculosis (**melioidosis**). The virulence of *B. pseudomallei* is well recognized, and this organism has been

Opportunistic Pathogens of Plants, Animals, and Humans

Bacteria	Historical Derivation
P. aeruginosa	*Pseudo*, false; *monas*, unit (refers to the Gram stain appearance of pairs of organisms that resemble a single cell); *aeruginosa*, full of copper rust or green (refers to the green color of colonies of this species due to production of blue and yellow pigments)
B. cepacia	*Burkholderia*, named after the microbiologist Burkholder; *cepacia*, like an onion (original strains isolated from rotten onions)
S. maltophilia	*Steno*, narrow; *trophos*, one who feeds; *monas*, unit (refers to the fact that these narrow bacteria require few substrates for growth); *malto*, malt; *philia*, friend (friend of malt [good growth with malt])

classified a 'select agent' for the risk of its use as an agent of bioterrorism. In contrast to *Pseudomonas* and *Burkholderia*, *S. maltophilia* is the only species in this genus of medical importance.

PSEUDOMONAS AERUGINOSA

This is the most common gram-negative rod responsible for opportunistic infections in hospitalized patients. *P. aeruginosa* produces a variety of adhesins, toxins, and tissue destroying enzymes, so it is amazing not that these organisms produce disease, but that infections are not more common in the hospital. The explanation for this is that the organism's virulence factors are not sufficient for disease (the susceptible host and opportunity for exposure define the risk for disease).

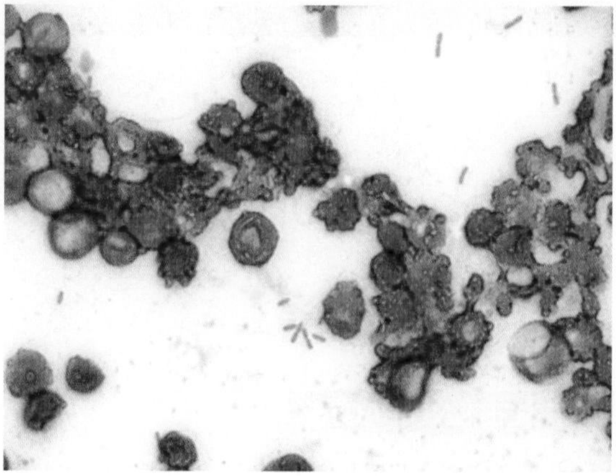

Pseudomonas aeruginosa in positive blood culture. Short gram-negative rods typically arranged in pairs.

PSEUDOMONAS AERUGINOSA	
Properties	• Bacterial surface components (i.e., pili, flagella, lipopolysaccharide, mucoid alginate capsule) bind to host cells • Alginate **capsule** protects for phagocytosis and antibiotic killing • **Exotoxin A** disrupts host protein synthesis (similar to diphtheria toxin) • Pigments (pyocyanin, pyoverdin) produce toxic forms of oxygen, stimulate cytokine release, and regulate toxin secretion • Elastase, phospholipase, and extracellular toxins mediate tissue destruction and inhibit neutrophil function • Innate and acquired **antibiotic resistance** make treatment difficult
Epidemiology	• Ubiquitous in nature and moist environmental hospital sites (e.g., flowers, sinks, toilets, mechanical ventilation, dialysis equipment) • No seasonal incidence of disease • Can transiently colonize the respiratory and gastrointestinal tracts of hospitalized patients, particularly those treated with broad-spectrum antibiotics, exposed to respiratory therapy equipment, or hospitalized for extended periods • Patients at high risk for developing infections include neutropenic or immunocompromised patients, cystic fibrosis patients, and burn patients
Clinical Disease	• **Pulmonary infection**: range from mild irritation of the bronchi (**tracheobronchitis**) to necrosis of the lung parenchyma (**necrotizing bronchopneumonia**) • **Primary skin infections**: opportunistic infections of existing wounds (e.g., burns) to localized infections of hair follicles (e.g., associated with immersion in contaminated waters such as hot tubs) • **Urinary tract infections**: opportunistic infections in patients with indwelling urinary catheters and following exposure to broad-spectrum antibiotics that select for these antibiotic-resistant bacteria • **Ear infections**: can range from mild irritation of external ear ("**swimmer's ear**") to invasive destruction of cranial bones adjacent to the infected ear ("**malignant otitis**") • **Eye infections**: opportunistic infections of mildly damaged corneas; can be very aggressive with complete vision loss • **Bacteremia**: dissemination of bacteria from primary infection to other organs and tissues; can be characterized by necrotic skin lesions (**ecthyma gangrenosum**)
Diagnosis	• Grows rapidly on common laboratory media and Gram stain morphology is characteristic • Identified by colonial characteristics (β-hemolysis on blood agar, green pigment, grapelike odor) and simple biochemical tests (positive oxidase reaction, oxidative utilization of carbohydrates)

PSEUDOMONAS AERUGINOSA—cont'd	
Treatment, Control, Prevention	• Treatment consists primarily of antibiotic combinations (e.g., aminoglycoside combined with active β-lactam antibiotic); monotherapy is generally ineffective; resistance to multiple antibiotics is common • Hospital infection-control efforts should concentrate on preventing contamination of sterile medical equipment and nosocomial transmission; unnecessary use of broad-spectrum antibiotics can select for resistant organisms • No vaccine is available for high-risk patients

CLINICAL CASE

Pseudomonas Folliculitis

Ratnam and associates[1] *described an outbreak of folliculitis caused by* P. aeruginosa *in guests at a Canadian hotel. A number of guests complained of a skin rash, which began as pruritic erythematous papules, and progressed to erythematous pustules distributed in the axilla and over the abdomen and buttocks. For most patients, the rash resolved spontaneously over a 5-day period. The local health department investigated the outbreak and determined the source was a whirlpool contaminated with a high concentration of* P. aeruginosa. *The outbreak was terminated when the whirlpool was drained, cleaned, and superchlorinated. Skin infections such as this are common in individuals with extensive exposure to contaminated water.*

BURKHOLDERIA CEPACIA

B. cepacia is a complex of a number of closely related species that colonize and produce disease in a select group of patients: those with cystic fibrosis, chronic granulomatous disease (CGD; a primary immunodeficiency in which white blood cells have defective intracellular microbial killing), or indwelling urinary or vascular catheters. In contrast to *P. aeruginosa*, *B. cepacia* has relatively few virulence factors, and infections can generally be treated with trimethoprim-sulfamethoxazole (TMP-SMX; a drug to which *Pseudomonas* is uniformly resistant).

BURKHOLDERIA CEPACIA	
Properties	• Relatively low level of virulence
Epidemiology	• Present in moist areas of hospital environment • Colonizes patients with increased susceptibility to infections
Clinical Disease	• **Pulmonary infections**: most worrisome infections are in patients with chronic granulomatous disease or cystic fibrosis, in whom infections can progress to significant destruction of pulmonary tissues • **Opportunistic infections**: urinary tract infections in catheterized patients; bacteremia in immunocompromised patients with contaminated intravascular catheters
Diagnosis	• Grows readily on common laboratory media • Can be classified in the *B. cepacia* complex by biochemical testing, but species identification requires gene sequencing with mass spectrometry
Treatment, Control, Prevention	• Generally susceptible to the sulfa drug, trimethoprim-sulfamethoxazole; may be susceptible *in vitro* to piperacillin, broad-spectrum cephalosporins, and ciprofloxacin, but the clinical response is poor • Avoid exposure of at risk patients, and carefully monitor colonized patients for progression to disease • No vaccine is available

CLINICAL CASE

Granulomatous Disease Caused by *Burkholderia*

Mclean-Tooke and associates[2] described a 21-year-old man with granulomatous lymphadenitis. The man presented with a history of weight loss, fevers, hepatosplenomegaly, and cervical lymphadenopathy. During the preceding 3 years he had presented on two occasions with enlarged lymph nodes that were biopsied, and histologic examination revealed granulomatous lymphadenitis. A clinical diagnosis of sarcoidosis was made, and the man was discharged on 20 mg prednisolone. Over the next 24 months, the patient remained clinically well; however, he developed pancytopenia, and granulomas were observed on a bone marrow biopsy. During the current hospitalization, the patient developed a cough. Chest radiograph revealed consolidation in the base of the lungs. A lung biopsy and bronchoalveolar lavage was submitted for culture, and B. cepacia *was isolated from both specimens. A subsequent immunologic evaluation of the patient confirmed that he had a genetic disease, Chronic Granulomatous Disease (CGD). This case illustrates the susceptibility of CGD patients to infections with* Burkholderia.

STENOTROPHOMONAS MALTOPHILIA

Much like *B. cepacia*, *S. maltophilia* is an opportunistic pathogen of immunocompromised patients, and the drug of choice for treating infections is TMP-SMX.

STENOTROPHOMONAS MALTOPHILIA	
Properties	• Primary virulence property is antibiotic resistance
Epidemiology	• Present in moist areas of hospital • Immunocompromised patients receiving broad-spectrum antibiotics, particularly carbapenems, are at greatest risk for disease • Infections traced to contaminated intravenous catheters, disinfectant solutions, mechanical ventilation equipment, and ice machines
Clinical Disease	• **Opportunistic infections**: a variety of infections (most commonly bacteremia and pneumonia) in immunocompromised patients
Diagnosis	• Grows readily on common laboratory media • Can be identified by biochemical tests or mass spectrometry
Treatment, Control, Prevention	• Generally susceptible to the sulfa drug, trimethoprim-sulfamethoxazole; uniformly resistant to carbapenem antibiotics • Avoid exposure of at-risk patients and carefully monitor colonized patients for progression to disease • No vaccine is available

CLINICAL CASE

Disseminated *Stenotrophomonas* Infections in a Neutropenic Patient

Teo and associates[3] described an 8-year-old Chinese girl with acute myeloid leukemia and a complex history of recurrent fungal and bacterial infections during treatment of her leukemia. Infections included pulmonary aspergillosis and septicemia with Klebsiella, Enterobacter, Staphylococcus, Streptococcus, *and* Bacillus. *While receiving treatment with meropenem (a carbapenem antibiotic) and amikacin (an aminoglycoside), and during a period of severe neutropenia, she became bacteremic with* S. maltophilia *that was sensitive to TMP-SMX. Over the next few days, she developed painful, erythematous, nodular skin lesions.* S. maltophilia *was isolated from a biopsy of one of the lesions. Treatment with intravenous TMP-SMX led to gradual resolution of the skin lesions. This case illustrates the predilection for* Stenotrophomonas *to cause disease in immunocompromised patients receiving a carbapenem antibiotic. Characteristically,* Stenotrophomonas *is one of the few gram-negative bacteria that is inherently resistant to carbapenems and susceptible to TMP-SMX.*

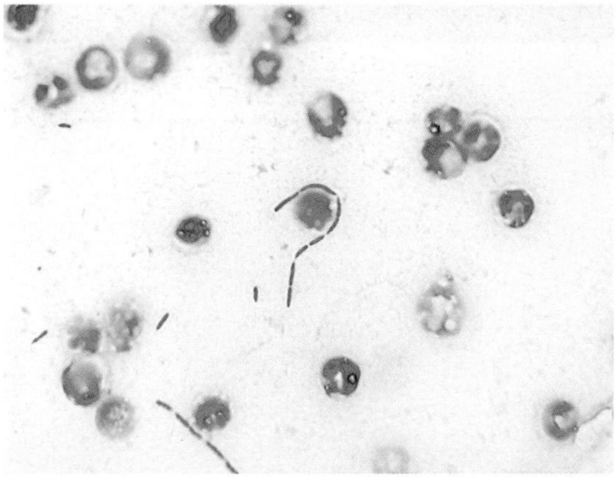

Stenotrophomonas maltophilia in positive blood culture. Like *Pseudomonas* and *Burkholderia, Stenotrophomonas* is typically arranged in pairs or occasionally short chains.

REFERENCES

1. Ratnam S, Hogan K, March SB, Butler RW. Whirlpool-associated folliculitis caused by *Pseudomonas aeruginosa*: report of an outbreak and review. *J Clin Microbiol.* 1986;23:655–659.
2. Mclean-Tooke APC, Aldridge C, Gilmour K, Higgins B, Hudson M, Spickett GP. An unusual cause of granulomatous disease. *BMC Clin Pathol.* 2007;7:1.
3. Teo WY, Chan MY, Lam CM, Chong CY. Skin manifestation of *Stenotrophomonas maltophilia* infection—a case report and review article. *Ann Acad Med Singapore.* 2006;35:897–900.

9

Anaerobic Bacteria

INTERESTING FACTS

- Although the clostridia that are responsible for tetanus, botulism, and gas gangrene are the most infamous members of the genus, *Clostridium difficile* is responsible for the most common clostridial infection: antibiotic-associated diarrheal disease
- Recovery from exposure to *Clostridium botulinum* toxin, which produces a flaccid paralysis, can occur with the regeneration of the damaged nerve endings. This is why repeated injections of this toxin for cosmetic purposes, Botox, are required
- It is recommended that infants do not eat honey because it can be contaminated with spores of *C. botulinum*. The intestines of older children and adults, but not infants, are populated with a mixture of bacteria that prevent the growth of *C. botulinum* and subsequent disease
- Anaerobes are prominent members of the gut that provide a wide variety of metabolic functions. Studies of germ-free rats have demonstrated that they require 30% more calories to maintain their body mass compared to normal rats

Anaerobic bacteria are the predominant population of microbes on humans, outnumbering the aerobic bacteria by 10-fold to 1000-fold in different anatomic sites. These organisms play an important role in maintaining human health by providing needed metabolic functions, such as digestion of food, stimulation of innate and regulatory immunity, and prevention of colonization with unwanted pathogens. The majority of infections with anaerobic bacteria are **endogenous**, resulting from transfer of the organisms from their normal residence on the skin or mucosal surfaces to normally sterile sites such as deep tissues and fluids (e.g., pleural fluid and peritoneal fluid). As might be expected, these endogenous infections are characteristically **polymicrobial** with a mixture of aerobic and anaerobic bacteria. The exceptions to this are infections caused by members of the genus ***Clostridium***. These bacteria are spore-forming organisms (the anaerobic counterpart to the aerobic spore-former, *Bacillus*). Because of their ability to form spores, clostridia are found in soil and other environmental sites, and typically cause monomicrobic, exogenous infections. The best known members of this genus are ***Clostridium tetani*** (cause of **tetanus**), ***C. botulinum*** (cause of **botulism**), and ***Clostridium perfringens*** (cause of **gas gangrene**). More recently ***C. difficile*** has gained prominence because it is the most important cause of **antibiotic-associated diarrheal disease** and is now recognized as one of the leading causes of hospital-acquired infections (not surprising with the aggressive use of antibiotics). Each of these pathogens has well-characterized virulence mechanisms and is fully capable of causing significant disease. In contrast, most other anaerobes are relatively avirulent and produce disease most effectively in a complex of different organisms. The one exception to this is *Bacteroides fragilis* which has a number of important virulence factors and, when present in a polymicrobial infection, is primarily responsible for the pathology.

Anaerobic Bacteria

Bacteria	Historical Derivation
Clostridium	*closter*, a spindle
C. tetani	*tetani*, related to tension (disease caused by this organism is characterized by muscle spasms)
C. botulinum	*botulus*, sausage (the first outbreak caused by this organism was associated with contaminated sausage)

Anaerobic Bacteria—cont'd

Bacteria	Historical Derivation
C. perfringens	*perfringens*, breaking through (this organism is highly virulent and associated with invasive tissue necrosis)
C. difficile	*difficile*, difficult (refers to the extreme oxygen sensitivity of this organism making it difficult to grow)
Bacteroides	*bacter*, staff or rod; *idus*, shape (rod shaped)
B. fragilis	*fragilis*, fragile (organism was believed to be fragile or rapidly killed by oxygen exposure)

A brief discussion of the other groups of anaerobic bacteria is appropriate. The **gram-positive cocci** consist of a number of genera that colonize the oral cavity, gastrointestinal tract, genitourinary tract, and skin. These bacteria are commonly present in polymicrobial infections and contribute to abscess formation and tissue destruction, but all can generally be treated with β-lactam antibiotics, such as penicillin. The anaerobic gram-positive rods are subdivided into the spore-forming rods (*Clostridium*) and non–spore-forming rods. The most common genera associated with disease are ***Actinomyces*** (actinomycosis, a chronic suppurative disease), ***Lactobacillus*** (endocarditis), and ***Propionibacterium*** (acne; also, a common contaminant of blood cultures). ***Veillonella*** is the most commonly isolated gram-negative cocci, but is rarely found in disease.

CLINICAL CASE

Pelvic Actinomycosis

Quercia and associates[1] described a classic presentation of pelvic actinomycosis associated with an intrauterine contraceptive device (IUD). The patient was a 41-year-old woman who presented with a 5-month history of abdominal and pelvic pain, weight loss, malaise, and a yellow vaginal discharge. She had used an IUD since 1994, and it was removed in June 2004. Her symptoms began soon after removal of the IUD. A computed tomography scan revealed a large pelvic mass involving the fallopian tubes, as well as numerous hepatic abscesses. A surgical biopsy was performed, and Actinomyces *was recovered in culture. She underwent surgical debridement and received oral therapy with a penicillin antibiotic for 1 year. The medical team thought the woman's pelvis was infected with* Actinomyces *at the time the IUD was removed. This episode illustrates the chronic nature of actinomycosis, and the need for surgical drainage and long-term antibiotic therapy.*

CLINICAL CASE

Lactobacillus Endocarditis

The following is a classical description of endocarditis caused by Lactobacillus.*[2] A 62-year-old woman was admitted for atrial fibrillation and a 2-week history of flulike symptoms. The patient had dental treatment 4 weeks before this admission and did not take antibiotic prophylaxis despite a history of rheumatic fever in childhood, with resultant mitral valve prolapse and regurgitation. On examination, the patient was afebrile, tachycardic, and mildly tachypneic. Cardiac examination was significant for a systolic murmur. Three blood cultures were collected, all of which yielded* Lactobacillus acidophilus *upon culture. The patient was treated with the combination of penicillin and gentamicin for a total of 6 weeks, resulting in complete recovery. This case illustrates the need for antibiotic prophylaxis during dental procedures for patients with underlying damaged heart valves, and the requirement for combined antibiotic therapy for successful treatment of serious infections caused by lactobacilli.*

CLINICAL CASE

Shunt Infected with *Propionibacterium*

Chu and associates[3] reported three patients with Propionibacterium acnes *infections of the central nervous system. The following patient illustrates the problems with this organism. A 38-year-old woman with congenital hydrocephalus presented with a 1-week history of decreased level of consciousness, headaches, and emesis. She had undergone numerous ventriculoperitoneal shunt placements in the past, with the last one placed 5 years before this presentation. The patient was afebrile and had no meningeal signs, but she was somnolent and arousable only by deep stimuli. Cerebrospinal fluid (CSF) collected from the shunt contained no erythrocytes but had 55 white blood cells; protein levels were high and glucose slightly low. Pleomorphic gram-positive rods were observed on Gram stain and* P. acnes *grew in the anaerobic culture of the CSF. After 1 week of therapy with high-dose penicillin, the CSF remained positive by Gram stain and culture. The patient was taken to surgery where all foreign material was removed, and the patient was treated with penicillin for an additional 10 weeks. This patient illustrates the chronic, relatively asymptomatic nature of this disease, the need to remove the shunt and other foreign bodies, and the need to treat for a prolonged period of time.*

The following is a summary for the most important anaerobic species.

CLOSTRIDIUM TETANI

C. tetani is ubiquitous, found in soil and transiently in the gastrointestinal tracts of many animals and humans. The vegetative (replicating) forms of *C. tetani* are extremely susceptible to oxygen toxicity, but the spores can survive in nature for many years. Disease is mediated by a plasmid-encoded, heat-labile neurotoxin (**tetanospasmin**). Tetanospasmin is an A-B toxin that inactivates proteins that regulate the release of the inhibitory neurotransmitters glycine and gamma-aminobutyric acid. This leads to unregulated excitatory synaptic activity in the motor neurons, resulting in **spastic paralysis**. Because the binding is irreversible, recovery from disease is prolonged even with aggressive therapy.

CLOSTRIDIUM TETANI	
Properties	• Tetanospasmin interferes with release of inhibitory neurotransmitters (glycine, gamma-aminobutyric acid)
Epidemiology	• Ubiquitous, spores found in most soils and can colonize gastrointestinal tract of humans and animals • Exposure to spores is common, but disease is uncommon except in developing countries where there is limited access to vaccine and medical care • Risk for disease is greatest for people with inadequate vaccine-induced immunity • Disease is uncommon in the United States, but it is estimated that more than 1 million cases occur worldwide annually with 30% to 50% mortality, particularly in neonates • Disease does not induce immunity
Clinical Disease	• **Generalized tetanus**: generalized musculature spasms and involvement of the autonomic nervous system in severe disease (e.g., cardiac arrhythmias, fluctuations in blood pressure, profound sweating, dehydration) • **Localized tetanus**: musculature spasms restricted to localized area of primary infection • **Neonatal tetanus**: neonatal infection primarily involving the umbilical stump; very high mortality
Diagnosis	• Diagnosis is based on clinical presentation and not laboratory tests (confirmatory) • Microscopy and culture are insensitive, and tetanus toxin and antibodies are not typically detected; culture of *C. tetani* is difficult because the organism rapidly dies after exposure to oxygen
Treatment, Control, Prevention	• Treatment requires debridement, antibiotic therapy (penicillin, metronidazole), passive immunization with antitoxin globulin to bind free toxin, and vaccination with tetanus toxoid to stimulate immunity • Prevention through use of vaccination, consisting of three doses of tetanus toxoid followed by booster doses every 10 years

CLINICAL CASE

Tetanus

The following is a typical history of a patient with tetanus.[4] An 86-year-old man saw a physician for care of a splinter wound in his right hand, acquired 3 days earlier while gardening. He was not treated with either a tetanus toxoid vaccine or tetanus immune globulin. Seven days later he developed pharyngitis, and after an additional 3 days, he presented to the local hospital with difficulty talking, swallowing, and breathing, and with chest pain and disorientation. He was admitted to the hospital with the diagnosis of stroke. On his 4th hospital day he had developed neck rigidity and respiratory failure, requiring tracheostomy and mechanical ventilation. He was transferred to the medical intensive care unit, where the clinical diagnosis of tetanus was made. Despite treatment with tetanus toxoid and immune globulin, the patient died 1 month after admission to the hospital. This case illustrates that C. tetani *is ubiquitous in soil and can contaminate relatively minor wounds. It also highlights the unrelenting progression of neurologic disease in untreated patients.*

CLOSTRIDIUM BOTULINUM

As with *C. tetani*, *C. botulinum* is commonly isolated from soil worldwide. Similar to tetanus toxin, *C. botulinum* produces a **heat-labile A-B toxin** that inactivates the proteins that regulate the release of acetylcholine, blocking neurotransmission at peripheral cholinergic synapses. Acetylcholine is required for excitation of muscle; therefore the resulting clinical presentation of botulism is a **flaccid paralysis**. As with tetanus, recovery of function after botulism is prolonged because regeneration of the nerve endings is required. Seven antigenically distinct botulinum toxins (A to G) are described, with human disease associated with types A, B, E, and F. Multiple bouts of botulism are theoretically possible.

CLOSTRIDIUM BOTULINUM	
Properties	• **Botulinum toxin** blocks neurotransmission at motor nerve synapses
Epidemiology	• *C. botulinum* spores are found in the soil worldwide • Classified as a 'select agent' because of concern for use as a bioterrorism agent • Relatively few cases of botulism in the United States but prevalent in developing countries • Infant botulism more common than other forms in the United States, but has significantly decreased in frequency following the recommendation not to give infants honey which can be contaminated with *C. botulinum* spores • Botulinum toxin is sensitive to heating but resistant to gastric acids
Clinical Disease	• **Food-borne botulism**: initial presentation of blurred vision, dry mouth, constipation, and abdominal pain; progresses to bilateral descending weakness of the peripheral muscles with flaccid paralysis • **Infant botulism**: initially nonspecific symptoms (e.g., constipation, weak cry, failure to thrive) that progresses to flaccid paralysis and respiratory arrest • **Wound botulism**: clinical presentation same as with food-borne disease, although the incubation period is longer and fewer gastrointestinal symptoms are reported • **Inhalation botulism**: rapid onset of symptoms (flaccid paralysis, pulmonary failure) and high mortality from inhalation exposure to botulinum toxin
Diagnosis	• Diagnosis is based on clinical presentation and not laboratory tests (confirmatory) • Culture of *C. botulinum* is difficult because the organism rapidly dies after exposure to oxygen • Food-borne botulism is confirmed if toxin activity is demonstrated in the implicated food or in the patient's serum, feces, or gastric fluid • Infant botulism is confirmed if toxin is detected in the infant's feces or serum, or the organism is cultured from feces • Wound botulism is confirmed if toxin is detected in the patient's serum or wound, or the organism is cultured from the wound
Treatment, Control, Prevention	• Treatment involves the combination of administration of metronidazole or penicillin, trivalent botulinum antitoxin, and ventilatory support • Spore germination in foods is prevented by maintaining food at an acid pH, by high sugar content (e.g., fruit preserves), or by storing the foods at 4°C or colder • Toxin is heat labile and therefore can be destroyed by heating the food for 10 minutes at 60°C to 100°C • Infant botulism associated with ingestion of contaminated soil or consumption of contaminated foods (particularly honey)

CLINICAL CASE

Foodborne Botulism with Commercial Carrot Juice

The CDC reported an outbreak of foodborne botulism associated with contaminated carrot juice.[5] On September 8, 2006, three patients went to a hospital in Washington County, GA, with cranial nerve palsies and progressive descending flaccid paralysis resulting in respiratory failure. The patients had shared meals on the previous day. They were treated with botulinum antitoxin because botulism was suspected. There was no progression of the patients' neurologic symptoms, but they remained hospitalized and on ventilators. An investigation determined that the patients had consumed contaminated carrot juice produced by a commercial vendor. Botulinum toxin type A was detected in the serum and stool of all three patients and in leftover carrot juice. An additional patient in Florida was also hospitalized with respiratory failure and descending paralysis after drinking carrot juice sold in Florida. Carrot juice has a low acid content (pH 6.0); therefore C. botulinum *spores can germinate and produce toxin if contaminated juice is left at room temperature.*

CLINICAL CASE

Infant Botulism

In January 2003, four children with infant botulism were reported by the CDC.[6] The following is a description of one of the children. A 10-week-old infant with a history of constipation in the 1st month of life was admitted to a hospital after having difficulty in sucking and swallowing for 2 days. The infant was irritable and had loss of facial expression, generalized muscle weakness, and constipation. Mechanical ventilation was required for 10 days because of respiratory failure. A diagnosis of infant botulism was established 29 days after the onset of symptoms by detection of C. botulinum *producing toxin type B in stool enrichment cultures. The patient was treated with botulism immune globulin intravenous (BIG-IV) and discharged fully recovered after 20 days. In contrast with foodborne botulism, diagnosis of infant botulism can be made by detecting the organism in the baby's stools.*

CLOSTRIDIUM PERFRINGENS

C. perfringens has a characteristic Gram stain morphology of large rectangular, gram-positive rods, and rarely forms spores in clinical specimens. These characteristics are important because they differentiate this species from other clostridia and make recognition of cells in clinical specimens easy for an experienced microbiologist. The species also grows rapidly in culture, forming characteristic large, spreading, β-hemolytic colonies. The production of one or more **"lethal" toxins** by *C. perfringens* (alpha, beta, epsilon, and iota toxins) is used to subdivide isolates into five types (A through E). Type A is most commonly associated with human diseases including soft-tissue infections, food poisoning, necrotizing enteritis, and septicemia.

CLOSTRIDIUM PERFRINGENS	

Properties	• Lethal toxins:
	  • **Alpha toxin** is a lecithinase that lyses erythrocytes, platelets, leukocytes, and endothelial cells; mediates massive hemolysis and tissue destruction characteristic of overwhelming disease
	  • **Beta toxin** is responsible for intestinal stasis, loss of mucosa with formation of necrotic lesions, and progression to necrotizing enteritis
	  • **Epsilon toxin** increases vascular permeability of the gastrointestinal wall
	  • **Iota toxin** has necrotic activity and increases vascular permeability
	• **Enterotoxin** binds to receptors on the brush border membrane of the small intestine epithelium in the ileum and jejunum, leading to altered membrane permeability and loss of fluids and ions; acts as a superantigen, stimulating T-lymphocyte activity and massive release of cytokines

CLOSTRIDIUM PERFRINGENS—cont'd	
Epidemiology	• Ubiquitous; present in soil, water, and intestinal tract of humans and animals • Type A strains are responsible for most human infections • Soft-tissue infections typically associated with bacterial contamination of wounds or localized trauma • Food poisoning associated with contaminated meat products (beef, poultry, gravy) held at temperatures between 5°C and 60°C, which allows the organisms to grow to large numbers
Clinical Disease	• **Cellulitis**: localized edema and erythema with gas formation in the soft tissues; generally not painful • **Suppurative myositis**: accumulation of pus in the muscle planes, without muscle necrosis or systemic symptoms • **Myonecrosis**: painful, rapid destruction of muscle tissue with rapid systemic spread and high mortality • **Food poisoning**: rapid onset of abdominal cramps and watery diarrhea with no fever, nausea, or vomiting; short duration and self-limited • **Necrotizing enteritis**: acute, necrotizing destruction of jejunum with abdominal pain, vomiting, bloody diarrhea, and peritonitis
Diagnosis	• Reliably seen in Gram-stained tissues (large rectangular gram-positive rods) although spores will not be observed • Grows rapidly in culture as a large, spreading colony surrounded by a zone of β-hemolysis and an outer zone of partial hemolysis
Treatment, Control, Prevention	• Rapid treatment is essential for serious infections • Severe infections require surgical debridement and high-dose penicillin therapy • Symptomatic treatment for food poisoning • Proper wound care and judicious use of prophylactic antibiotics will prevent most infections

CLINICAL CASE

Clostridium perfringens Gastroenteritis

The Centers for Disease Control and Prevention (CDC) reported two outbreaks of C. perfringens *gastroenteritis associated with corned beef served at St Patrick's Day celebrations.*[7] *On March 18, 1993, the Cleveland City Health Department received telephone calls from 15 persons who became ill after eating corned beef purchased from one delicatessen. After publicizing the outbreak, 156 persons contacted the Health Department with a similar history. In addition to a history of diarrhea, 88% complained of abdominal cramps and 13% with vomiting, which developed an average of 12 hours after eating the implicated meat. An investigation revealed the delicatessen had purchased 1400 pounds of raw, salt-cured meat, and beginning on March 12, portions of the corned beef were boiled for 3 hours, allowed to cool at room temperature, and then refrigerated. On March 16 and 17, the meat was removed from the refrigerator, heated to 48.8°C, and served. Cultures of the meat yielded greater than* 10^5 *colonies of* C. perfringens *per gram. The Health Department recommended that if the meat could not be served immediately after cooking, it should be rapidly cooled in ice and refrigerated. Before it is served, it should be warmed to at least 74°C to destroy the heat-sensitive enterotoxin.*

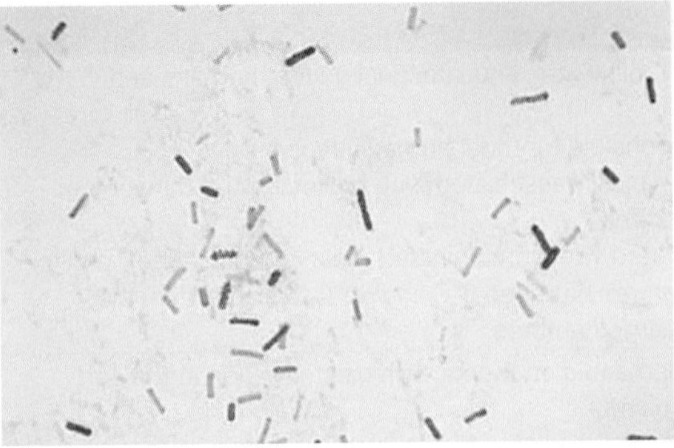

Gram stain of *Clostridium perfringens* in a wound specimen. Cells are uniformly rectangular in shape, may decolorize and appear gram negative; spores are rarely observed with this species.

CLOSTRIDIUM DIFFICILE

C. difficile is currently the most commonly encountered clostridial pathogen, responsible for antibiotic-associated gastrointestinal diseases ranging from self-limited diarrhea to life-threatening colitis. The disease is mediated by two toxins: an **enterotoxin** (toxin A) and a **cytotoxin** (toxin B). The enterotoxin is chemotactic for neutrophils, stimulating the infiltration of polymorphonuclear neutrophils into the ileum with release of cytokines. The cytotoxin causes destruction of the epithelial cytoskeleton. The cytotoxin alone is sufficient for producing disease but not the enterotoxin. Highly virulent stains have been observed and were initially thought to be due to increased toxin production. More recent studies have discounted this explanation although it is widely cited. Disease is widespread in hospitals, particularly in patients treated with clindamycin, broad-spectrum β-lactam antibiotics, and other agents. It is now recognized that a significant proportion of infections recognized in the hospital were acquired in the community; that is, the patients are colonized with *C. difficile* at the time of hospitalization. In many cases, this is related to previous hospitalization in a healthcare facility.

CLOSTRIDIUM DIFFICILE	
Properties	• **Enterotoxin (toxin A)** stimulates infiltration of neutrophils and release of cytokines • **Cytotoxin (toxin B)** causes destruction of the intestinal epithelium
Epidemiology	• Colonizes the intestines of a small proportion of healthy individuals • Exposure to antibiotics is associated with depletion of the normal intestinal population of bacteria, overgrowth of *C. difficile*, and subsequent disease (endogenous infections) • Spores can be detected in hospital rooms of infected patients (particularly around beds and bathrooms); these can be an exogenous source of infection • Highly virulent stains periodically circulate in the hospital and community
Clinical Disease	• **Antibiotic associated diarrhea**: acute diarrhea generally developing 5 to 10 days after initiation of antibiotic treatment (particularly clindamycin, penicillins, cephalosporins, fluoroquinolones); may be brief and self-limited or more protracted • **Pseudomembranous colitis**: most severe form of *C. difficile* disease with profuse diarrhea, abdominal cramping, and fever; whitish plaques (pseudomembranes) form over intact colonic tissue (seen on colonoscopy)
Diagnosis	• Diagnosis of *C. difficile* disease is by detection of the genes encoding the bacterial toxins or direct detection of the toxin in stool specimens • Use of culture is slow, and isolation of *C. difficile* must be further validated by demonstrating that the isolate produces toxin B, so culture is rarely done for routine diagnostic purposes • Immunoassays for toxins in stool specimens are insensitive and not reliable • Tests for detection of *C. difficile* cytoplasmic antigens (i.e., glutamine dehydrogenase) is sensitive but not specific so should only be used as a screening assay • Nucleic acid amplification tests for the toxin genes are the most sensitive and specific diagnostic tests

CLOSTRIDIUM DIFFICILE—cont'd	
Treatment, Control, Prevention	• The implicated antibiotic should be discontinued • Treatment with metronidazole or vancomycin should be used in severe disease; fecal transplants (repopulation of the bowel with the indigenous population of bacteria) has been used to treat recurrent disease • Relapse is common because antibiotics do not kill spores; a second course of therapy is usually successful but multiple courses may be required • The hospital room should be carefully cleaned after the infected patient is discharged

CLINICAL CASE

Clostridium difficile Colitis

Limaye and colleagues[8] presented a classic presentation of C. difficile *disease in a 60-year-old man. He had received a transplanted liver 5 years previous to his hospital admission for evaluation of crampy abdominal pain and severe diarrhea. Three weeks prior to admission he received a 10-day course of oral trimethoprim-sulfamethoxazole for sinusitis. On physical examination, the patient was febrile and had moderate abdominal tenderness. Abdominal computed tomography scan revealed right-colon thickening but no abscess. Colonoscopy showed numerous whitish plaques and friable erythematous mucosa consistent with pseudomembranous colitis. Empiric therapy with oral metronidazole and intravenous levofloxacin was initiated. A stool immunoassay for* C. difficile *toxin A was negative, but* C. difficile *toxin was detected by both culture and cytotoxicity assay (demonstration stool filtrate causes cytotoxicity to cell cultures that is neutralized by specific antisera against* C. difficile *toxins). Therapy was changed to oral vancomycin and the patient responded with resolution of diarrhea and abdominal pain. This is an example of severe* C. difficile *disease following antibiotic exposure in an immunocompromised patient, with a characteristic presentation of pseudomembranous colitis. The diagnostic problems with immunoassays are well known and have now been replaced by polymerase chain reaction assays that target the toxin genes. Treatment with metronidazole is currently preferred, although vancomycin is an acceptable alternative.*

BACTEROIDES FRAGILIS

B. fragilis is the most important member of a complex of closely related species (***B. fragilis* group**). The bacteria are pleomorphic in size and shape and resemble a mixed population of gram-negative rods in a casually examined Gram stain. *B. fragilis* grows rapidly in culture and is stimulated by the presence of bile; both features serve the bacteria well *in vivo* because *B. fragilis* is found most commonly in the intestines. The most important structural feature of this species is an antiphagocytic **polysaccharide capsule** that stimulates abscess formation.

BACTEROIDES FRAGILIS	
Properties	• Polysaccharide capsule is the primary virulence factor, responsible for abscesses characteristic of infections with *B. fragilis* • Fimbriae on cell surface are responsible for adherence to host cells • Production of fatty acids (e.g., succinic acid) inhibits phagocytosis and intracellular killing • Catalase and superoxide dismutase protect the bacteria by inactivating hydrogen peroxide and superoxide free radicals • Heat-labile toxin (*B. fragilis* toxin) stimulates chloride secretion and fluid loss in the small intestine, and induces interleukin-8 secretion which contributes to the inflammatory damage of the intestinal epithelium

Continued

BACTEROIDES FRAGILIS **—cont'd**	
Epidemiology	• Colonizes the gastrointestinal tract of animals and humans as a minor member of the microbiome; rare or absent from the oropharynx or genital tract of healthy individuals • Endogenous infections are most commonly polymicrobial, involving both aerobic and anaerobic bacteria
Clinical Disease	• **Intraabdominal infections**: characterized by abscess formation and associated with leakage of bowel contents or dissemination by bacteremia • **Skin and soft-tissue infections**: associated with trauma and can progress from localized colonization to life-threatening **myonecrosis** • **Gynecologic infections**: include pelvic inflammatory disease, abscesses, endometritis, and surgical wound infections; abscess formation is characteristic of *B. fragilis* infections • **Gastroenteritis**: presents as a self-limited watery diarrhea when caused by enterotoxin-producing *B. fragilis*; primarily in children younger than 5 years old
Diagnosis	• Characteristic Gram stain (pleomorphic gram-negative rods) from clinical specimens • Grows rapidly in cultures incubated anaerobically • Easily identified by biochemical tests, gene sequencing, or mass spectrometry laser desorption/ionization mass spectrometry
Treatment, Control, Prevention	• Resistant to penicillin and 25% of isolates are resistant to clindamycin; uniformly susceptible to metronidazole and most strains are susceptible to carbapenems and piperacillin-tazobactam • Prevention is difficult because infections are endogenous • No vaccine is available

CLINICAL CASE

Retroperitoneal Necrotizing Fasciitis

Pryor and associates[9] described an unfortunate patient with a polymicrobic fasciitis. A 38-year-old man with a 10-year history of human immunodeficiency virus infection underwent an uncomplicated hemorrhoidectomy. Over the next 5 days, thigh and buttock pain developed with nausea and vomiting. At the time that the man presented to the hospital with a heart rate of 120 beats/minute, blood pressure of 120/60 mmHg, respiratory rate of 22 respirations/minute, and temperature of 38.5°C. Physical examination revealed extensive erythema around the surgical site, flank, thighs, and abdominal wall. Gas was observed in the tissues underlying the areas of erythema and extended to his upper chest. At surgery, extensive areas of tissue necrosis and foul-smelling brownish exudates were found. Multiple surgeries to aggressively debride the involved tissues were necessary. Cultures obtained at surgery grew a mixture of aerobic and anaerobic organisms, with Escherichia coli, *β-hemolytic streptococci, and* B. fragilis *predominating. This clinical case illustrates the potential complications of rectal surgery—aggressive destruction of tissue, polymicrobic etiology with* B. fragilis *as a prominent organism, and foul-smelling necrotic tissue with gas production.*

Bacteroides fragilis in positive blood culture. Cells are faintly staining, pleomorphic gram-negative rods.

REFERENCES

1. Quercia R, Bani Sadr F, Cortez A, Arlet G, Pialoux G. Genital tract actinomycosis caused by *Actimyces israëlii*. *Med Mal Infect*. 2006;36:393–395.
2. Salvana EM, Frank M. *Lactobacillus endocarditis*: case report and review of cases reported since 1992. *J Infect*. 2006;53:e5–10.
3. Chu RM, Tummala RP, Hall WA. Focal intracranial infections due to *Propionibacterium acnes*: report of three cases. *Neurosurgery*. 2001;49:717–720.
4. Centers for Disease Control and Prevention. Tetanus—Puerto Rico, 2002. *MMWR Morb Mortal Wkly Rep*. 2002;51:613–615.
5. Centers for Disease Control and Prevention. Botulism associated with commercial carrot juice—Georgia and Florida, September 2006. *MMWR Morb Mortal Wkly Rep*. 2006;55:1098–1099.
6. Centers for Disease Control and Prevention. Infant botulism—New York City, 2001–2002. *MMWR Morb Mortal Wkly Rep*. 2003;52:21–24.
7. Centers for Disease Control and Prevention. *Clostridium perfringens* gastroenteritis associated with corned beef served at St. Patrick's Day meals—Ohio and Virginia, 1993. *MMWR Morb Mortal Wkly Rep*. 1994;43:137,143–144.
8. Limaye AP, Turgeon DK, Cookson BT, Fritsche TR. Pseudomembranous colitis caused by a toxin A(–) B(+) strain of *Clostridium difficile*. *J Clin Microbiol*. 2000;38:1696–1697.
9. Pryor JP, Piotrowski E, Seltzer CW, Gracias VH. Early diagnosis of retroperitoneal necrotizing fasciitis. *Crit Care Med*. 2001;29:1071–1073.

10

Spiral-Shaped Bacteria

INTERESTING FACTS

- *Campylobacter jejuni* is the most common cause of bacterial gastroenteritis
- *Helicobacter pylori* is the most common cause of bacterial gastritis and peptic ulcer disease
- *Treponema pallidum* is the most common cause of painless genital ulcers
- Lyme disease caused by *Borrelia burgdorferi* is the most common arthropod-transmitted bacterial disease

The bacteria discussed in this chapter are neither cocci nor rods; rather, they are spiral- or helical-shaped. Five organisms will be discussed in detail:

There are a number of related bacteria that should be mentioned because they are important human pathogens, but will not be discussed further:

Spiral- or Helical-Shaped Bacteria

Bacteria	Historical Derivation
C. jejuni	*kampylos*, curved; *bacter*, rod; *jejuni*, of the jejunum (curved rod of the jejunum [site of disease])
H. pylori	*helix*, spiral; *bacter*, rod; *pylorus*, lower part of the stomach (spiral rod in the lower part of the stomach)
T. pallidum	*trepo*, turn; *nema*, a thread; *pallidum*, pale (refers to very thin, spiral rods that do not stain with traditional dyes)
B. burgdorferi	named after A. Borrel and W. Burgdorfer
Leptospira species	*lepto*, thin; *spira*, a coil (refers to the thin coiled morphology of the bacteria)

Related Bacteria

Related Bacteria	Human Diseases
Campylobacter coli	Gastroenteritis
Campylobacter upsaliensis	Gastroenteritis
Campylobacter fetus	Vascular infections (e.g., septicemia, septic thrombophlebitis, endocarditis)
Helicobacter cinaedi	Gastroenteritis, proctocolitis
Helicobacter fennelliae	Gastroenteritis, proctocolitis
Borrelia afzelii	Lyme disease (in Europe and Asia)
Borrelia garinii	Lyme disease (in Europe and Asia)
Borrelia recurrentis	Epidemic (louse-borne) relapsing fever
Borrelia, many species	Endemic (tick associated) relapsing fever

CAMPYLOBACTER JEJUNI

Campylobacters, primarily *C. jejuni* and *C. coli*, are the most common causes of **bacterial gastroenteritis** in both developed and developing countries. The role of these gram-negative bacteria in human disease was not recognized for many years because they are small (0.2 to 0.5 μm wide and 0.5 to 5.0 μm long) and grow best in reduced oxygen, increased carbon dioxide, and at 42°C. They were initially discovered when stool specimens were processed for viruses by filtration through 0.45 μm filters.

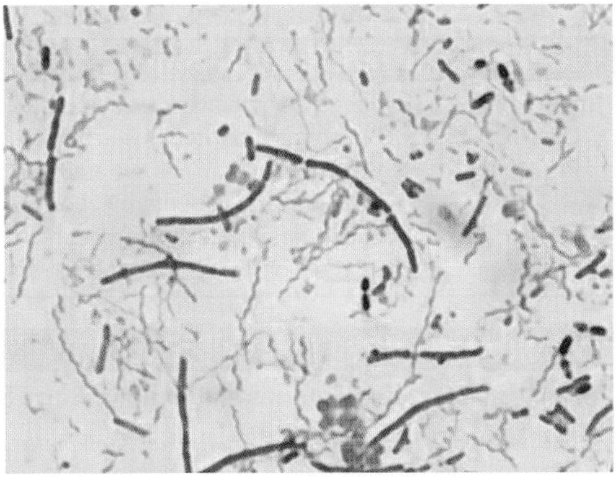

Campylobacter jejuni in stool specimen. *C. jejuni* is the thin, curved, gram-negative bacteria in the midst of larger gram-negative rods and gram-positive diplococci.

CAMPYLOBACTER JEJUNI	
Properties	• Polysaccharide capsule provides protection from phagocytosis • Lipopolysaccharide with endotoxin is absent in these gram-negative bacteria • Adhesins, cytotoxic enzymes, and enterotoxins are detected in *C. jejuni*, but specific role in disease is poorly defined • Cross-reactivity with host tissues responsible for autoimmune complications of *Campylobacter* infections (Guillain-Barré syndrome, reactive arthritis)
Epidemiology	• Zoonotic infection; improperly prepared **poultry** is a common source of human infections • Infections acquired by ingestion of contaminated food, unpasteurized milk, or contaminated water • Person-to-person spread is unusual • Dose required to establish disease is high because the organism is susceptible to gastric acids • Previous exposure provides partial immunity and results in less severe disease • Worldwide distribution with enteric infections seen throughout the year
Clinical Disease	• **Gastroenteritis**: damage to mucosal surfaces of jejunum, ileum, and colon; acute enteritis with diarrhea, fever, and severe abdominal pain; can mimic acute appendicitis, particularly in children and young adults • **Guillain-Barré syndrome**: well-recognized complication of *Campylobacter* infection; autoimmune disorder of peripheral nervous system characterized by development of symmetric weakness over several days, with recovery requiring months or longer • **Reactive arthritis**: complication of *Campylobacter* infection; characterized by joint pain and swelling involving the hands, ankles, and knees; persisting from 1 week to several months
Diagnosis	• Microscopic detection of thin, "S-shaped" gram-negative rods in stool specimens is specific but insensitive • Commercial multiplex, nucleic acid amplification tests are highly sensitive and specific for enteric pathogens, and particularly useful for detection of *C. jejuni* and *C. coli* infections • Culture requires use of specialized media incubated with reduced oxygen, increased carbon dioxide, and elevated temperatures; requires incubation for 2 or more days and is relatively insensitive unless fresh media are used • Detection of *Campylobacter* antigens in stool specimens is moderately sensitive and very specific compared with culture

Continued

CAMPYLOBACTER JEJUNI—cont'd	
Treatment, Control, Prevention	• For gastroenteritis, infection is self-limited and is managed by fluid and electrolyte replacement • Severe gastroenteritis and septicemia are treated with erythromycin or azithromycin • Gastroenteritis is prevented by proper preparation of food and consumption of pasteurized milk; preventing contamination of water supplies also controls infection • Experimental vaccines targeting the outer capsular polysaccharides are promising for control of infections in animal reservoirs

CLINICAL CASE

Campylobacter jejuni Enteritis and Guillain-Barré Syndrome

Scully and associates[1] described the clinical history of a 74-year-old woman who developed Guillain-Barré syndrome following an episode of C. jejuni *enteritis. After 1 week of fever, watery diarrhea, nausea, abdominal pain, weakness, and fatigue, the patient's speech was noted to be severely slurred. She was taken to the hospital where it was noted she was unable to speak, although she was oriented and able to write coherently. She had perioral numbness, bilateral ptosis, and facial weakness, and her pupils were nonreactive. Neurologic examination revealed bilateral muscle weakness in her arms and chest. On the 2nd hospital day, the muscle weakness extended to her upper legs. On the 3rd hospital day, the patient's mental status remained normal, but she could only move her thumb minimally and could not lift her legs. Sensation to light touch was normal, but deep-tendon reflexes were absent.* C. jejuni *was recovered from this patient's stool culture, collected at the time of admission, and the clinical diagnosis of Guillain-Barré syndrome was made. Despite aggressive medical treatment, the patient had significant neurologic deficits 3 months after discharge to a rehabilitation facility. This woman illustrates one of the significant complications of* Campylobacter *enteritis.*

HELICOBACTER PYLORI

Like *C. jejuni*, *H. pylori* is a relatively recently appreciated human pathogen. Helicobacters are similar in size and shape to campylobacters, and growth requires complex media supplemented with blood, serum, charcoal, starch or egg yolk, and microaerophilic conditions. *H. pylori* was initially associated with gastritis in 1983, and subsequently implicated as a cause of peptic ulcers, gastric adenocarcinomas, and gastric mucosa-associated lymphoid tissue lymphomas. Helicobacters are subdivided into species that primarily colonize the stomach (**gastric helicobacters**) and those that colonize the intestines (**enterohepatic helicobacters**). *H. pylori* is a gastric helicobacter.

HELICOBACTER PYLORI	
Properties	• Initial colonization facilitated by blockage of acid production and neutralization of gastric acids with ammonia produced by bacterial **urease** activity. • Actively motile, permitting migration through gastric mucosa to gastric epithelial cells where attachment is mediated by bacterial adhesin proteins • Localized tissue damage caused by urease byproducts, mucinase, phospholipases, and the activity of vacuolating cytotoxin A. • Type VI secretion system injects bacterial proteins into epithelial cells, which interferes with normal cytoskeletal structure
Epidemiology	• Infections are common, particularly in people in a low socioeconomic class or in developing nations, and colonization can be lifelong • **Humans** are the primary reservoir • Person-to-person spread is important (typically fecal-oral) • Ubiquitous and worldwide, with no seasonal incidence of disease

HELICOBACTER PYLORI—cont'd	
Clinical Disease	• **Gastritis**: inflammation of gastric mucosa, characterized by feeling of fullness, nausea, vomiting, and hypochlorhydria (decreased acid production; can progress to chronic disease • **Peptic ulcers**: development of ulcers, commonly at the junction between the corpus and antrum of stomach or the proximal duodenum (duodenal ulcer) • **Gastric adenocarcinoma**: progression of chronic gastritis to stomach cancer • **Mucosa-associated lymphoid tissue B-cell lymphomas**
Diagnosis	• Microscopy: histologic examination of biopsy specimens is sensitive and specific • Urease test relatively sensitive and highly specific; urea breath test is a noninvasive test • *H. pylori* antigen test is sensitive and specific; performed with stool specimens • Culture requires incubation in microaerophilic conditions; growth is slow; relatively insensitive unless multiple biopsies are cultured • Serology useful for demonstrating exposure to *H. pylori* but not disease
Treatment, Control, Prevention	• Multiple regimens have been evaluated for treatment of *H. pylori* infections. Combined therapy with a proton pump inhibitor (e.g., omeprazole), a macrolide (e.g., clarithromycin) and a β-lactam (e.g., amoxicillin) for 2 weeks has had a high success rate • Recommended to only treat symptomatic patients because prophylactic treatment of colonized individuals has not been useful and potentially has adverse effects, such as predisposing patients to adenocarcinomas of the lower esophagus • Human vaccines are not currently available

TREPONEMA PALLIDUM

T. pallidum is the organism responsible for the sexually transmitted disease, **syphilis**. Although this disease has been recognized for centuries, diagnosis by traditional tests such as microscopy and culture are not useful because *T. pallidum* and related treponemes are small (0.1–0.2 μm × 6–20 μm), tightly coiled spirochetes that are too thin to be seen by light microscopy and *T. pallidum* has not been cultured in the laboratory. **Serology** remains the primary diagnostic test for syphilis, with **nontreponemal** tests (measurement of antibodies that develop against lipids released from damaged host cells during the early stages of disease) used for screening patients, and **treponemal** tests (antibodies specifically directed against *T. pallidum*) used as confirmatory tests.

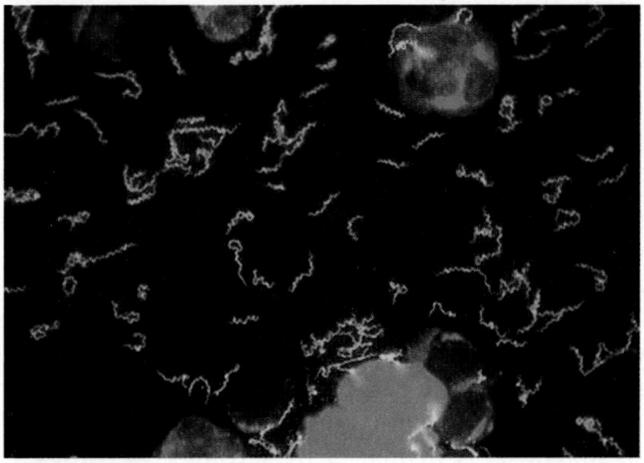

Treponema pallidum observed in an ulcer specimen using fluorescein-labeled antibodies for *T. pallidum*.

TREPONEMA PALLIDUM	
Properties	• Outer membrane proteins promote adherence to host cells • Hyaluronidase facilitates perivascular infiltration • Coating of fibronectin protects against phagocytosis • Tissue destruction primarily results from host's immune response to infection
Epidemiology	• **Humans** are the only natural host • Venereal syphilis transmitted by sexual contact or congenitally from mother to fetus • Syphilis occurs worldwide with no seasonal incidence • Third most common sexually transmitted bacterial disease in the United States (after *Chlamydia* and *Neisseria gonorrhoeae* infections) • Patients with genital ulcers at increased risk for acquiring and transmitting HIV

Continued

TREPONEMA PALLIDUM—cont'd	

Clinical Disease	• **Syphilis** develops in stages:
	  • **Primary disease**: **painless ulcer** or **chancre** at site of infection with regional lymphadenopathy and bacteremia
	  • **Secondary syphilis**: flulike syndrome with generalized mucocutaneous rash and bacteremia
	  • **Late stage syphilis**: diffuse chronic inflammation and destruction of any organ or tissue
	• **Neurosyphilis**: neurologic symptoms, primarily **meningitis**, can develop in early or late stages of disease
	• **Congenital syphilis**: may result in fetal death; child born with multiorgan malformations; or latent disease that initially presents as rhinitis followed by a widespread desquamating maculopapular rash; teeth and bone malformation, blindness, deafness, and cardiovascular syphilis are common in untreated infants

Diagnosis	• Darkfield or direct fluorescent antibody microscopy useful if mucosal ulcers are observed in primary or secondary stages of syphilis • Serology is very sensitive in secondary and late stages of syphilis • Nucleic acid amplification tests have been developed but are not widely used
Treatment, Control, Prevention	• Penicillin is drug of choice; doxycycline or azithromycin is administered if the patient is allergic to penicillin • Safe sex practices should be emphasized, and sexual partners of infected patients should be treated • No vaccine is available

BORRELIA BURGDORFERI

Borreliae are large spirochetes (0.2–0.5 μm × 830 μm) that stain best with aniline dyes (e.g., Giemsa or Wright stain). *B. burgdorferi* and related organisms are responsible for **Lyme disease**, named after Lyme, Connecticut, where the disease was first described. Typically few organisms are present in skin lesions or the patient's blood, and borreliae are microaerophilic with complex nutritional needs, so diagnosis is primarily by serology. **Serology** is relatively insensitive during the early stage of disease, but is uniformly positive in late stages of disease. False-positive tests can occur so tests should only be performed in patients with the appropriate history and clinical presentation, a fact that is frequently overlooked and is responsible for many misdiagnosed patients.

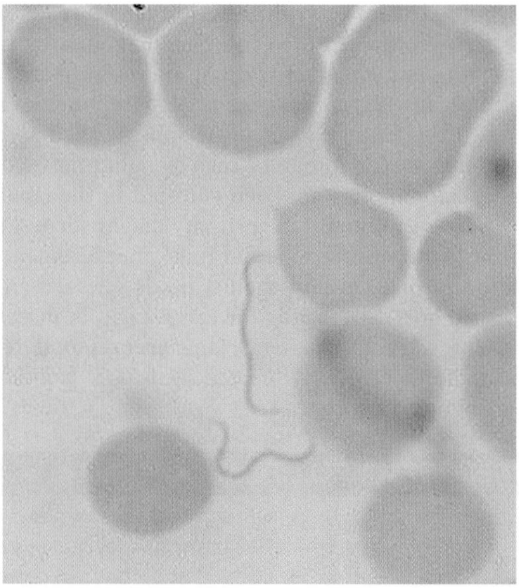

Giemsa stain of *Borrelia* spp. in the blood of a patient with endemic relapsing fever. Although *Borrelia burgdorferi* observed in tissues has the same appearance, it is rarely seen in clinical specimens.

BORRELIA BURGDORFERI	
Properties	• Immune reactivity against the Lyme disease agents may be responsible for the clinical disease
Epidemiology	• *B. burgdorferi* causes disease in the United States and Europe; *B. garinii* and *B. afzelii* cause disease in Europe and Asia • Transmitted by hard **ticks** from mice to humans; reservoir: mice, deer, and ticks • Most common tick-borne disease in the United States • Nymph stage of tick responsible for more than 90% of human disease so, although the ticks must feed for more than 2 days, the tick may not be noticed because of its small size • In the United States, 95% of Lyme disease cases are from two principle foci: Northeast and mid-Atlantic states (Maine to Virginia) and Upper Midwest states (Minnesota, Wisconsin) • Worldwide distribution • Seasonal incidence corresponds to feeding patterns of vectors; most cases of Lyme disease in the United States occur in late spring and early summer (feeding pattern of nymph stage of ticks); peak in June and July

Clinical Disease	• **Lyme disease** develops in stages:
	  • **Early localized disease**: small macule or papule develops at the site of the tick bite and then enlarges to a lesion with a flat, red border and central clearing (**erythema migrans**)
	  • **Early disseminated disease**: hematogenous dissemination is characterized by systemic signs (severe fatigue, headache, fever, malaise), arthritis and arthralgia, myalgia, erythematous skin lesions, and cardiac and neurologic symptoms
	  • **Late stage** manifestations include **arthritis** and **chronic skin involvement**

Diagnosis	• Microscopy and culture of limited value • Nucleic acid amplification tests are available for Lyme disease but are relatively insensitive • Serology is test of choice for Lyme disease
Treatment, Control, Prevention	• For early localized or disseminated Lyme disease, treatment is with amoxicillin, tetracycline, or cefuroxime; late manifestations are treated with intravenous penicillin or ceftriaxone • Reduced exposure to hard ticks through use of insecticides, application of insect repellents to clothing, and wearing protective clothing that reduces exposure of skin to insects • Vaccines are not available

CLINICAL CASE

Lyme Disease in Lyme, Connecticut

In 1977, Steere and associates[2] reported an epidemic of arthritis in eastern Connecticut. The authors studied a group of 39 children and 12 adults who developed an illness characterized by recurrent attacks of swelling and pain in a few large joints. Most attacks were for a week or less, but some attacks lasted for months. Twenty-five percent of the patients remembered they had an erythematous cutaneous lesion 4 weeks before the onset of their arthritis. This was the first report of Lyme disease, named after the town in Connecticut where the disease was first recognized. We now know the erythematous lesion (erythema migrans) is the characteristic presentation of early Lyme disease. A few years after this report, the Borrelia *responsible for Lyme disease,* B. burgdorferi, *was isolated.*

CLINICAL CASE

Outbreak of Tick-Borne Relapsing Fever

In August 2002, the New Mexico Department of Health was notified of an outbreak of tick-borne relapsing fever.[3] Approximately 40 people attended a family gathering held in a cabin in the mountains of northern New Mexico. Half of the family members slept overnight in the cabin. Some of the family arrived 3 days before the event to clean the unoccupied cabin. Four days after the event, one of the individuals who arrived ear-

ly sought care at a local hospital with a 2-day history of fever, chills, myalgia, and a raised pruritic rash on the forearms. Spirochetes were observed on a peripheral blood smear. As many as 14 individuals who attended the family gathering developed symptoms consistent with relapsing fever and had either positive serology or spirochetes observed in blood smears. The majority had a history of fever, headache, arthralgia, and myalgia. Rodent nesting material was found inside the interior walls of the cabin. This outbreak of endemic relapsing fever illustrates the risks associated with exposure to ticks that feed on infected rodents, the fact that tick bites are generally not remembered because the feeding is for a short duration at night, and the relapsing nature of this febrile illness caused by Borrelia *species.*

LEPTOSPIRA SPECIES

The taxonomy of this genus is a source of confusion in the literature. It is sufficient to recognize that a number of species of *Leptospira* can cause the human disease, **leptospirosis**. The organisms are very thin (0.1 μm × 6–20 μm) so brightfield microscopy is not useful. Additionally, they have complex nutritional requirements and grow slowly in culture, so most diagnoses are based on serology.

LEPTOSPIRA SPECIES	
Properties	• Immune reactivity against *Leptospira* may be responsible for the clinical disease
Epidemiology	• US reservoirs: rodents (particularly rats), dogs, farm animals, and wild animals • **Humans: accidental end-stage host** • Organism can penetrate the skin through minor breaks in the epidermis • People are infected with leptospires through exposure to water contaminated with urine from an infected animal or handling of tissues from an infected animal • People at risk are those exposed to urine-contaminated streams, rivers, and standing water; occupational exposure to infected animals for farmers, meat handlers, and veterinarians • Infection is rare in the United States but has worldwide distribution • Disease is more common during warm months (recreational exposure)

Clinical Disease	• Most human infections are clinically unapparent and detected only through demonstration of specific antibodies
	• Symptomatic infections (**leptospirosis**) develop in two stages:
	  • Initial phase is flulike symptoms with fever, muscle pain, chills, headache, vomiting, or diarrhea
	  • Second phase characterized by more severe disease with sudden onset of headache, myalgia, chills, abdominal pain
	• May present as **aseptic meningitis**
	• **Icteric form** of disease (**Weil disease**) characterized by jaundice, vascular collapse, thrombocytopenia, hemorrhage, and hepatic and renal dysfunction

Diagnosis	• Microscopy not useful because too few organisms are generally present in fluids or tissues • Culture: leptospires detected in blood or cerebrospinal fluid in the first 7 to 10 days of illness; urine after the 1st week • Serology using the microscopic agglutination test is relatively sensitive and specific but not widely available in resource-limited countries; enzyme-linked immunosorbent assay tests are less accurate but can be used to screen patients
Treatment, Control, Prevention	• Treatment with penicillin or doxycycline • Doxycycline but not penicillin is used for prophylaxis • Herds and domestic pets should be vaccinated • Rats should be controlled

CLINICAL CASE

Leptospirosis in Triathlon Participants

There are a number of reports of leptospirosis in athletes participating in water sports events. In 1998, public health officials reported leptospirosis in triathlon participants in Illinois and Wisconsin.[4] A total of 866 athletes participated in the Illinois event on June 21, 1998, and 648 participated in the Wisconsin event on July 5, 1998. The case definition of leptospirosis used for this investigation was onset of fever, followed by at least two of the following symptoms or signs: chills, headache, myalgia, diarrhea, eye pain, or red eyes. Nine percent of the participants met this case definition, two-thirds sought medical care, including one-third who were hospitalized. Leptospirosis was confirmed in a portion of these patients by serologic tests. These outbreaks illustrate the potential danger of swimming in contaminated water, the presentation of leptospirosis in a previously healthy population, and the severity of disease that can be experienced.

REFERENCES

1. Case records of the Massachusetts General Hospital. Case 39-1999. A 74-year-old woman with acute, progressive paralysis after diarrhea for one week. *N Engl J Med*. 1999;341:1996–2003.
2. Steere AC, Malawista SE, Snydman DR, et al. Lyme arthritis: an epidemic of oligoarticular arthritis in children and adults in three Connecticut communities. *Arthritis Rheum*. 1977;20:7–17.
3. Centers for Disease Control and Prevention. Tickborne relapsing fever outbreak after a family gathering—New Mexico, August 2002. *MMWR Morb Mortal Wkly Rep*. 2003;52:809–812.
4. Centers for Disease Control and Prevention. Update: leptospirosis and unexplained acute febrile illness among athletes participating in triathlons—Illinois and Wisconsin, 1998. *MMWR Morb Mortal Wkly Rep*. 1998;47:673–676.

11

Intracellular Bacteria

INTERESTING FACTS

- *Rickettsia rickettsii*, the bacteria responsible for Rocky Mountain spotted fever, was named after Howard Ricketts who died from another rickettsial disease, typhus
- Humans are the accidental hosts of all the intracellular pathogens discussed in this chapter with one exception, *Chlamydia trachomatis*, the most common sexually transmitted pathogen in the United States (then again, humans are certainly not willing hosts)
- The incidences of ehrlichiosis and anaplasmosis have increased every year since the diseases were first reported in 1998 as a result of improved diagnosis and spread of the pathogens
- Many chlamydia infections are asymptomatic, which facilitates person-to-person transmission

The bacteria discussed in this chapter are obligate aerobic, intracellular organisms with a gram-negative cell wall structure. Beyond those features they are taxonomically unrelated and classified in four separate families:

- Rickettsiaceae: *Rickettsia* and *Orientia*
- Anaplasmataceae: *Ehrlichia* and *Anaplasma*
- Coxiellaceae: *Coxiella*
- Chlamydiaceae: *Chlamydia* and *Chlamydophila*

Four Species of Intracellular Bacteria of Interest

Bacteria	Historical Derivation
R. rickettsii	*Rickettsia*, named after Howard Ricketts who implicated the wood tick as the vector of Rocky Mountain spotted fever
Ehrlichia chaffeensis	*Ehrlichia*, named after the German microbiologist Paul Ehrlich; *chaffeensis*, bacteria first isolated in a soldier at Fort Chaffee, Arkansas
Coxiella burnetii	*Coxiella burnetii*, named after Herald Cox and F.M. Burnet who isolated the bacterium from ticks in Montana and patients in Australia, respectively
C. trachomatis	*Chlamydis*, a cloak; *trachomatis*, of trachoma or rough (disease characterized by rough granulations on the conjunctival surfaces that lead to chronic inflammation and blindness)

CLINICAL CASE

Rocky Mountain Spotted Fever

Oster and associates[1] described a series of patients who acquired Rocky Mountain spotted fever after working with R. rickettsii *in the laboratory. One patient, a 21-year-old veterinary technician, presented to a clinic with complaints of myalgia and a nonproductive cough. He was treated with penicillin and discharged. Over the next few days, he developed chills and a headache. When he returned to the hospital, he had a temperature of 40.0°C and a macular rash on his extremities and trunk. Intramuscular tetracycline was started but he remained febrile, and the rash evolved to petechia on his truck, extremities, and soles of his feet. Bilateral pleural effusions developed, and intravenous tetracycline was begun. Over the next 2 weeks, the effusions resolved and the patient made a slow but uneventful recovery. Although this patient was not working directly with* R. rickettsii*, he had visited a laboratory that was processing the bacterium. This patient illustrates the characteristic presentation of Rocky Mountain spotted fever—headache, fever, myalgias, and a macular rash that can evolve into a petechial or spotted rash.*

There are a number of related bacteria that should be mentioned because they are important human pathogens:

Related Bacteria

Related Bacteria	Human Diseases
Rickettsia akari	Rickettsialpox: spotted fever transmitted by infected mites in urban areas such as New York
Rickettsia prowazekii	Typhus (three forms: epidemic, recrudescent, sporadic)
Rickettsia typhi	Endemic or murine typhus
Orientia tsutsugamushi	Scrub typhus is transmitted by mites ("chiggers")
Anaplasma phagocytophilum	Human granulocytic anaplasmosis
Chlamydophila psittaci	Psittacosis (Parrot fever): asymptomatic colonization to severe bronchopneumonia
Chlamydophila pneumoniae	Asymptomatic or mild disease to severe atypical pneumonia

CLINICAL CASE

Rickettsialpox in New York City

Koss and associates[2] described 18 patients with rickettsialpox who were diagnosed at Columbia Presbyterian Medical Center in New York City during a 20-month period after the anthrax bioterrorism attack in the fall of 2001. The patients presented to the hospital because they had a necrotic eschar and were thought to have cutaneous anthrax. The patients also had fever, headache, and a papulovesicular rash. Many patients also complained of myalgias, sore throat, arthralgias, and gastrointestinal symptoms. Immunohistochemical staining of eschar and skin biopsies confirmed the diagnosis of rickettsialpox and not cutaneous anthrax. The etiologic agent of rickettsialpox is R. akari*, and the disease is transmitted from rodents to human by mites ("chiggers"). These patients illustrate the diagnostic difficulties of recognizing uncommon diseases, even when the clinical presentation is characteristic.*

CLINICAL CASE

Psittacosis in a Previously Healthy Man

Scully and associates[3] described a 24-year-old man who was admitted into a local hospital in acute respiratory distress. Several days before his hospitalization, he developed nasal congestion, myalgia, dry cough, mild dyspnea, and a headache. Immediately before admission, the cough became productive and he developed pleuritic pain, fever, chills, and diarrhea. Radiographs demonstrated consolidation of the right upper lobe of the lungs and patchy infiltrates in the left lower lobe. Despite the fact his antibiotic treatment included erythromycin, doxycycline, ceftriaxone, and vancomycin, his pulmonary status did not begin to improve for 7 days, and he was not discharged from the hospital until a month after his admission. A careful history revealed the man had been exposed to parrots in a hotel lobby while vacationing. The diagnosis of Chlamydophila psittaci *pneumonia was made by growing the organism in cell culture and serologic tests.*

RICKETTSIA RICKETTSII

The genus *Rickettsia* is subdivided into two groups of diseases:

- **Spotted fever** group: many species of *Rickettsia* in the spotted fever group are associated with human disease, although *R. rickettsii* and *R. akari* are the most important. *R. prowazekii* is the etiologic agent of **epidemic or louse-borne typhus**, with **humans the principal reservoir** and the human body louse as the vector. Recrudescent disease can occur years after the initial infection.
- **Typhus** group: *R. typhi* is responsible for **endemic or murine typhus**, with rodents as the primary reservoir and the rat flea and cat flea as the principal vectors.

Members of the family Rickettsiaceae are small, and grow only in the cytoplasm of eukaryotic cells. Although they have a gram-negative cell wall, they stain poorly with the Gram stain. The following is a summary of *R. rickettsii*:

RICKETTSIA RICKETTSII	
Properties	• Outer membrane protein A on surface of bacteria responsible for attachment to endothelial cells; after penetration into cell, *R. rickettsii* is released from the phagosome and multiplies in the cell • Endothelial cell damage related to bacterial replication resulting in vasculitis
Epidemiology	• *R. rickettsii* is the most common rickettsial pathogen in the United States • Hard ticks (e.g., dog tick, wood tick) are the primary reservoirs and vectors • Transmission requires prolonged contact • Distribution in Western Hemisphere; in the United States, primarily in North Carolina, Oklahoma, Arkansas, Tennessee, and Missouri • Disease is most common in April to September
Clinical Disease	• **Rocky Mountain spotted fever** develops an average of 7 days after the tick bite; onset heralded by high fever and headache, associated with malaise, myalgias, nausea, vomiting, abdominal pain, and diarrhea; macular rash develops after 3 days, evolving to petechial form • Complications include neurologic manifestations, pulmonary and renal failure, and cardiac abnormalities
Diagnosis	• Serology (e.g., microimmunofluorescence tests) is used most commonly • Gram stain and culture are of no value; staining of infected tissues with fluorescein labeled antibodies useful but generally available only in reference laboratories • Nucleic acid amplification tests are insensitive
Treatment, Control, Prevention	• Doxycycline is drug of choice • Should avoid tick-infected areas, wear protective clothing, and use effective insecticides • Should remove attached ticks immediately • No vaccine is available

EHRLICHIA CHAFFEENSIS

The genera *Ehrlichia* and *Anaplasma* (formerly all in the genus *Ehrlichia*) are small intracellular bacteria that parasitize blood cells (e.g., granulocytes, monocytes, erythrocytes, and platelets). Three species are important human pathogens: *E. chaffeensis* (infects monocytes), *Ehrlichia ewingii* (infects granulocytes), and *A. phagocytophilum* (infects granulocytes). In contrast with the Rickettsiaceae, these bacteria remain in the phagosome and prevent fusion with lysosomes. The masses of replicating bacteria in the phagosome (called **morulae**) can be detected by staining infected cells with Giemsa or Wright stains. *E. chaffeensis* is a model for infections with these organisms:

EHRLICHIA CHAFFEENSIS	
Properties	• Replicates in infected cells and is protected from the host's immune response • Initiates host inflammatory response that contributes to pathology
Epidemiology	• Infections predominantly in Midwestern United States (Missouri, Arkansas, Oklahoma) and coastal Atlantic states (Maryland, Virginia, New Jersey, New York) • White tail deer is the primary reservoir and Lone Star tick is the vector • Humans are not natural hosts (accidental hosts) • Infects blood monocytes and mononuclear phagocytes in tissues and organs
Clinical Disease	• **Human monocytic ehrlichiosis**: 1 to 2 weeks after the tick bite, patient develops high fever, headache, malaise, and myalgias; late-onset rash develops in less than half the patients; leucopenia, thrombocytopenia, and elevated serum transaminases develop in majority of patients and recovery is prolonged

EHRLICHIA CHAFFEENSIS—cont'd	
Diagnosis	• Microscopy is of limited value; bacteria stain poorly with Gram stain and Giemsa-stained intracytoplasmic inclusions are detected only early in infection • Bacteria are not cultured • Nucleic acid amplification tests are useful but not widely available • Serology is useful but antibodies develop slowly (3–6 weeks after initial presentation)
Treatment, Control, Prevention	• Doxycycline is the drug of choice; rifampin is an acceptable alternative • Prevention involves avoidance of tick-infested areas, use of protective clothing and insect repellents, and prompt removal of embedded ticks • Vaccine is not available

CLINICAL CASE

Human Anaplasmosis

Heller and associates[4] described a 73-year-old man who presented to their hospital with fever, weakness, and leg myalgias. Six days before his admission he had traveled to South Carolina, and 3 days later he developed intense leg pains, a high fever, and generalized weakness. Upon admission he was febrile, tachycardic, and hypertensive; the liver and spleen could not be palpated and no cutaneous rash was noted. Cultures for bacteria, fungi, and viruses were negative. A peripheral blood smear showed rare intracytoplasmic inclusions in the granulocytes suggestive of morulae. Polymerase chain reaction analysis of blood samples collected on the second and third hospital days were positive for A. phagocytophilum *DNA, confirming the diagnosis of anaplasmosis. The patient was treated successfully with a 14-day course of doxycycline, although residual muscle weakness and residual pain persisted. Serum collected during the convalescent period was positive for* Anaplasma. *It is noteworthy that the patient did not remember a tick bite during his South Carolina trip, consistent with the observation that the early tick stages (larva and nymphs) are most commonly associated with human disease.*

COXIELLA BURNETII

C. burnetii is a gram-negative bacterium that stains weakly with the Gram stain, grows intracellularly in eukaryotic cells, and causes the disease **Q (query) fever**, so named because the causal organism was not identified in the original Australian outbreak. Two structural forms of the bacterium develop: small cell variants that are stable in the environment, and large cell variants that are the metabolically active, replicating form. The small cell variants can also undergo phase variation (**phase I** and **phase II**). Small cell variants attach to macrophages and monocytes and are internalized in a phagocytic vacuole. If phase II variants are internalized, then the vacuole will fuse with lysosomes resulting in bacterial death. This is avoided if phase I variants are internalized. Most disease is asymptomatic but symptomatic disease can present acutely and persist into chronic infections. The following is a summary of *C. burnetii*:

COXIELLA BURNETII	
Properties	• Replicating bacteria are protected in their intracellular location • Chronic infections develop if persistent intracellular survival occurs; mediated by overproduction of interleukin-10 that interferes with phagosome-lysosome fusion
Epidemiology	• Many reservoirs including mammals, birds, and ticks • Most human infections associated with contact with infected cattle, sheep, goats, dogs, and cats • Bacteria in high concentrations in placenta; soil becomes contaminated with dried placentas left on the ground after parturition, feces, and urine • Most disease acquired through inhalation of aerosolized bacteria; possible exposure from consumption of contaminated milk; ticks are not an important vector for human disease • Worldwide distribution • No seasonal incidence

Continued

COXIELLA BURNETII—cont'd	
Clinical Disease	• Most human infections are **asymptomatic** or mild, with exposure confirmed by serology • **Q fever**: symptomatic infections present with nonspecific flulike symptoms with an abrupt onset, high fever, fatigue, headache, and myalgias. More severe disease progresses to include hepatitis or pneumonia • **Chronic Q fever**: can develop months to years after the initial exposure, with **subacute endocarditis** the most common presentation
Diagnosis	• Microscopy is not useful and culture is rarely performed • Serology is the test of choice with detection of the antibody response to phase I and phase II antigens; antibodies against phase II detected in acute disease; antibodies against both phase I and II antigens develop in chronic disease • Nucleic acid amplification tests are not sensitive and not widely available
Treatment, Control, Prevention	• Doxycycline is drug of choice for acute infections; hydroxychloroquine combined with doxycycline is used to treat chronic infections • Phase I antigen vaccine is protective and safe if administered in a single dose before the animal or human has been exposed to *Coxiella*; not available in the United States

CLINICAL CASE

Coxiella burnetii Endocarditis

Karakousis and associates[5] described a 31-year-old man from West Virginia who developed chronic endocarditis caused by C. burnetii. *At the time the patient was admitted to the hospital, he described an 11-month history of fevers, night sweats, paroxysmal coughing, fatigue, and weight loss. He had received various antibiotic treatments for bronchitis, with no relief. His past medical history was significant for congenital heart disease, with placement of a shunt as an infant. He lived on a farm and participated in birthing his calves. His cardiac examination upon admission revealed a murmur, no hepatosplenomegaly or peripheral stigmata of endocarditis were noted, and his liver enzymes were elevated. All bacterial and fungal blood cultures were negative; however, serology for* Coxiella *phase I and phase II antibodies were markedly elevated. Treatment with doxycycline and rifampin was initiated, and the patient rapidly defervesced. Although prolonged treatment was recommended, the patient was unreliable, and he rapidly became symptomatic every time he discontinued one or both antibiotics. He also refused to take hydroxychloroquine because of his concerns about retinal toxicity. This patient typifies the risk for patients with underlying heart disease and the difficulties in treating this infection.*

CHLAMYDIA TRACHOMATIS

Members of the family Chlamydiaceae are obligate intracellular parasites that have a unique developmental cycle, forming metabolically inactive infectious forms (**elementary bodies**, EBs) and metabolically active, replicating forms (**reticulate bodies**, RBs). EBs are extremely stable in the environment. EBs bind to receptors on the surface of host cells, are internalized, prevent fusion of phagosomes with lysosomes, and convert to the replicating RBs. After about 24 hours of replication, the RBs are reorganized into EBs, the host cell ruptures, and the infectious EBs are released. The following is a summary for *C. trachomatis*:

CHLAMYDIA TRACHOMATIS	
Properties	• Receptors for elementary bodies are restricted to nonciliated columnar, cuboidal, and transitional epithelial cells • Intracellular survival because bacteria prevent fusion of phagosome with lysosomes
Epidemiology	• **Most common sexually transmitted bacteria in the United States** • Leading cause of preventable **blindness** worldwide • Ocular trachoma primarily in North and sub-Saharan Africa, the Middle East, South Asia, and South America • Lymphogranuloma venereum prevalent in Africa, Asia, and South America
Clinical Disease	• **Trachoma**: chronic inflammatory granulomatous process of eye surface, leading to corneal ulcerations, scarring, pannus formation, and blindness • **Adult inclusion conjunctivitis**: acute process with mucopurulent discharge, dermatitis, and corneal infiltrates; corneal vascularization in chronic disease • **Neonatal conjunctivitis**: acute process characterized by a mucopurulent discharge • **Infant pneumonia**: after a 2- to 3-week incubation period the infant develops rhinitis, followed by bronchitis with a characteristic dry cough • **Urogenital infections**: acute process involving the genitourinary tract with characteristic mucopurulent discharge; asymptomatic infections common in women • **Lymphogranuloma venereum**: a **painless ulcer** develops at the site of infection that spontaneously heals, followed by inflammation and swelling of lymph nodes draining the area, then progression to systemic symptoms
Diagnosis	• Culture is highly specific but relatively insensitive and not widely available • Antigen tests are insensitive • Nucleic acid amplification tests are the most sensitive and specific tests currently available
Treatment, Control, Prevention	• Ocular and genital infections are treated with azithromycin or doxycycline • Newborn conjunctivitis and pneumonia treated with erythromycin • Lymphogranuloma venereum treated with doxycycline or erythromycin • Safe sex practices and prompt treatment of patient and sexual partners help control infections • Vaccine not available

CLINICAL CASE

Reiter Syndrome and Pelvic Inflammatory Disease

Serwin and associates[6] described a 30-year-old man who presented to a university hospital with complaints of dysuria for a 3-year duration, penile inflammation, joint swelling, and fever. Skin lesions and nail changes were also noted. High levels of Chlamydia *antibodies were present, but antigen tests and nucleic acid amplification tests of the urethral exudates and conjunctiva were negative for* C. trachomatis. *A diagnosis of Reiter syndrome was made, and treatment with ofloxacin was initiated. Complete remission of the skin lesions and urethral symptoms was achieved. The patient's wife was also admitted to the hospital with a history of 2 years of lower abdominal pain and vaginal bleeding and discharge. The diagnosis of pelvic inflammatory disease was made, and* C. trachomatis *infection was confirmed by positive cervical and urethral antigen tests (direct fluorescent antibody). The vaginal smear was also positive for* Trichomonas vaginalis. *These patients illustrate two complications of* C. trachomatis *urogenital infections: Reiter syndrome and pelvic inflammatory disease.*

CLINICAL CASE

Chlamydia trachomatis Pneumonia in Newborn Infants

Niida and associates[7] described two female infants with C. trachomatis *pneumonia. The first infant was born by vaginal delivery after 39 weeks' gestation and the second by caesarean section at 40 weeks' gestation because of fetal distress. The infants were in good condition until fever and tachypnea developed at 3 and 13 days, respectively. Chest radiographs showed infiltrates over the whole lungs. Cultures of blood, urine, throat, feces, and cerebrospinal fluid were negative, but antigen tests for* C. trachomatis *were positive from conjunctival and nasopharyngeal swabs. These cases illustrate the presentation of pneumonia in infants infected with* C. trachomatis *at or near birth, although the characteristic staccato cough was not described.*

REFERENCES

1. Oster CN, Burke DS, Kenyon RH, Ascher MS, Harber P, Pedersen Jr CE. Laboratory-acquired Rocky Mountain spotted fever. The hazard of aerosol transmission. *N Engl J Med.* 1977;297:859–863.
2. Koss T, Carter EL, Grossman ME, et al. Increased detection of rickettsialpox in a New York City hospital following the anthrax outbreak of 2001: use of immunohistochemistry for the rapid confirmation of cases in an era of bioterrorism. *Arch Dermatol.* 2003;139:1545–1552.
3. Case records of the Massachusetts General Hospital. Weekly clinicopathological exercises. Case 16-1998. Pneumonia and the acute respiratory distress syndrome in a 24-year-old man. *N Engl J Med.* 1998;338:1527–1535.
4. Heller HM, Telford 3rd SR, Branda JA. Case records of the Massachusetts General Hospital. Case 10-2005. A 73-year-old man with weakness and pain in the legs. *N Engl J Med.* 2005;352:1358–1364.
5. Karakousis PC, Trucksis M, Dumler JS. Chronic Q fever in the United States. *J Clin Microbiol.* 2006;44:2283–2287.
6. Serwin AB, Chodynicki MP, Porebski P, Chodynicka B. Reiter's syndrome and pelvic inflammatory disease in a couple. *J Eur Acad Derm Vener.* 2006;20:735–736.
7. Niida Y, Numazaki K, Ikehata M, Umetsu M, Motoya H, Chiba S. Two full-term infants with *Chlamydia trachomatis* pneumonia in the early neonatal period. *Eur J Pediatr.* 1998;157:950–951.

12

Introduction to Viruses

OVERVIEW

Viruses are the simplest and generally smallest microbe. They are obligate intracellular parasites, dependent on their host cell for survival and replication. In many ways these are the most efficient microbes, carrying the minimum amount of genetic information as DNA or RNA (but not both), possessing a simple protein shell (called capsid) and in some cases surrounded by a membranous envelope. Their life cycle consists of finding the right host cell (defined by specific receptors for the different viruses), penetrating into the cell, and then either remaining dormant in the cell by integrating into the host DNA or taking over the host metabolic machinery to direct viral replication. After a period when many viral particles have been produced, the particles can either be slowly released from the host cell (to preserve the cell integrity and survival) or essentially explode from the cell in search of new cellular targets.

The replication and pathology of most viral infections is restricted to specific host cell types (e.g., cells of the hematopoietic system, respiratory tract, gastrointestinal tract, central nervous system, liver, etc.); therefore virology is best understood by focusing on the viruses that infect specific target cells or organs. This is in contrast with bacteria where a single species can infect many tissues (consider infections caused by *Staphylococcus aureus*), or a bacterial infection at a specific site can be caused by many bacteria (consider all the bacteria that can cause pneumonia). Therefore for the presentations in the virology chapters the focus will be on the viruses associated with specific disease states. This section is not a comprehensive review of all viruses of medical importance. Rather, the focus is on the viruses that will be encountered most commonly in medical practice.

CLASSIFICATION

The classification of viruses has traditionally been done based on their structural properties:

- Presence of DNA or RNA
- Presence of nucleic acids in a single strand or double strand
- Shape of the protein shell (icosahedral, spherical, other)
- Presence or absence of an envelope
- Overall size

The following is a list of the 7 DNA and 13 RNA virus families organized by their structural properties and examples of some of the important human pathogens.

DNA and RNA Virus Families

Structure[a]	Family	Most Important Members
DNA Viruses		
DS, brick-shaped, envelope	Poxviridae	Smallpox virus Vaccinia virus Monkeypox Molluscum contagiosum

Continued

DNA and RNA Virus Families—cont'd

Structure[a]	Family	Most Important Members
DS, icosahedral, envelope	Herpesviridae	Herpes simplex virus 1, 2 (HSV-1, HSV-2)
		Varicella-zoster virus (VZV)
		Epstein-Barr virus (EBV)
		Cytomegalovirus (CMV)
		Human herpesvirus 6, 7, 8 (HHV-6, HHV-7, HHV-8)
DS, spherical, envelope	Hepadnaviridae	Hepatitis B virus (HBV)
DS, icosahedral, no envelope	Adenoviridae	Adenovirus
	Papillomaviridae	Human papillomavirus
	Polyomaviridae	JC virus
		BK virus
SS, icosahedral, no envelope	Parvoviridae	Parvovirus B19
RNA Viruses		
DS, icosahedral, no envelope	Reoviridae	Rotavirus
SS, bullet-shaped, no envelope	Rhabdoviridae	Rabies virus
SS, filamentous, envelope	Filoviridae	Ebola virus
		Marburg virus
SS, icosahedral, no envelope	Picornaviridae	Rhinovirus
		Poliovirus
		Echovirus
		Coxsackievirus
		Hepatitis A virus
SS, icosahedral, envelope	Caliciviridae	Norovirus
		Sapovirus
	Togaviridae	Rubella virus
		Equine encephalitis viruses
		Chikungunya virus
SS, spherical, envelope	Orthomyxoviridae	Influenza virus
	Paramyxoviridae	Parainfluenza virus
		Respiratory syncytial virus (RSV)
		Human metapneumovirus
		Measles virus
		Mumps virus
	Coronaviridae	Human coronavirus
		SARS-CoV[b]
		MERS-CoV[b]
	Arenaviridae	Lassa virus
		Lymphocytic choriomeningitis virus
	Bunyaviridae	Hantaan virus
	Retroviridae	Human immunodeficiency virus (HIV)
		Primate T-lymphotropic virus
	Flaviviridae	Dengue virus
		Yellow fever virus
		West Nile virus
		Zika virus
		Hepatitis C virus

[a]*DS,* Double-strand nucleic acids; *SS,* single-strand nucleic acids.
[b]*SARS-CoV,* Severe acute respiratory syndrome coronavirus; *MERS-CoV,* Middle East respiratory syndrome coronavirus.

ROLE IN DISEASE

The clinical presentation of viral infections can be complex. For example, a primary respiratory pathogen could initially present with a diffuse rash and progress to later complications such as meningitis or encephalitis. The following is a summary of important presentations for many viral infections.

Viruses Responsible for Cutaneous Manifestations

Virus	Macules/ Papules	Vesicles	Petechiae
DNA Viruses			
Herpes viruses			
• HSV		X	
• VZV		X	
• CMV	X		X (congenital)
• EBV	X		X
• HHV-6, HHV-7, HHV-8	X		
Poxviruses			
• Variola		X	
• Vaccinia		X	
• Monkeypox	X		
• Molluscum contagiosum virus	X		
Other DNA viruses			
• Adenovirus	X		X
• Human papillomavirus	X		
• Parvovirus B19	X		
• HBV	X		

Virus	Macules/ Papules	Vesicles	Petechiae
RNA Viruses			
Flaviviridae			
• Dengue virus	X		X
• Yellow fever virus	X		
• Zika virus	X		
Arenaviridae			
• Lassa virus			
• Lymphochorio-meningitis virus	X		
Bunyaviridae			
• Hantaan virus			X
Filoviridae			
• Ebola virus			X
• Marburg virus			X
Picornaviridae			
• Coxsackievirus	X	X	X
• Echovirus	X	X	X
Other RNA viruses			
• HIV	X		
• Rubella virus	X	X	X
• Rubeola virus	X		

Viruses Responsible for Respiratory Infections

Virus	Rhinorrhea	Pharyngitis	Laryngitis	Croup	Bronchitis	Pneumonia
Rhinovirus	X	X	X		X	
Influenza virus	X	X	X	X	X	X
Paramyxoviruses						
• Parainfluenza virus	X	X	X	X	X	X
• RSV	X	X	X	X	X	X
• Human metapneumovirus	X	X	X		X	X
• Measles virus					X	X
Coronavirus	X	X	X		X	X
HIV		X				
Adenovirus	X	X	X	X	X	X

Continued

Viruses Responsible for Respiratory Infections—cont'd

Virus	Rhinorrhea	Pharyngitis	Laryngitis	Croup	Bronchitis	Pneumonia
Herpesviruses						
• HSV		X				X
• CMV		X				X
• EBV		X				

Viruses Responsible for Meningitis and Encephalitis

Virus	Meningitis	Encephalitis
Herpesviruses[a]	X	X (common)
Adenovirus	X	
Enteroviruses[b]	X (common)	X
Arboviruses[c]	X	X (common)
Paramyxoviruses		
• Parainfluenza virus	X	X
• Mumps virus	X	X (uncommon)
• Measles virus		X
Rubella virus		X
Arenaviruses		
• Lymphochorio-meningitis virus	X	X
• Lassa virus		X
Rabies virus		X
HIV	X	X

[a]Primarily HSV-2; other members include HSV-1, CMV, EBV, VZV.
[b]Include echovirus, coxsackievirus, and (now rare) poliovirus.
[c]"Arboviruses" is a historic term still used commonly to refer to the many viruses transmitted by arthropods (primarily mosquitos); these include eastern equine encephalitis virus, western equine encephalitis virus, La Crosse virus, California encephalitis virus, Venezuelan equine encephalitis virus, St. Louis encephalitis virus, Murray Valley encephalitis virus, Japanese encephalitis virus, Hendra virus, Chikunguna virus, West Nile virus, and many others of restricted geographic regions.

Viruses Responsible for Pericarditis and Myocarditis

Virus	Pericarditis	Myocarditis
Herpesviruses	X	
Adenovirus	X	X
HBV	X	
Enteroviruses	X (common)	X
Influenza viruses	X	X
Mumps virus	X	X
Measles virus		X
Rubella virus		X
Lymphochoriomeningitis virus	X	
Arboviruses		X

Gastrointestinal symptoms can be a prominent presentation of many viral infections, but the gastrointestinal tract is the primary site of replication for the following viruses:

- Norovirus (most common)
- Rotavirus
- Sapovirus
- Adenovirus
- Astrovirus

It is well recognized that human immunodeficiency virus (HIV) is transmitted by sexual contact but genital lesions are not observed. In contrast, three sexually transmitted viruses characteristically produce genital lesions:

- Herpes simplex virus types 1 and 2
- Human papilloma virus
- Molluscum contagiosum virus

Although a number of viruses produce hepatitis, five viruses are primary pathogens of the liver: hepatitis A, B, C, D, and E virus (HAV, HBV, HCV, HDV, and HEV). These will be discussed in a later chapter.

Infection of the eye, particularly keratitis, is observed with adenovirus and herpes simplex virus. Less commonly involved are other members of the herpes virus group and enteroviruses.

ANTIVIRAL AGENTS

In contrast with antibacterial agents, where relatively few new antibiotics have been introduced in recent years, there has been a proliferation of antivirals with more than 50 agents currently available. More than half of these are for the treatment of infections caused by three viruses: HIV and hepatitis B and C viruses. A number of antivirals have also been developed to treat respiratory infections and herpesvirus group infections. The antivirals listed in this section are in current use, recognizing a number of other antivirals are in development and some will be introduced to the market within the next few years.

The spectrum of antiviral agents for treatment of HIV infections is impressive, as well as bewildering. Any discussion here will most likely be rapidly outdated. Rather than a comprehensive summary, I will present the mode of action and some specific examples. The student should recognize that these antivirals are administered in carefully considered combinations.

Antiviral Agents for HIV Infections

Mode of Action	Antivirals
Nucleoside and nucleotide reverse transcriptase inhibitors	Zidovudine, didanosine, stavudine, lamivudine, abacavir, tenovovir, emtricitabine
Non-nucleoside reverse transcriptase inhibitors	Nevirapine, delavirdine, efavirenz, etravirine, rilpivirine
Protease inhibitors	Saquinavir, ritonavir, indinavir, nelfinavir, fosamprenavir
Viral entry inhibitors	Enfuvirtide, maraviroc
Integrase strand inhibitors	Raltegravir, elvitegravir, dolutegravir

Antiviral Agents for Hepatitis Virus Infections

Antivirals	Mode of Action	Viral Targets
Adefovir	Analog of adenosine monophosphate; inhibitor of viral DNA polymerases and reverse transcriptase	HBV; also HIV, poxviruses, and herpesviruses
Entecavir	Deoxyguanosine analog; inhibits DNA polymerase and reverse transcriptase	HBV
Lamivudine	Analog of dideoxy-thiacytidine; inhibits DNA synthesis	HBV; also HIV
Tenofovir	Adenosine 5′-monophosphate analog; inhibits DNA polymerase and reverse transcriptase	HBV
Boceprevir	Inhibitor of NS3/NS4A protease	Hepatitis C virus
Telaprevir	Inhibitor of NS3/NS4A protease	Hepatitis C virus
Simeprevir	Inhibitor of NS3/NS4A protease	Hepatitis C virus
Sofosbuvir	Uridine nucleoside polymerase inhibitor	Hepatitis C virus

Antiviral Agents for Respiratory Infections

Antivirals	Mode of Action	Viral Targets
Amantadine, Rimantadine	Tricyclic amines; inhibit viral uncoating and assembly	Influenza A virus
Oseltamivir, Zanamivir	Sialic acid analog; inhibitor of neuraminidase	Influenza A and B viruses
Ribavirin	Guanosine analog; inhibits viral replication	RSV, as well as hepatitis C and E viruses

Antiviral Agents for Herpesvirus Infections		
Antivirals	**Mode of Action**	**Viral Targets**
Acyclovir Valacyclovir	Deoxyguanosine analog; inhibitors of viral DNA polymerase; inhibits DNA synthesis; valacyclovir converted to acyclovir	HSV-1, HSV-2 VZV
Penciclovir Famciclovir	Acyclic guanosine analog; inhibits DNA synthesis; famciclovir converted to penciclovir	HSV-1, HSV-2 VZV
Ganciclovir Valganciclovir	Deoxyguanosine analog; inhibits DNA synthesis; valganciclovir converted to ganciclovir	CMV
Foscarnet	Pyrophosphate analog; inhibits DNA polymerase and HIV reverse transcriptase	All herpesviruses, as well as HIV
Cidofovir	Deoxycytidine monophosphate analog; inhibits DNA synthesis	All herpesviruses, as well as papilloma virus, polyoma virus, poxviruses, and some adenoviruses
Idoxuridine	Thymidine analog; inhibits DNA synthesis	Topical treatment of HSV keratitis
Trifluridine	Pyrimidine nucleoside; inhibits DNA synthesis	Topical treatment of HSV keratitis

13

Human Immunodeficiency Viruses

INTERESTING FACTS

- More than 1.2 million persons in the United States are infected with HIV, including more than 10% that are unaware of their infection
- Despite widespread educational efforts about risk factors for infection, there are approximately 50,000 newly acquired infections in the United States annually with approximately two-thirds of the infections in men who have sex with men
- One in four newly infected individuals in the United States is between the ages of 13 and 24 years
- Currently, almost 40 million people worldwide are infected with HIV, including 2.6 million children
- More than 25 million people in sub-Saharan Africa are infected with HIV and 70% of newly acquired infections are in this region
- It is estimated that 35 million people have died of acquired immunodeficiency syndrome (AIDS)

In the 35 years since the first infections by HIV were recognized, knowledge of the biology and pathology of these viruses has increased at an exponential rate. We have moved from fear of the unknown to the reality that scientific knowledge and countless hours of investigations have brought us to the conversion of an untreatable infection to a chronic, manageable disease and to the belief that we will see preventive vaccines and therapeutic cures in the future. Despite this optimism, HIV and AIDS pose a daunting medical challenge. The World Health Organization estimates that by the beginning of 2015, 37 million people were living with HIV, 2 million acquired their infection in 2014, and there were 1.2 million AIDS-related deaths in 2014. The highest incidences of disease are in the poorest countries of the world in sub-Saharan Africa and in south, southeast, and eastern Asian countries. AIDS-related morbidity and mortality in these regions is further complicated by the high coprevalence of malnutrition and infectious disease such as hepatitis B and C, malaria, and tuberculosis. The reality is that a great deal of human suffering will occur before our dreams of conquering this disease are realized.

To provide a focus for this chapter, it is important to know the members of the Retroviridae family of viruses and an understanding of what will be discussed:

Retroviridae Family of Viruses

Virus	Disease
Lentivirus	
• Human immunodeficiency virus 1 (HIV-1)	Acquired immunodeficiency syndrome
• Human immunodeficiency virus 2 (HIV-2)	Acquired immunodeficiency syndrome
Delta retrovirus	
• Human T-cell lymphotropic virus 1 (HTLV-1)	Adult T-cell leukemia/lymphoma; tropical spastic paraparesis
• Human T-cell lymphotropic virus 2 (HTLV-2)	Atypical hairy cell leukemia

Additional delta retroviruses have been described but not conclusively associated with human disease. HIV-2 causes a disease similar to HIV-1 but is geographically restricted to west Africa, progresses more slowly, and is less transmissible. The focus of this chapter will be restricted to HIV-1.

HUMAN IMMUNODEFICIENCY VIRUS 1 (HIV-1)

HIV-1 is subdivided into four groups (M, N, O, and P) based on the origin of the parent virus. Group M is responsible for the global spread of HIV-1 while the other groups have remained restricted to western Africa. Group M is subdivided further into nine subtypes with:

- Subtype B predominant in western Europe, the Americas, and Australia
- Subtype C predominant in Africa and India

The methods for transmission of HIV-1 are well known: genital contact with infectious body fluids such as semen, vaginal secretions, and blood; contact with contaminated blood or tissues; and infant exposure to infected mother. Risk factors for transmission include unprotected sex, sexual exposure to multiple partners, sexual exposure to genital ulcers (e.g., due to syphilis or herpes simplex virus), men who have sex with men, intravenous drug abuse, and transfusion with unscreened blood products. The likelihood of transmission is directly related to the viral concentration in the infectious fluids or tissues, so risk is highest when contact is with an individual with active, advanced disease.

Following exposure to HIV, the virus binds and penetrates into CD4 T lymphocytes and other cells with the appropriate receptors. This is followed by rapid viral replication that induces inflammatory cytokines and chemokines. Viral replication is balanced by HIV-specific CD8 T-cell killing of the infected cells, thus depleting the CD4 T-cell population with resulting compromised T-cell immune response. Innate immunity mediated by natural killer cells is also important for containing the infection. Although viral exposure can progress to unrelenting immune suppression and associated complications, most infections are characterized by an extended period of latency where slow viral replication can occur; most infected cells remain dormant, only to reactivate months or years later.

The central role of the CD4 T cells is the initiation and regulation of the innate and immune responses. Activated cells initiate immune responses by the release of cytokines required for the activation of epithelial cells, neutrophils, macrophages, other T cells, B cells, and natural killer cells. Initially this is manifested by increased susceptibility to infections with fungi (e.g., *Candida*, *Cryptococcus*, *Histoplasma*, *Pneumocystis*, and *Microsporidia*) and bacteria. Further depletion of immune responsiveness is associated with opportunistic infections with intracellular bacteria (e.g., mycobacteria and nocardia), parasites (e.g., *Toxoplasma*, *Cryptosporidium*, and *Cystoisospora*), and viruses (e.g., herpesvirus group and JC polyomavirus), as well as some viral related neoplasms (e.g., Epstein-Barr virus lymphoma and human herpesvirus 8 Kaposi sarcoma). These opportunistic infections and malignancies are the hallmark of AIDS and the primary contributor to AIDS-related mortality.

Laboratory diagnosis of HIV infections is complex with many different approaches in use. Rapid point-of-care immunoassays are widely used as screening tests for assessment of patients with active infections. Generally the tests are simple to use, test for antibody response to multiple viral antigens, and provide results within 30 minutes. The disadvantage of these tests is relatively poor sensitivity, particularly when used shortly following exposure to HIV. Laboratory-based immunoassays are also available, with significantly better analytic performance. The most recently designed tests detect both immunoglobulin M and immunoglobulin G antibodies to recombinant HIV antigens as well as expression of the HIV p24 antigen. Although these tests are an improvement over the point-of-care tests, they are unreliable for detection of early infections. For this purpose, detection of viral RNA by nucleic acid amplification tests is used to screen blood products or to assess the quantity of viral particles in the blood of an infected patient (for staging disease or monitoring response to therapy).

Therapy has made remarkable progress since the first antivirals were developed, providing more manageable drug regiments, less toxicity, and better therapeutic outcomes. More than 25 drugs or combinations of drugs currently exist. Although treatment options are rapidly changing, current practice is the use of two nucleoside reverse transcriptase inhibitors with a non-nucleoside reverse transcriptase inhibitor, protease inhibitor, or integrase inhibitor. Prophylactic treatment of pregnant women and individuals exposed to contaminated blood (e.g., needlestick) is recommended. Use of vaginal microbicides to prevent male-to-female acquisition has not been demonstrated to be effective. Likewise, prophylactic use of antiviral for individuals engaged in high-risk activities is not recommended. An HIV vaccine is not currently available. The following is a summary of HIV:

HUMAN IMMUNODEFICIENCY VIRUS	
Properties	• Enveloped RNA virus • Primary target for HIV is activated **CD4 T lymphocytes**; entry into cell is via binding to CD4 receptor and then binding to the CCR5 or CXCR4 coreceptor; other susceptible cells include resting CD4 T cells, monocytes, macrophages, and dendritic cells, as well as astrocytes (responsible for neurologic disorders) and renal epithelial cells (resulting neuropathy)
Epidemiology	• Worldwide distribution with the greatest prevalence in the poorest countries • Transmission via direct contact with contaminated fluids (e.g., blood, semen, vaginal fluid) and tissues • Recognition of HIV infection frequently occurs with the development of opportunistic bacterial, fungal, viral, or parasitic infections
Clinical Disease	• Acute disease develops 2 to 4 weeks after infections, presenting with flulike symptoms or as infectious mononucleosis; aseptic meningitis may develop within the first 3 months; symptoms subside within 2 to 3 weeks although the virus continues to replicate with resultant CD4 cell death • When the CD4 T cells fall below 500 cells/μL, and the viral concentration (viral load) is >75,000 copies/mL, the onset of more severe disease occurs with weight loss and diarrhea (HIV wasting syndrome) and opportunistic infections, malignancies, and dementia • Opportunistic infections include oral candidiasis (thrush), *Pneumocystis* pneumonia, *Cryptococcus* meningitis, cerebral toxoplasmosis, tuberculosis, diarrheal disease (caused by mycobacteria, *Salmonella*, *Shigella*, *Campylobacter*, *Cryptosporidia*, and other agents)
Diagnosis	• Initial screening of patients can be performed by point-of-care immunoassays or more sensitive laboratory-based immunoassays • Detection of viral nucleic acids by nucleic acid amplification tests is the most sensitive method for screening blood products, assessment of the stage of infection, or monitoring response to antiviral therapy
Treatment, Control, Prevention	• Antiviral treatment of HIV infections is rapidly evolving with the use of multiple agents to inhibit viral reverse transcriptase, protease, and integrase; refer to Infectious Diseases Society of America and World Health Organization treatment guidelines for current recommendations • Prevention of disease is by avoidance of high-risk activities • Prophylaxis with antiviral agents after the first trimester recommended for HIV-infected pregnant women; antiviral prophylaxis recommended for accidental exposure to HIV-contaminated blood • No HIV vaccine currently exists although clinical trials of candidate vaccine are underway

CLINICAL CASE

First Report of AIDS in Los Angeles

On June 5, 1981, the Centers for Disease Control and Prevention published the first report of five homosexual men in Los Angeles with Pneumocystis carinii (Pneumocystis jiroveci) *pneumonia with concurrent cytomegalovirus (CMV) infections and candida mucosal infection. Patient 1 was a previously healthy 33-year-old man who developed* P. carinii *pneumonia and oral mucosal candidiasis after a 2-month history of fever associated with elevated liver enzymes, leukopenia, and CMV viruria. The patient's condition continued to deteriorate despite treatment with trimethoprim-sulfamethoxazole (TMP-SXT), pentamidine, and acyclovir, and he died on May 3. Patient 2 was a 30-year-old man who developed* P. carinii *pneumonia in April 1981 after a 5-month history of daily fevers and of elevated liver function tests and CMV viruria. He also had leukopenia and mucosal candidiasis. His pneumonia responded to TMP-SXT but his fevers persisted. He was lost to follow up. Patient 3 was well until January 1981 when he developed esophageal and oral candidiasis that responded to amphotericin B treatment. He was hospitalized in February for* P. carinii *pneumonia that responded to TMP-SXT. His esophageal candidiasis recurred and was again treated with amphotericin B. An esophageal biopsy was positive for CMV. Patient 4 was a 29-year-old man who developed* P. carinii *pneumonia in February 1981. His pneumonia did not respond to TMP-SXT and he died in March. Both* P. carinii *and CMV were found in the lung tissue. Patient 5 was a previously healthy 36-year-old man, clinically diagnosed with CMV infection in September 1980. He was seen in April 1981 because of a 4-month history of fever, dyspnea, and cough. On admission he was found to have* P. carinii *pneumonia, oral candidiasis, and CMV retinitis. His pneumonia was treated with TMP-SXT and topical nystatin was used to treat the* Candida *infection. All five patients had profound immunosuppression and multiple opportunistic infections. This report documented not an isolated focal epidemic but rather the first patients of the AIDS pandemic.*

14

Human Herpesviruses

INTERESTING FACTS

- Herpesvirus infections typically occur early in life and have lifelong persistence
- Most people have been exposed to herpes simplex virus, varicella-zoster virus (VZV), and Epstein-Barr virus (EBV); 25% or more have been exposed to cytomegalovirus (CMV)
- Vaccines are only available for VZV and primarily to prevent zoster, a reactivation of dormant varicella virus primarily in individuals >50 years of age
- Seventy percent of genital herpes infections are acquired from a partner who is asymptomatic; this is logical because symptoms include an intense burning sensation
- Infectious mononucleosis caused by EBV can be acquired by kissing and use of shared utensils, toothbrushes, and cups, but not by coughing or sneezing
- About 1 in 150 infants are born with congenital CMV infection and 80% never develop symptoms; the most severe symptoms are in infants infected during the first trimester of pregnancy

The herpesvirus group is an important collection of eight human pathogens:

Eight Human Pathogens of Human Herpesviruses

	INFECTIONS IN:	
Virus	**Immunocompetent Persons**	**Immunocompromised Persons**
Herpes simplex virus, type 1 (HSV-1)	Gingivostomatitis* Keratoconjunctivitis Cutaneous herpes Genital herpes	Gingivostomatitis Keratoconjunctivitis Cutaneous herpes Disseminated infection
Herpes simplex virus, type 2 (HSV-2)	Genital herpes* Cutaneous herpes Gingivostomatitis Encephalitis* Neonatal herpes	Genital herpes Cutaneous herpes Disseminated infection
Varicella-zoster virus (VZV)	Chickenpox (varicella)* Herpes zoster (shingles)*	Disseminated infection
Cytomegalovirus (CMV)	Mononucleosis Hepatitis Congenital disease*	Hepatitis Retinitis Disseminated infection
Epstein-Barr virus (EBV)	Mononucleosis* Hepatitis Encephalitis	Lymphoproliferative syndromes* Oral hairy leukoplakia

Continued

Eight Human Pathogens of Human Herpesviruses—cont'd

	INFECTIONS IN:	
Virus	**Immunocompetent Persons**	**Immunocompromised Persons**
Human herpesvirus 6 (HHV-6)	Exanthem subitum* Childhood febrile seizures Encephalitis	Fever and rash Encephalitis Bone marrow suppression
HHV-7	Exanthem subitum Childhood febrile seizures Encephalitis	Encephalitis
HHV-8	Febrile exanthema	Kaposi sarcoma* Castleman disease Primary effusion lymphoma

*Virus is the most common cause.

HHVs are divided into three subfamilies:

- Alpha herpesviruses: herpes simplex virus 1 and 2 (HSV-1, HSV-2), VZV; latent infections established in neurons of sensory ganglia
- Beta herpesviruses: CMV, HHV-6, HHV-7; latent infections established in mononuclear cells
- Gamma herpesviruses: EBV, HHV-8; latent infections established in lymphoid cells

The ability to establish latent infections means that recurrent diseases can occur when natural immunity wanes or during times of immunosuppression. Most infections with these viruses are asymptomatic or mild, with the exception of VZV (chickenpox) and HHV-6 (fever and rash). In the following section, HSV-1, HSV-2, VZV, CMV, and EBV are discussed in detail.

HERPES SIMPLEX VIRUS, TYPES 1 AND 2

HSV-1 and HSV-2 are ubiquitous viruses transmitted person-to-person by contact with infectious secretions. Infections include mucocutaneous lesions, involvement of the central nervous system, and disseminated infections, particularly in immunocompromised patients. The viruses establish lifelong latent infections with periodic asymptomatic and symptomatic episodes of virus production. These viruses are particularly important causes of some specific diseases:

Herpes Simplex Virus, Types 1 and 2

Virus	Disease
HSV-1	Most common cause of viral orofacial lesions ("cold sores")
HSV-1	Most common cause of acute viral encephalitis in the United States
HSV-1	Most common cause of corneal blindness in the United States
HSV-2	Most common cause of painful genital ulcers

CLINICAL CASE

Neonatal HSV

Parvey and Ch'ien[1] reported a case of neonatal HSV contracted during birth. During a breech presentation, a fetal monitor was placed on the buttocks of the baby, and because of the greatly prolonged labor, the baby was delivered by cesarean section. The 5-lb boy had minor difficulties that were successfully treated, but on the 6th day, vesicles with an erythematous base appeared at the site where the fetal monitor had been placed. HSV was grown from the vesicle fluid and from spinal fluid, corneal scraping, saliva, and blood. The baby became moribund, with frequent apneic episodes and seizures. Intravenous treatment with adenosine arabinoside (ara-A; vidarabine) was initiated. The baby also developed bradycardia and occasional vomiting. The vesicles spread to cover the lower extremities and were also on the back, palm, nares, and right eyelid. Within 72 hours of ara-A treatment, the baby's condition started to improve. Treatment was continued for 11 days but discontinued because of a low platelet count. The baby was discharged on the 45th day after his birth, and normal development was reported at 1 and 2 years of age. At 6 weeks after birth, a herpes lesion was found on the mother's vulva. The baby was successfully treated with ara-A and was able to overcome the damage caused by infection. The virus, most likely HSV-2, was probably acquired through an abrasion caused by the fetal monitor while the neonate was in the birth canal. Ara-A has since been replaced with antiviral drugs that are better, less toxic, and easier to administer: acyclovir, valacyclovir, and famciclovir.

The following is a summary of HSV-1 and HSV-2:

HERPES SIMPLEX VIRUS, TYPES 1 AND 2	
Properties	• Enveloped DNA viruses • Infection initiated in abraded skin or mucosal surfaces; replication in epithelial cells precedes infection of sensory or autonomic nerve endings, followed by migration of the virus to nerve cell bodies in ganglia where latency is established • Reactivation of virus replication can be caused by a number of stimuli (e.g., heat, cold, stress) and can be characterized by either asymptomatic or symptomatic (i.e., presence of vesicular lesions) shedding of virus
Epidemiology	• Worldwide distribution; HSV-1 typically acquired earlier in life than HSV-2; HSV-2 generally acquired when sexual activity is initiated • Both viruses inactivated rapidly in the environment so infection requires close contact • HSV-1 most common cause of orofacial lesions ("**cold sores**") and acute **viral encephalitis** in the United States; HSV-2 is the most common cause of **genital ulcers**; both viruses overlap in sites of clinical disease
Clinical Disease	• **Orofacial infections** present most commonly as gingivostomatitis and pharyngitis; lesions may be present on palate, gingiva, tongue, lip, and adjacent areas of face; symptomatic reactivated disease typically with vesicular lesions at the edge of the lips (**herpes labialis**); recurrent lesions more frequent with HSV-1 • Primary **genital infections** characterized by up to 2 weeks of symptoms with painful ulcerative lesions and viral shedding; mucoid discharge and dysuria may be present; recurrent lesions more frequent with HSV-2 • **Eye infections**: HSV infection of the eye is the most frequent cause of **corneal blindness** in the United States • **Encephalitis**: HSV-1 infection is the most common cause of acute, viral encephalitis in the United States • **Disseminated disease**: complication of immunosuppression
Diagnosis	• HSV-1 and HSV-2 can be readily detected by culture of cutaneous lesions or corneal scrapings; nucleic acid amplification test (NAAT) of these specimens available for rapid diagnosis • NAAT is the test of choice for CNS or disseminated diseases • Serologic response to infections can be measured but does not distinguish between active primary infections and past or recurrent disease
Treatment, Control, Prevention	• Acyclovir, valacyclovir, or famciclovir is used for mucocutaneous and disseminated infections; encephalitis is treated with acyclovir; foscarnet or cidofovir is used to treat acyclovir-resistant strains • Prevention of disease is difficult because infected patients may be shedding virus asymptomatically; condom use is partially protective • No vaccine is currently available

CLINICAL CASE

Aseptic Meningitis Complicating Acute HSV-2 Proctitis

Atia and colleagues[2] reported the clinical history of a male homosexual patient who developed aseptic meningitis during the course of acute proctitis due to HSV-2. The 23-year-old man was seen at a health care clinic 4 days after passive homosexual contact. On examination the rectal tissue was inflamed and with purulent discharge. Bacteria consistent with Neisseria gonorrhoeae *were observed on Gram stain, but the culture was negative. Ampicillin was administered but 2 days later the patient was readmitted with complaints of anal discomfort and pain on defecation. Multiple clusters of herpetiform vesicles were observed around the anus and cultures were positive for HSV-2. Three days later the patient returned to the hospital with symptoms of malaise, headache, photophobia, hesitancy of micturition, and pain radiating down his legs. His temperature and pulse rate were elevated and the patient had signs of meningitis. Cerebrospinal fluid was collected and was consistent with the diagnosis of aseptic lymphocytic meningitis. No viral cultures were performed with the cerebrospinal fluid, but the anorectal lesions were again positive for HSV-2. Despite the fact that antiviral therapy was not available (in the early 1980s), this patient had an uneventful recovery. This case illustrates the significant risk for sexually transmitted diseases in male homosexuals practicing unsafe sexual activities and the limited diagnostic and therapeutic options that were available in the 1980s during the early years of the AIDS epidemic.*

VARICELLA-ZOSTER VIRUS

VZV is responsible for two distinct diseases: the primary infection is **varicella** or **chickenpox**, and the recurrent infection is **zoster** or **shingles**. Chickenpox is characterized by a generalized maculopapular or vesicular rash and is generally a benign disease except in immunocompromised patients. Zoster is a disease where a painful vesicular rash develops along the nerve track where the virus reactivates. This can also present as a disseminated disease in an immunocompromised patient.

VARICELLA-ZOSTER VIRUS	
Properties	• Enveloped DNA virus • Initial replication in upper respiratory tract, followed by lymphatic spread to the reticuloendothelial system, viremia, and widespread infection of epithelial cells in the epidermis • Epithelial cells degenerate with viral replication, forming fluid-filled vesicles
Epidemiology	• Worldwide distribution with humans only host • Person-to-person spread primarily by the respiratory route; the virus is not stable in the environment so close contact is required for transmission • Chickenpox is primarily a disease of school-aged children, except in populations where vaccination of children is widely used
Clinical Disease	• **Chickenpox**: rash, low-grade fever, and malaise develops following a 2-week incubation period; the rash develops over a 3- to 5-day period and is characterized as maculopapular and vesicular lesions with an erythematous base in different stages of development; the lesions resolve over a 1- to 2-week period; disease is generally benign and self-limited, although a more prolonged and severe rash occurs in immunocompromised patients and complications (**acute cerebellar ataxia, encephalitis,** or **pneumonia**) may occur and are associated with significant morbidity and mortality • **Zoster**: characterized by development of vesicular lesion along a dermatome, with thoracic and lumbar dermatomes most commonly involved; if the fifth cranial nerve is involved, **herpes zoster ophthalmicus** can develop and threaten vision; onset of disease is identified by pain along the dermatome followed by the development of the lesion over a 3- to 5-day period; relief may take as long as 1 month; infections in immunocompromised patients (particularly HIV patients) may involve more chronic development of lesions
Diagnosis	• Clinical diagnosis is confirmed by culture (infrequently done), microscopy (specific stain is the Tzanck smear), detection of infected cells in lesions by immunofluorescent microscopy, or NAAT (test of choice because it is rapid, sensitive, and specific)
Treatment, Control, Prevention	• Treatment is symptomatic and with the antiviral **acyclovir**; valacyclovir and famciclovir can also be used to treat chickenpox and zoster • Varicella-zoster immune globulin can be used as a prophylaxis in high-risk patients • Two doses of a live, attenuated **vaccine** is recommended for children for the prevention of vaccinia, and a high titer attenuated vaccine is recommended for adults over the age of 50 to prevent zoster; inactivated vaccines are under evaluation for immunocompromised patients

CYTOMEGALOVIRUS

CMV is a ubiquitous virus that causes a wide spectrum of clinical diseases. The following are some of the most noteworthy.

Following the initial infection with CMV, which can frequently be asymptomatic or present with mild nonspecific symptoms, latency is established in a number of cells including polymorphonuclear cells, T lymphocytes, endothelial cells, renal epithelial cells, and the salivary glands. It is not surprising that this virus is the most significant cause of complications following immunosuppression for transplantation or by disease.

Cytomegalovirus

Population	Disease
Unborn child	Congenital CMV syndrome
Healthy teenager	Infectious mononucleosis syndrome
Solid organ transplant patient	Disseminated infection with associated organ rejection
Bone marrow transplant patient	CMV pneumonia
HIV AIDS patient	CMV retinitis

CYTOMEGALOVIRUS

Properties	• Enveloped DNA virus; genetic variability similar to that seen with RNA viruses • Largest herpesvirus (genome 236 kb, encodes 164 proteins) compared with VZV (125 kb), HSV-1 and HSV-2 (155 kb), and EBV (172 kb)
Epidemiology	• Worldwide distribution • Asymptomatic primary infections are common in healthy individuals • Twenty percent of cases of infectious mononucleosis are caused by CMV
Clinical Disease	• **Infectious mononucleosis**: characterized with fever, lymphadenopathy, and lymphocytosis (lymphocytes >50% of peripheral white blood cells); pharyngitis less common than with EBV infections; symptoms persist for 1 month or longer; **Guillain-Barré syndrome** (progressive inflammatory polyneuropathy with muscle weakness and distal sensory loss) is a well-recognized complication of CMV mononucleosis • **Congenital CMV**: generally asymptomatic if mother is immune; fulminant disease for child of nonimmune mother with multiorgan involvement including CNS with microcephaly, chorioretinitis, and cerebral calcification; death *in utero* or soon after birth; surviving infants with significant defects including mental retardation, retinitis, and hearing disorders • **CMV pneumonia**: interstitial pneumonia following infectious mononucleosis is typically mild and self-limited; in contrast, in bone marrow transplant patients, this is rapidly progressive and associated with a high mortality despite aggressive treatment • **CMV retinitis**: CMV is a common opportunistic infection in patients with advanced HIV infections and retinitis is the most common manifestation
Diagnosis	• Culture of CMV in epithelial cells can be done but replication is slow and not practical for diagnostic purposes • Detection of CMV protein pp65 (protein in outer layer beneath the envelope) by immunofluorescent staining of neutrophils in peripheral blood was widely used but has more recently been replaced by NAAT • Quantitative assessment of blood-borne CMV is useful for monitoring transplant patients (rising titers are an early indicator of disease)
Treatment, Control, Prevention	• Antivirals used for treating CMV infections include ganciclovir, foscarnet (used to treat ganciclovir-resistant CMV), and cidofovir (not associated with ganciclovir or foscarnet resistance) • Ganciclovir and valganciclovir are used for CMV prophylaxis for high-risk immunocompromised patients • No vaccine is currently available

CLINICAL CASE

CMV Pneumonia Post–Bone Marrow Transplant

Nagafuji and associates[3] reported a 52-year-old woman who developed fatal CMV interstitial pneumonia following autologous bone marrow transplantation for amyeloblastic leukemia. The woman was documented to be CMV-serology positive before transplantation. Following transplantation, her leukocytosis resolved at day 11. On day 25, bone marrow aspiration showed marked hemophagocytosis; treatment with prednisolone was initiated. On day 35, she was noted to be febrile and her CMV antigenemia assay was strongly positive. Ganciclovir and anti-CMV hyperimmune globulin was administered. On day 48, ganciclovir was withdrawn because of myelotoxicity. On day 56, hemorrhagic cystitis developed and CMV was cultured from the urine. Foscarnet was administered and the CMV antigenemia resolved. Foscarnet was discontinued on day 84, but the CMV-associated hemophagocytic syndrome was again documented on day 116. This was again managed with foscarnet, but on day 158 progressive CMV pneumonia developed and the patient died on day 171. The case illustrates the difficulty of managing CMV infections in immunocompromised bone marrow transplant patients.

EPSTEIN-BARR VIRUS

EBV is the most common cause of infectious mononucleosis and is associated with a number of malignant diseases.

EPSTEIN-BARR VIRUS	
Properties	• Enveloped DNA virus • Initial replication of virus in oral epithelial cells with subsequent spread to B lymphocytes; replication of viral DNA (but not intact virus particles) is synchronized with host cell DNA replication and limited gene products are produced in the infected cell (markers for identifying these cells)
Epidemiology	• Worldwide distribution with most infections occurring early in life • Asymptomatic infections occur most commonly in the very young • Person-to-person transmission through oral secretions (kissing, sharing utensils); close contact required for transmission • Virus can be cultured from the oral secretions of 10% to 20% of healthy adults and a higher proportion of immunocompromised patients
Clinical Disease	• **Infectious mononucleosis**: acute infections characterized by pharyngitis, fever, fatigue, lymphadenopathy, and leukocytosis with monocytes and atypical lymphocytes observed in peripheral blood; symptoms typically resolve within 1 month • **Burkitt lymphoma**: undifferentiated B-cell lymphoma of the jaw that is observed in Central Africa • **Lymphoproliferative disease**: uncontrolled proliferation of infected B lymphocytes observed in immunocompromised patients (solid organ and bone marrow transplants) • **Nasopharyngeal carcinoma**: proliferation of EBV-infected epithelial cells in nasopharynx; disease in South Chinese and Alaskan Inuit Eskimo populations • **Central nervous system lymphoma**: EBV lymphoma in the brains of HIV AIDS patients and stem cell transplant patients
Diagnosis	• Diagnosis of infectious mononucleosis is based on clinical presentation and presence of **heterophile antibodies** (positive reaction: ability to agglutinate sheep erythrocytes as absorption of serum with guinea pig kidney cells) • Diagnosis of infections also performed by measuring the antibody response to structural proteins (viral capsid antigens), nonstructural proteins expressed early in lytic cycle (early antigens), and nuclear proteins expressed in latently infected cells (EBV nuclear antigens) • Diagnosis now commonly performed with NAAT

EPSTEIN-BARR VIRUS—cont'd	
Treatment, Control, Prevention	• Treatment of infectious mononucleosis is supportive • Acyclovir and ganciclovir are active against replicating EBV; however, most disease manifestations are the result of the immune response to EBV-infected cells, so antiviral agents will be ineffective • No vaccine is currently available

CLINICAL CASE

EBV Infectious Mononucleosis Associated with Agranulocytosis

Hammond and colleagues[4] described a series of patients with unusually severe infections with EBV. One patient was a 32-year-old man who developed sore throat, malaise, myalgias, and headaches. The symptoms persisted for 3 months before the patient saw a physician, who documented tender regional lymph nodes and an injected pharynx but no hepatosplenomegaly. The leukocyte count was 6600 cells/mm^3, with 2000 atypical lymphocytes and 660 monocytes. A monospot test was positive. The patient's symptoms persisted and he returned to his physician 1 month later. He appeared acutely ill with an elevated temperature, severe exudative pharyngitis, and tender cervical and submandibular adenopathy. Hematology tests demonstrated severe leukocytopenia and thrombocytopenia. The monospot test was positive, as was specific EBV serology; CMV serology was negative. For the first 4 days of hospitalization, fever and agranulocytosis persisted, with the total leukocyte count remaining less than 2000 cells/mm^3 and no polymorphonuclear cells seen on smear. Thereafter the total leukocyte count slowly increased (patient was discharged after hospitalization for 1 week), and although the malaise and fatigue persisted over the next 3 months, the adenopathy gradually resolved. This case illustrates the potential severity of primary EBV infection in an adult patient.

HUMAN HERPESVIRUSES 6, 7, AND 8

HHV-6 is responsible for infantile fevers (frequently associated with **febrile seizures**) and a common pediatric disease, **exanthema subitum** or roseola infantum (also called sixth disease). This is a disease that presents with a high fever after a 1-week incubation period, persisting for 3 to 4 days. At the time of defervescence, a maculopapular rash will develop and spread from the trunk to the extremities. This will last for up to 2 days. HHV-7 is also associated with infantile fevers and exanthema subitum, although less commonly than HHV-6. HHV-8 is responsible for **Kaposi sarcoma**, typically manifested as cutaneous plaques or nodules in immunocompromised patients (e.g., highly advanced HIV disease).

REFERENCES

1. Parvey LS, Ch'ien LT. Neonatal herpes simplex virus infection introduced by fetal-monitor scalp electrodes. *Pediatrics.* 1980;65:1150–1153.
2. Atia WA, Ratnatunga CS, Greenfield C, Dawson S. Aseptic meningitis and herpes simplex proctitis. A case report. *Br J Vener Dis.* 1982;58:52–53.
3. Nagafuji K, Eto T, Hayashi S, Tokunaga Y, Gondo H, Niho Y. Fatal cytomegalovirus interstitial pneumonia following autologous peripheral blood stem cell transplantation. Fukuoka Bone Marrow Transplantation Group. *Bone Marrow Transpl.* 1998;21:301–303.
4. Hammond WP, Harlan JM, Steinberg SE. Severe neutropenia in infectious mononucleosis. *West J Med.* 1979;131:92–97.

15

Respiratory Viruses

INTERESTING FACTS

- Rhinoviruses are the most common cause of acute upper respiratory viral infections ("common cold")
- Although most coronavirus infections are mild common colds, the severe acute respiratory syndrome coronavirus (SARS-CoV) and Middle East respiratory syndrome coronavirus (MERS-CoV) are responsible for up to 50% mortality in infected individuals
- Most mortality associated with influenza virus infections is not caused by influenza virus but by secondary bacterial pneumonias caused by *Staphylococcus aureus* and *Streptococcus pneumoniae*
- Vaccines are only available for influenza virus infections because many serotypes of the other respiratory viruses exist and infection is associated with only partial, short-term immunity to reinfection

A large collection of viruses produce upper and/or lower respiratory tract infections, ranging from the "common cold" to life-threatening overwhelming pneumonia. This chapter focuses on six RNA virus groups to illustrate the range of respiratory infections produced by viruses. Most infections caused by these viruses occur during the cold months of the year and frequently produce symptoms indistinguishable from each other. This is generally not a problem because neither antiviral treatment nor vaccines are available for most of these pathogens. The one notable exception is for influenza virus infections, where a rapid diagnosis is important for the prompt initiation of antiviral treatment and to monitor the effectiveness of the vaccine in the population.

RHINOVIRUSES

Although most rhinovirus infections are not severe and complications are rare, the prevalence of infections and duration of symptoms result in prolonged periods of feeling miserable (and the coughing and sneezing is not welcomed by anyone). The following is a summary of key facts about rhinoviruses.

RHINOVIRUSES	
Properties	• Nonenveloped RNA viruses; more than 100 serotypes described • Symptoms caused by infection of respiratory ciliated epithelial cells stimulates cellular inflammatory response with expression of cytokines and chemokines
Epidemiology	• Worldwide distribution, with infections in both children and adults • Infections occur throughout the year but typically peak in the fall and spring, with decreased activity during the winter and summer months • Transmission most common with large droplets (cough, sneeze) where hands are contaminated and then transfer to nose or eyes • Transmission most efficient when symptoms are most severe (high virus concentration in respiratory secretions) • Multiple serotypes and short-lived immunity make recurrent disease inevitable

RHINOVIRUSES—cont'd	
Clinical Disease	• Primarily an upper respiratory tract infection • Initiated with sore, "scratchy" throat followed closely with rhinorrhea and nasal obstruction; cough, sneezing, headache, and low-grade fever (particularly in children) also develop • Symptoms can persist for 1 week or more
Diagnosis	• Definitive diagnosis cannot be made based on clinical parameters • Virus can be grown in culture but this is rarely performed • Antigen tests have been replaced in recent years by nucleic acid amplification tests (NAATs)
Treatment, Control, Prevention	• No specific antiviral therapy is available • Vaccines are not available

CORONAVIRUSES

Human coronaviruses primarily cause respiratory infections. A number of strains of coronaviruses are recognized, most of which are responsible for the common cold. However, in 2002 a new strain emerged in China that rapidly spread in the region, then to Hong Kong, Vietnam, and Singapore. Focal outbreaks were also reported in other countries by travelers from the endemic region who became ill when they returned home. The virus was named **SARS-CoV**. Two facts about this virus are critical: person-to-person spread occurred readily, including in the health care workers exposed to the patients, and the disease was responsible for a high mortality rate, particularly for patients with underlying pulmonary disease (i.e., 50% mortality) and in the elderly. The outbreak ended 18 months later but in 2012 a new coronavirus infection erupted in the Middle East, again associated with a high mortality rate. This strain, **MERS-CoV**, has spread from the initial focus in the Kingdom of Saudi Arabia through the Middle East and to other countries via travelers. In contrast with the SARS-CoV strain, this coronavirus is only intermittently spread person-to-person; however, coronaviruses have a high mutation rate so this can change rapidly. In addition, the strain continues to circulate in the Middle East. It is interesting that both the SARS-CoV and MERS-CoV strains are related to bat coronavirus strains. The SARS-CoV strain was isolated in bats, and there is epidemiologic evidence to implicate bats in the MERS-CoV. This is one more reason to dislike bats.

Fortunately, most coronavirus infections are not caused by the more virulent strains. The following is a summary of coronaviruses.

CORONAVIRUSES	
Properties	• Enveloped RNA virus • Replicate in ciliated and nonciliated epithelial cells of the nasopharynx • Stimulate production of cytokines and chemokines resulting in cold symptoms; hyperproduction of this inflammatory response is responsible for the pathology with SARS-CoV and MERS-CoV
Epidemiology	• Responsible for about 15% of common colds; infections in pediatric and adult patients primarily in winter and spring • Common cold coronaviruses with worldwide distribution; SARS-CoV and MERS-CoV with more restricted geographic distribution (the former initially in China, latter in Kingdom of Saudi Arabia)
Clinical Disease	• Infections with the common cold coronaviruses have a 2-day incubation period, with peak symptoms 3 to 4 days after exposure; symptoms similar to rhinovirus infections (sore throat, rhinorrhea, cough, headache) • SARS-CoV infections not typically associated with coldlike symptoms; typically present with fever, headache, myalgia, followed by a nonproductive cough; progression to severe pulmonary disease most likely in older adults and patients with underlying disease (e.g., diabetes, cardiac disease, hepatitis, chronic pulmonary disease) • MERS-CoV infections can be restricted to mild upper respiratory tract symptoms, but more likely progresses to respiratory and multiorgan failure

Continued

CORONAVIRUSES—cont'd	
Diagnosis	• Although the viruses can be grown with some difficulty in culture, this is rarely done except in public health laboratories • Diagnosis most commonly by NAATs
Treatment, Control, Prevention	• No specific antiviral therapy is available • Vaccines are not available • Rigorous infection control practices used to control infections with SARS-CoV and MERS-CoV

CLINICAL CASE

Previously Healthy Patient with SARS Infection

Luo and colleagues[1] described a previously healthy patient who was transferred to his hospital after a 9-day history of persistent fevers, myalgias, and headache. The patient presented with a fever of 39.4°C, chills, a dry cough, shortness of breath, and diarrhea. Chest x-ray showed inflammation in the right upper lung fields. White blood cells and chemistries were normal. The patient failed to respond to antibiotic treatment and on day 3 he developed a deep cough and dyspnea along with diffuse pulmonary inflammation. The diagnosis of SARS was made in view of his severe hypoxemia with Pa_{O_2} *of 60 mmHg and* Pa_{O_2}/Fi_{O_2} *of 150 mmHg, and a clinical picture consistent with other hospitalized patients with SARS. The patient was transferred to the intensive care unit and placed on ventilatory support, but continued to deteriorate into multiorgan dysfunction syndrome involving the kidney, liver, and heart. The medical staff initiated molecular adsorbent recirculating system therapy (extracorporeal liver support utilizing albumin dialysis for 8 hours) and after 4 consecutive days of therapy, clinical improvement was noted. After 13 days, ventilatory support was withdrawn and the patient continued to improve. The patient was discharged after 44 days of hospitalization. This case illustrates the severe infection caused by SARS-CoV. It is remarkable that within the same virus family, most strains are responsible for mild upper respiratory infections while others such as SARS and MERS can cause devastating pneumonia with multiorgan involvement.*

INFLUENZA VIRUSES

These are the oldest recognized respiratory viruses producing epidemic disease every few years. The structural properties of these viruses are important to understand. The genetic information is encoded in single-stranded RNA. Single-stranded nucleic acids (as with the other respiratory viruses discussed in this chapter) are more susceptible to mutations during replication, so gene products such as the surface proteins (in the case of influenza these would be hemagglutinin [H] and neuraminidase [N]) can be altered. This can create a previously unrecognized virus (new virus: little or no immunity). The influenza viruses have the RNA arranged in discrete segments, so if a cell is infected with two different influenza viruses, rearrangement can occur creating a unique third virus. This is the reason novel viruses can be created every few years and produce epidemics. A worldwide pandemic can occur if the virus is both unique and highly infectious and, if the strain is highly virulent, a pandemic associated with high mortality can occur. There are three distinct influenza groups: A, B, and C. Influenza A and B viruses are responsible for epidemic disease, with influenza A causing more severe disease; and influenza C virus causes milder upper respiratory infections. The circulating strain of influenza virus is identified by its type and surface proteins, such as A (H3N2). Influenza A strains circulate in bird populations ("avian flu") so the opportunity for a new strain to emerge is great. In some cases these strains will also circulate in pig populations ("swine flu") further increasing their genetic uniqueness and virulence. The following is a summary of these viruses.

INFLUENZA VIRUSES	
Properties	• Enveloped RNA viruses with genome divided into 8 segments • Three types of influenza viruses: A, B, C; A and B associated with epidemics; A is the most virulent • Strains identified by their surface proteins: hemagglutinin (H), neuraminidase (N) • Virus infects ciliated columnar epithelial cells of the trachea and bronchials

INFLUENZA VIRUSES—cont'd	
Epidemiology	• Worldwide distribution with infections primarily in the cold months • Person-to-person spread either by airborne route (sneezing, coughing) or by contact with infectious particles on contaminated surfaces (hand to nose) • Severity of disease determined by the virulence of the virus strain and immunity to the circulating strain
Clinical Disease	• After a 1- to 2-day incubation period, onset is acute with fever, chills, myalgias, and headache, as well as cough, chest pain, and nasal discharge; symptoms may last 1 week or longer • Complications include primary viral pneumonia or secondary bacterial pneumonia (most commonly with *Staphylococcus aureus* and *Streptococcus pneumoniae*)
Diagnosis	• Viral culture has generally been replaced with immunoassays or NAATs • Specific diagnosis is important for guiding antiviral therapy
Treatment, Control, Prevention	• Treatment and prophylaxis of influenza A and B infections with neuraminidase inhibitors zanamivir or oseltamivir; must be initiated early in infection • Previously influenza A but not B was treated with amantadine or rimantadine, but resistance is now widespread • Multiplex vaccines widely used to control disease; however, if the circulating strain is not included in the vaccine it will be ineffective

CLINICAL CASE

H5N1 Avian Influenza

The first case of H5N1 avian influenza in a human was described by Ku and Chan.[2] *After a 3-year-old boy from China developed a fever of 40°C and abdominal pain, he was given antibiotics and aspirin. On the third day, he was hospitalized with a sore throat, and his chest radiograph demonstrated bronchial inflammation. Blood studies showed a left shift with 9% band forms. On the sixth day the boy was still febrile and fully conscious, but on the seventh day his fever increased, he was hyperventilating, and his blood oxygen levels decreased. A chest radiograph indicated severe pneumonia. The patient was intubated. On the eighth day, the boy was diagnosed with fulminant sepsis and acute respiratory distress syndrome. Therapy for acute respiratory distress syndrome and other attempts to improve oxygen uptake were unsuccessful. He was treated empirically for sepsis, herpes simplex virus infection (acyclovir), methicillin-resistant* S. aureus *(vancomycin), and fungal infection (amphotericin B), but his condition deteriorated further, with disseminated intravascular coagulation and liver and renal failure. He died on the 11th day. Laboratory results indicated evaluated influenza A antibody on the eighth day, and influenza A was isolated from a tracheal isolate taken on the ninth day. The isolate was sent to the Centers for Disease Control and Prevention and elsewhere, where it was typed as H5N1 avian influenza and named* A/Hong Kong/156/97 (H5N1). *The child may have contracted the virus while playing with pet ducklings and chickens at his kindergarten. Although the H5N1 virus still has difficulty infecting humans, this case demonstrates the speed and severity of the respiratory and systemic manifestations of avian influenza H5N1 disease.*

PARAMYXOVIRIDAE

Paramyxoviridae is an important family of respiratory pathogens of both children and adults. Three members are discussed below: parainfluenza virus, respiratory syncytial virus (RSV), and human metapneumovirus (HMV), and two other members of this family, measles virus and mumps virus, can also present with respiratory symptoms.

PARAINFLUENZA VIRUSES

Parainfluenza viruses are the most important cause of **croup** in children and a significant cause of severe lower respiratory tract viral disease in immunocompromised patients.

PARAINFLUENZA VIRUSES	
Properties	• Enveloped RNA virus with four major human serotypes: parainfluenza virus-1 (PIV-1), PIV-2, PIV-3, PIV-4 • Preferentially infect ciliated epithelial cells of the upper and lower respiratory tract
Epidemiology	• Worldwide distribution with infections in both children and adults • Person-to-person spread by exposure to respiratory droplets or contact with contaminated surfaces • PIV-1 and PIV-2 cause seasonal outbreaks in fall; PIV-3 and PIV-4 causes outbreaks in spring
Clinical Disease	• Most pediatric infections limited to upper respiratory tract with cold symptoms developing about 1 day after exposure to the virus and persisting for a week or more; involvement of the sinuses and middle ear occurs in up to half of children • PIV-1 and PIV-2 associated with laryngotracheobronchitis (**croup**) with initial development of fever, rhinorrhea, and pharyngitis, and then progressing to a barking cough associated with stridor and difficulty breathing; PIV-1 disease is generally more severe than PIV-2 disease • PIV-3 disease is more commonly associated with pneumonia and bronchiolitis in children, and PIV-4 primarily causes mild upper respiratory infections • PIV infections in adults are generally asymptomatic or mild upper respiratory infections, except in immunocompromised patients where severe lower respiratory tract disease can develop and is associated with high mortality
Diagnosis	• Although PIV can be grown in culture, most clinical diagnoses are by NAATs
Treatment, Control, Prevention	• No specific antiviral treatment • Croup is managed symptomatically with glucocorticoids and nebulized epinephrine • Vaccine is not available

RESPIRATORY SYNCYTIAL VIRUS

RSV infections are most severe in infants; they are responsible for the majority of infections due to bronchial disease (**bronchiolitis**) and as many as half of hospitalizations due to pneumonia. The majority of middle ear infections (**otitis media**) in young children are caused by RSV. Mild disease is widespread in adults but severe complications can occur in high-risk patients, particularly those with underlying pulmonary disease.

RESPIRATORY SYNCYTIAL VIRUS	
Properties	• Enveloped RNA virus; two major antigenic groups (A and B) with multiple subgroups; both groups circulate in populations simultaneously • RSV infects the ciliated columnar epithelial cells of the lower airways as well as pneumocytes
Epidemiology	• Worldwide distribution with infections in both children and adults • Person-to-person spread by exposure to respiratory droplets or contact with contaminated surfaces • Infections occur annually from late fall through early spring; may extend throughout the year in warmer climates • Initial infections early in life, followed by milder recurrent infections throughout life
Clinical Disease	• Infection in infants primarily involves the lower respiratory tract, presenting after a 2- to 5-day incubation period as bronchiolitis; pneumonia can develop but croup occurs less commonly • RSV infections in children and adults present initially as an upper respiratory tract infection with nasal congestion and cough • Otitis media is associated with pediatric disease and co-infections with bacterial pathogens are responsible for more severe otitis • Adult disease is primarily mild, although severe lower respiratory disease is well-recognized in elderly, immunocompromised adults and those with underlying cardiopulmonary disease (chronic obstructive pulmonary disease, congestive heart failure)

RESPIRATORY SYNCYTIAL VIRUS—cont'd	
Diagnosis	• Although RSV can be grown in culture, most clinical diagnoses are by NAATs • Virus shedding in adult patients, even with severe disease, is quantitatively lower than in infants which makes diagnosis more challenging
Treatment, Control, Prevention	• Mild infections are treated symptomatically • Bronchiolitis is generally managed with bronchodilators and corticosteroids • Ribavirin is approved for treatment of hospitalized infants with lower respiratory tract disease, although benefits have not been consistently demonstrated for this population or for older children or adults with RSV infections • Vaccine is not available

HUMAN METAPNEUMOVIRUS

HMV was recently discovered, although serologic evidence demonstrates this virus is widely disseminated in the population and is an important human pathogen.

HUMAN METAPNEUMOVIRUS	
Properties	• Enveloped RNA virus closely related to RSV • Two genotypes with multiple subgroups; genetic diversity observed with two surface glycoproteins, resulting in a number of novel circulating strains of virus • Immunity to HMV is incomplete and reinfections occur throughout life • Infection of bronchial epithelial cells results in a prolonged inflammatory response
Epidemiology	• Worldwide distribution with infections most common in winter and spring in temperate climates, as with RSV and influenza virus • Primary infections by 5 years of age • Severity of HMV infections related to co-infections with RSV or *S. pneumoniae*
Clinical Disease	• Diseases range from mild upper respiratory infections to bronchitis and severe pneumonia • Infections in children characterized by fever, cough, wheezing, and rhinorrhea; conjunctivitis, pharyngitis, laryngitis, and otitis may occur; involvement of the bronchial airways and lungs may develop • Adult disease is similar to that in children, with lower respiratory complications more common in patients with underlying respiratory disease or immunosuppression
Diagnosis	• Although HMV can be grown in culture, most clinical diagnoses are by NAATs
Treatment, Control, Prevention	• No specific antiviral treatment • Vaccine is not available

ADENOVIRUS

Although most respiratory infections are caused by RNA viruses, the nonenveloped DNA virus, adenovirus, has been associated with outbreaks of severe respiratory infections.

CLINICAL CASE

Pathogenic Adenovirus 14

The Centers for Disease Control and Prevention3 reported that analysis of isolates from trainees during an outbreak of febrile respiratory infection at Lackland Air Force Base showed 63% resulted from adenovirus, and 90% of these were adenovirus 14. Of the 423 cases, 27 were hospitalized with pneumonia, 5 required admission to the intensive care unit, and 1 patient died. In an analogous case reported by Cable News Network,4 and 18-year-old high-school athlete complained of flulike symptoms with vomiting, chills, and fever of 40°C that progressed to life-threatening pneumonia within days. The adenovirus causing these infections is a mutant of the adenovirus 14 that was identified in 1955. The adenovirus 14 mutant has spread around the United States, putting adults at risk for severe disease. Adenovirus 14 infection usually causes a benign respiratory infection in adults, with newborns and the elderly at higher risk for severe outcomes. Although most virus mutations produce a weaker virus, occasionally a more virulent antibody-escape or antiviral drug-resistant virus may occur.

REFERENCES

1. Luo HT, Wu M, Wang MM. Case report of the first Severe Acute Respiratory Syndrome patient in China: successful application of extracorporeal liver support MARS therapy in multiorgan failure possibly induced by Severe Acute Respiratory Syndrome. *Artif Organs.* 2003;27:847–849.
2. Ku AS, Chan LT. The first case of H5N1 avian influenza infection in a human with complications of adult respiratory distress syndrome and Reye's syndrome. *J Paediatr Child Health.* 1999;35:207–209.
3. Centers for Disease Control and Prevention. Acute respiratory disease associated with adenovirus serotype 14—four states, 2006-2007. *MMWR Morb Mortal Wkly Rep.* 2007;56:1181–1184.
4. www.cnn.com/2007/HEALTH/conditions/12/19/killer.cold/index.html.

Hepatitis Viruses

INTERESTING FACTS

- Hepatitis A (HAV) is the primary hepatitis virus that is spread person-to-person by fecal contamination; hepatitis B virus (HBV) is spread primarily via contaminated blood products or sexually
- HBV and hepatitis C virus (HCV) are primarily associated with chronic, progressive disease leading to cirrhosis and liver cancer
- HBV is 100-fold more infectious than HIV and almost 250 million people are infected worldwide
- HCV infection is the leading reason for liver transplantation in the United States
- Approximately 150 million people worldwide live with chronic HCV virus infections and 500,000 die annually

A number of viruses can infect the liver (e.g., herpesvirus group, adenoviruses, paramyxovirus group, and enteroviruses) but five viruses are responsible for primary infections:

Virus	Genus	Nucleic Acid	Exposure
Hepatitis A virus (HAV)	Hepatovirus (*hepa*, liver)	RNA	Fecal–oral
Hepatitis B virus (HBV)	Orthohepadnavirus (*hepa* DNA virus)	DNA	Sexual, blood
Hepatitis C virus (HCV)	Hepacivirus (*hepa* C virus)	RNA	Blood
Hepatitis D virus (HDV)	Delta virus (*delta*, D virus)	RNA	Sexual, blood
Hepatitis E virus (HEV)	Hepevirus (*hep* E virus)	RNA	Fecal–oral

The viruses can present with acute symptoms of hepatitis ranging from mild disease to fulminant, rapidly fatal disease. Additionally, HBV, HCV, and hepatitis D virus (HDV) are the most common causes of chronic hepatitis worldwide, increasing the risk of cirrhosis and hepatocellular carcinoma. The enteric hepatitis viruses (HAV and hepatitis E virus [HEV]) are not associated with chronic disease, with the exception of HEV infections in immunosuppressed patients. The clinical presentation of acute disease can be indistinguishable for the hepatitis viruses, with the majority of infections resulting in asymptomatic or mild disease. Progression to fulminant disease is primarily observed with HBV and HCV, with HAV progressing less often. Chronic infections are most troublesome because the infected patients serve as a reservoir for viral transmission and this population is at risk for long-term hepatic complications. The following is a summary for the five hepatitis viruses:

	HAV	HBV	HCV	HDV	HEV
Acute disease	+	+	+	+	+*
Fulminant disease	–	+	+	–	–
Chronic disease	–	+	+*	+	–
Antiviral treatment available	–	+	+	–	+
Vaccine available	+	+	–	–	+†

*Most common cause.

†Currently only licensed for China.

The following are summaries for each pathogen.

HEPATITIS A VIRUS

HAV is a member of the Picornavirus family (*pico*, small RNA virus) and related to rhinovirus (cause of common cold), echovirus and coxsackievirus (causes of viral meningitis), and poliovirus (cause of paralytic disease). HAV causes acute, self-limited infections and is not responsible for chronic liver disease.

HEPATITIS A VIRUS	
Properties	• Nonenveloped RNA virus; three genotypes are responsible for human infections • In the absence of an envelope, these viruses are resistant to heat, organic solvents, and detergents; they are inactivated by bleach and quaternary ammonium compounds • Infects hepatocytes; pathology believed to be related to cellular immune response, while humoral immunity limits cell-to-cell spread
Epidemiology	• Worldwide distribution although vaccine programs have reduced the risk of transmission • Fecal–oral transmission; highest concentration of virus in stools during the 2 weeks before jaundice develops; although stool concentrations decrease after jaundice develops, viruses are in stool specimens for as long as 6 months (particularly in infants) • Virus can remain stable and infectious in the environment for prolonged periods
Clinical Disease	• Asymptomatic disease more common in young children than in older children and adults • Onset of symptomatic disease with dark urine (bilirubinuria) with development of pale stools and jaundice a few days later; hepatomegaly and elevated liver enzymes; about half of patients will experience itching due to cholestasis; resolution of symptoms typically within 1 month
Diagnosis	• Majority of patients have elevated anti-HAV immunoglobulin M antibodies at the time symptoms develop • Immunoassay for HAV antigens or nucleic acid amplification test (NAATs) also useful
Treatment, Control, Prevention	• No specific antiviral treatment • Inactivated **HAV vaccines** have effectively controlled this infection; should be administered to children at 1 year of age • Immunoglobulins were administered following exposure but now have been replaced with the HAV vaccine • Transmission is difficult to control because peak shedding of virus is before symptoms develop, and shedding can occur for months after symptoms disappear

HEPATITIS B AND D VIRUSES

HBV is the only DNA virus that primarily infects hepatic cells. Hepatitis D virus (delta virus or HDV) is a defective RNA virus that requires the envelope of HBV for viral assembly. Infections with HBV range from asymptomatic to icteric, including both fulminant acute disease and chronic progressive disease.

HEPATITIS B AND D VIRUSES	
Properties	• Replication of HBV is distinguished by the production of large quantities of defective particles without viral DNA but with viral surface antigen (HBsAg) expressed on the surface; this antigen is highly immunogenic • Two other viral antigens of importance: core antigen (HBcAg) that forms the protein shell around the viral DNA, and soluble "e" antigen (HBeAg) that is secreted from infected cells; antibody response to the antigens are important markers for infection • HDV expresses a protein antigen (HDAg) that is an important marker for infection • Pathology in acute and chronic disease related to host cellular and humoral immune response to infection

HEPATITIS B AND D VIRUSES—cont'd	
Epidemiology	• Worldwide distribution; vaccination programs have modified prevalence • HDV found only in patients with HBV infections • Transmission by contact with blood (very high concentrations of virus) or sexual contact; virus not found in urine or stool • Highest incidence of chronic disease in Africa, the Middle East, southeast Asia, China, northern Canada, and Greenland • Populations at risk include intravenous drug abusers, male homosexuals, and HIV-infected individuals • Risk of chronic disease greatest with infants
Clinical Disease	• Incubation period of 1 to 4 months before symptoms develop • Acute disease may be subclinical or initiated with flulike symptoms; jaundice is uncommon in infants, more common in older children and most common in adults; jaundice and elevation of liver enzymes (serum aminotransferases) typically resolve by 4 months; persistence of elevated enzymes indicative of chronic disease • Fulminant hepatitis occurs in <1% of HBV infected patients, but is more common in patients co-infected with HDV • Chronic hepatitis is defined as persistence of HBsAg for more than 6 months; patients are at significant risk for cirrhosis, liver failure, hepatocarcinoma, and death • Co-infection with HDV or HCV increases the risk of adverse outcomes
Diagnosis	• Diagnosis of HBV infection is by detection of HBsAg, HBcAg, and HBeAg and the host antibody response to these proteins (see below) • Presence of HDAg is indicative of co-infection with HDV
Treatment, Control, Prevention	• Management of acute HBV infection is supportive • Acute fulminant disease treated with lamivudine or entecavir • Active chronic disease treated with entecavir, lamivudine, or tenofovir • Widespread use of recombinant **vaccine** expressing HBsAg provides long-lasting immunity following three doses (at 0, 1–2, and 6–12 months) or two doses (11–15 years and 6 months later) • Postexposure immunization recommended for nonimmune individuals

Serologic diagnosis of HBV infection and disease:

Test	Acute HBV Disease	Active Chronic HBV Disease	Inactive Chronic HBV Disease
HBsAg	+	+	+
Anti-HBs	–	–	–
HBeAg	+	+/–	–
Anti-HBe	–	+/–	+
HBcAg	+	+	+
Anti-HBc	+	–	–
Alanine aminotransferase	Elevated	Elevated	Normal

HEPATITIS C VIRUS

HCV is a member of the Flaviviridae family (*flavi*, yellow) which include yellow fever virus (jaundice is a prominent feature of this disease), dengue virus (hemorrhagic fever), and a number of arthropod-transmitted viruses responsible for encephalitis including West Nile virus, St. Louis encephalitis virus, Japanese encephalitis virus, and Murray Valley encephalitis virus. HCV is the **most common cause of chronic hepatitis** worldwide.

HEPATITIS C VIRUS	
Properties	• Small, enveloped RNA virus; six genotypes and significant strain differences
Epidemiology	• Worldwide distribution with highest prevalence in northern Africa, the Middle East, southeast Asia, and China • Transmission by exposure to contaminated blood through intravenous drug abuse or unsafe medical practices; sexual contact uncommon • Virus detected within days of exposure and remains elevated for the first 2 to 3 months of infection; low-level viremia can be detected intermittently in persistent infections • HCV is the leading cause of chronic hepatitis
Clinical Disease	• Acute infections are typically asymptomatic; if symptoms are present they are indistinguishable from other acute hepatitis virus infections • Development of fulminant disease is determined by virus genotype, host factors, and co-infection with other hepatitis viruses (e.g., HAV) • Chronic disease is associated with long-term persistence of virus production, development of cirrhosis and metabolic disorders, and hepatocellular carcinoma
Diagnosis	• Patients initially screened for antibodies to HCV; confirmation of active disease by detection of viral RNA with NAAT
Treatment, Control, Prevention	• Treatment of HCV infections is rapidly evolving; please consult the Infectious Disease Society of America and American Association for the Study of Liver Diseases guidelines • Prevention by reduced exposure to contaminated blood • Anti-HCV vaccines are not available because of the rapid development of strain variations

CLINICAL CASE

Hepatitis C Virus

In a case reported by Morsica and associates,[1] a 35-year-old woman was admitted with malaise and jaundice. Elevated blood levels of bilirubin (71.8 μmol/L; normal value <17 μmol/L) and alanine amino transferase (410 IU/L; normal value <30 IU/L) indicated liver damage. Serology was negative for antibodies to HAV, HBV, HCV, Epstein-Barr virus, cytomegalovirus, and HIV-1. However, HCV genomic RNA sequences were detected by RT-PCR (reverse transcriptase polymerase chain reaction analysis). Alanine amino transferase levels peaked on the 3rd week after admission and returned to normal by the 8th week. Anti-HCV antibody was also detected by the 8th week. It was suspected that she was infected by her sexual partner and this was confirmed by genotyping virus obtained from both individuals. Conformation was provided by partial sequence analysis of the E2 gene from the two viral isolations. The 5% genetic divergence detected between the isolates was less than the 20% divergence expected from unrelated strains. Before analysis, the sexual partner was unaware of his chronic HCV infection. Even more than HBV, which is also transmitted by sexual and parenteral means, HCV causes inapparent and chronic infections. Inapparent transmission of the virus, as in this case, enhances spread of the virus. The molecular analysis demonstrates the genetic instability of the HCV genome, a possible mechanism for facilitating its chronic infection by changing its antigenic appearance to promote escape from the immune response.

HEPATITIS E VIRUS

HEV is an enteric RNA virus that causes acute, self-limited hepatitis in immunocompetent individuals and chronic disease in immunocompromised patients. Although HEV infections are uncommon in developed countries, this is the most common cause of **acute hepatitis** in developing countries with poor sanitary controls.

HEPATITIS E VIRUS	
Properties	• Nonenveloped RNA virus stable on environmental surfaces and resistant to many disinfectants (similar to HAV) • Four genotypes with many subtypes
Epidemiology	• Worldwide distribution with greatest prevalence in India, China, and northern Africa • Transmission fecal–oral route; most commonly from ingestion of fecal-contaminated water or foods; person-to-person transmission uncommon because low levels of virus in stools (in contrast with HAV) • Outbreaks common in developing countries but not developed countries • Prevalence of infection more common in older children and adults than in infants (in contrast to HAV)
Clinical Disease	• Acute disease indistinguishable from other forms of acute viral hepatitis • HEV infection of pregnant women associated with a high risk of fulminant disease and mortality • HEV genotype 3 has been associated with chronic hepatitis in immunocompromised patients (solid organ transplants, stem cell transplants, HIV-infections)
Diagnosis	• Serology is used but NAATs are more sensitive and specific
Treatment, Control, Prevention	• Acute HEV infections managed with supportive care • Fulminant disease can be managed with ribavirin but this is contraindicated in pregnant women so an alternative is needed • Ribavirin used in immunosuppressed patients with chronic HEV infections • Recombinant **vaccine** currently available in China • Prevention by implementation of appropriate sanitary conditions to prevent fecal contamination of water supplies

REFERENCE

1. Morsica G, Sitia G, Bernardi MT, et al. Acute self-limiting hepatitis C after possible sexual exposure: sequence analysis of the E-2 region of the infected patient and sexual partner. *Scand J Infect Dis*. 2001;33:116–120.

17

Gastrointestinal Viruses

INTERESTING FACTS

- The "stomach flu" is not caused by influenza virus (this virus does not cause gastrointestinal symptoms) but by one of the gastrointestinal viruses, most commonly norovirus
- Infections with norovirus are easily transmitted because the virus can survive for days on environmental surfaces, relatively few viral particles can cause disease, and infected individuals shed the virus for days to weeks after the symptoms resolve
- Specific antiviral agents are not available for gastrointestinal viruses, and vaccines are only available for rotavirus infections
- Viruses are responsible for nearly half of all infectious diarrheas, although diagnostic tests for viruses are performed by only a small proportion of laboratories

Five viruses are responsible for primary gastrointestinal disease:

- Rotavirus
- Norovirus
- Sapovirus
- Astrovirus
- Adenovirus

Of these viruses, **rotavirus and norovirus are the most common**, with the other viruses far less important. Before rotavirus was detected in the mid-1970s, no virus had been demonstrated to cause gastroenteritis. Part of the reason the role of viruses was not appreciated was because most of these viruses cannot be grown *in vitro* in cell cultures. Early diagnosis required observation of viral particles in stool specimens by electron microscopy. This problem has been overcome, first by the use of immunoassays to detect viral antigens and then more recently by detecting viral nucleic acids using nucleic acid amplification techniques (e.g., polymerase chain reaction [PCR]).

ROTAVIRUS

Rotavirus was the first virus demonstrated to cause human gastrointestinal disease by observing large numbers of viral particles in the stool of symptomatic children. Despite the recognition of the importance of this virus and the introduction of vaccines to control spread of the pathogen, rotaviruses are still the **most common cause of viral diarrhea** in most countries.

ROTAVIRUS	
Properties	• Nonenveloped RNA virus that binds to cell surface carbohydrates of epithelial cells of the small intestinal villi • Absence of envelope renders these viruses stable in the environment • Mucosal damage leads to malabsorption and a secretory diarrhea

ROTAVIRUS—cont'd	
Epidemiology	• Exposure is worldwide with most children infected by age 2 or 3 years • Severe disease most common in children between 6 months and 2 years of age • Most common cause of severe, dehydrating viral diarrhea in children in all countries; mortality highest in developing countries • Multiple strains can circulate in a community simultaneously • Reinfections with milder disease due to partial immunity occur throughout life • Major route of person-to-person spread is fecal-oral
Clinical Disease	• Asymptomatic infections can occur, particularly in previously exposed individuals • Following a 1- to 3-day incubation period, onset of disease is characterized by vomiting and fever lasting 2 to 3 days, progressing to profuse watery diarrhea that can last up to 1 week • Severe dehydration and electrolyte abnormalities can occur
Diagnosis	• Clinical diagnosis is confirmed by detection of viral antigens in stool specimens by immunoassays (generally positive for the first week or longer after onset); more recently, nucleic acid amplification tests (NAATs) by polymerase chain reaction have come into widespread use
Treatment, Control, Prevention	• Therapy is supportive with maintenance of hydration; no antivirals are currently available • Live, attenuated **rotavirus vaccines** are available and associated with a significant decrease in symptomatic disease

CLINICAL CASE

Severe Rotavirus Infection in an Infant

Bharwani and colleagues[1] described a 10-month-old infant who developed a severe rotavirus infection. The previously healthy girl presented to the hospital emergency department with two brief generalized tonic-clonic convulsions after 2 days of vomiting, diarrhea, and a low-grade fever. Upon arrival her blood pressure was 102/54 mmHg, heart rate was 150 beats/minute, respiratory rate was 34 breaths/minute, body temperature was 37.8°C and oxygen saturation was 94% on room air. She was lethargic and dehydrated. Blood tests revealed hyponatremia, hypoproteinemia, leukocytosis, and thrombocytosis. After initial stabilization (hydration, correction of electrolyte imbalances, seizure control), bacterial cultures of blood, cerebrospinal fluid, and urine were performed (all were negative). Over the next 24 hours the patient developed generalized edema with ascites and pleural effusion. Because of labored breathing, dyspnea, and continued acidosis, the patient was transferred to the intensive care unit where thoracentesis was performed to relieve the accumulated fluids. Stool tested positive for red and white blood cells and for rotavirus; no bacterial pathogens were recovered. Methylprednisolone was administered on day 4 due to persistent hypoalbuminemia and on day 6 because the patient was tachycardiac and hypotensive. Blood tests showed neutropenia, thrombocytopenia, anemia, and coagulopathy, with increased prothrombin and partial prothrombin times. Bacterial cultures remained negative throughout the hospitalization, and over the next 2 weeks the patient gradually improved. The infant was fully recovered at follow-up at 2 months postdischarge. This case demonstrates a severe episode of rotavirus infection that would have been fatal without the aggressive medical support that was available. This is a reminder that rotavirus is responsible for many of the fatalities associated with infant diarrhea.

CLINICAL CASE

Acute Rotavirus Infection

Mikami and associates[2] described an outbreak of acute gastroenteritis that occurred over a 5-day period in 45 of 107 children (aged 11 to 12 years) after a 3-day school trip. The source person for the outbreak was ill at the start of the trip. A case of acute gastroenteritis caused by rotavirus is defined as three or more episodes of diarrhea and/or two or more episodes of vomiting per day. Other symptoms included fever, nausea, fatigue, abdominal pain, and headache. The rotavirus responsible for the outbreak was identified from stools of several individuals as serotype G2 group A rotavirus by comparison of the genomic RNA migration pattern by electrophoresis, by reverse transcriptase-PCR, and by enzyme-linked immunosorbent assay of virus obtained from stool samples. Although rotavirus is the most common cause of infantile diarrhea, this virus, especially the G2 strain, also causes gastroenteritis in adults.

NOROVIRUS AND SAPOVIRUS

Two members of the Caliciviridae family, norovirus and sapovirus, are important enteric pathogens. A number of genetic variants of both viruses exist, so reinfection and disease can occur, particularly with norovirus. Because norovirus is far more common than sapovirus and clinical disease is similar, the following comments refer to norovirus.

NOROVIRUS	
Properties	• Nonenveloped RNA virus that is relatively heat- and acid-stable • Produces damage to the microvilli of the small intestine
Epidemiology	• Worldwide distribution • Major viral enteric pathogen in both children and adults • **Most common cause of outbreaks of viral gastroenteritis**, e.g., cruise ships, schools, hospitals, long-care facilities • Commonly responsible for sporadic disease • Exposure occurs throughout life • Major route of person-to-person spread is fecal-oral, although food-borne disease can also occur
Clinical Disease	• Following a 1- to 2-day incubation period, the initial symptoms include abdominal cramping and nausea, followed by vomiting and diarrhea • Symptoms generally resolve after 2 to 3 days
Diagnosis	• Virus is present in the stool of symptomatic patients for 2 to 3 days, although elderly patients and immunocompromised patients may shed virus for weeks to months • Virus cannot be cultured • Immunoassays to detect viral antigens in stool are widely used, although NAATs are more sensitive and are considered the test of choice
Treatment, Control, Prevention	• No specific antiviral therapy is available • Symptomatic treatment including fluid replacement is generally sufficient • Vaccines are not currently available • Use of bleach to clean potentially contaminated surfaces such as in health care institutions, schools, or cruise ships can help control outbreaks

CLINICAL CASE

Norovirus Outbreak

Evans and associates[3] described an outbreak of gastroenteritis in children who attended a concert; infection was traced back to contamination of a specific seating area, bathrooms, and other areas visited by one individual. The male individual was ill before attending a concert and then vomited four times in the concert hall: in a waste bin in the corridor, into the toilets, onto the floor of the fire escape, and on a carpeted area in the walkway. His family members showed symptoms within 24 hours. A children's concert for several schools was held the next day. Children sitting in the same section as the incident case and those who traversed the contaminated carpet had the highest incidence of disease, characterized by watery diarrhea and vomiting for approximately 2 days. Reverse transcriptase-PCR analysis of fecal samples from two ill children detected norovirus genomic RNA. Infected vomit may have up to a million viruses per milliliter, and only 10 to 100 viruses are required to transmit the disease. Contact with contaminated shoes, hands, clothing, or aerosols may have infected the children. Norovirus is resistant to routine cleansers; disinfection usually requires freshly prepared hypochlorite bleach–containing solutions or steam cleaning.

ASTROVIRUS

Astroviruses were initially detected in stool specimens by electron microscopy.

ASTROVIRUS	
Properties	• Nonenveloped RNA virus • Multiple genotypes are recognized
Epidemiology	• Worldwide distribution • Disease most common in young child but can occur in adults • Transmission by fecal-oral route
Clinical Disease	• Incubation period is 3 to 4 days • Symptomatic disease characterized by diarrhea, headache, malaise, and nausea; vomiting less prominent and dehydration not as severe as with rotavirus; symptoms persist for less than 5 days
Diagnosis	• Diagnosis by immunoassay or more recently NAATs
Treatment, Control, Prevention	• Illness is self-limited and treatment is supportive • Antivirals are not available

ADENOVIRUS

Adenovirus is the only DNA virus responsible for gastrointestinal diseases. Although many serotypes have been described, types 40 and 41 are most commonly associated with diarrheal disease.

ADENOVIRUS	
Properties	• Nonenveloped DNA virus
Epidemiology	• Adenovirus exposure is common and worldwide, with most initial exposures in childhood and reexposure throughout life • Enteric adenovirus types 40 and 41 associated with infantile diarrhea • Outbreak-related adult disease can occur
Clinical Disease	• Majority of infections are subclinical • Acute infantile disease presents as a watery diarrhea that lasts 8 to 12 days, accompanied by fever and vomiting
Diagnosis	• The enteric viruses cannot be cultured • Diagnosis by immunoassay or, more commonly, by NAATs
Treatment, Control, Prevention	• No approved antiviral treatment is available • Vaccines for the enteric adenovirus is not available

REFERENCES

1. Bharwani SS, Shaukat Q, Basak RA. 10-month-old with rotavirus gastroenteritis, seizures, anasarca and systemic inflammatory response syndrome and complete recovery. *BMJ Case Rep*. 2011:2011.
2. Mikami T, Nakagomi T, Tsutsui R, et al. An outbreak of gastroenteritis during school trip caused by serotype G2 group A rotavirus. *J Med Virol*. 2004;73:460–464.
3. Evans MR, Meldrum R, Lane W, et al. An outbreak of viral gastroenteritis following environmental contamination at a concert hall. *Epidemiol Infect*. 2002;129:355–360.

18

Introduction to Fungi

OVERVIEW

Fungi are more complex than the bacteria and viruses. These are eukaryotic organisms that contain a well-defined nucleus, mitochondria, Golgi bodies, and endoplasmic reticulum. They are distinguished from other eukaryotic organisms by a rigid cell wall composed of **chitin** and **glucan** and a cell membrane in which **ergosterol** is substituted for cholesterol as the major sterol component. These unique structural properties are exploited both for diagnosis and as targets for antifungal treatment.

As with the word of caution in the Introduction of the Bacteriology Section, the student should not be intimidated by the lists of fungi, diseases, and antifungal agents found in this chapter. Rather, I felt it was important to provide a structure to organize the information presented in this Section, and I encourage the students to return to this chapter as they master the information in the other chapters on fungi.

CLASSIFICATION

Fungi are classified in their own separate kingdom, Kingdom Fungi, and exist either as unicellular organisms (**yeasts**) that can replicate asexually, or as multicellular filamentous organisms (**molds**) that replicate sexually and asexually. Although most fungi exist in only one of the two forms, some clinically important fungi can assume either morphology (**dimorphic fungi**). A few other morphologic features are important for the student to understand. Fundamentally, molds consist of filaments called **hyphae** with budding forms or **spores**. Molds have been historically identified by the morphology of these structures. The hyphae can be subdivided into a string of individual compartments or cells separated by a **septum** or wall, and are either pigmented (**dematiaceous mold**) or nonpigmented (**hyaline mold**). Thus the molds can be subdivided into three groups: nonseptate (generally nonpigmented) molds; septate, dematiaceous molds; and septate, hyaline molds. Although this may be a bit confusing, it has a practical application in classifying some of the fungal diseases, as will be seen in the subsequent chapters.

The taxonomy of fungi is complex and, frankly, beyond the interest of most students and physicians. Suffice to say that the asexual form of molds (**anamorph**) and the sexual form of molds (**teleomorph**) have different morphologies and have historically had different names. For the purpose of this textbook, only the commonly recognized names (primarily the anamorph names) will be used.

In contrast with the chapters on bacteria and later chapters on parasites, this section of the textbook has been organized based on the clinical presentation of disease: cutaneous and subcutaneous fungi, systemic dimorphic fungi, and opportunistic fungi. The following table is a list of the most common diseases and associated genera of fungi in each group. It should be recognized that this is not an exhaustive list; rather, these are the fungi that a physician is likely to see.

Superficial, Cutaneous, and Subcutaneous Fungi	Dimorphic Fungi	Opportunistic Fungi
Pityriasis versicolor • *Malassezia furfur* Dermatophytoses • *Microsporum* spp. • *Trichophyton* spp. • *Epidermophyton floccosum*	Blastomycosis • *Blastomyces dermatitidis* Histoplasmosis • *Histoplasma capsulatum* Coccidioidomycosis • *Coccidioides immitis* • *Coccidioides posadasii*	Candidiasis • *Candida albicans* • *Candida glabrata* • *Candida*, other spp. Cryptococcosis • *Cryptococcus neoformans* • *Cryptococcus gattii*
Onychomycosis • *Candida* spp. • *Aspergillus* spp. • *Trichosporon* spp. • *Geotrichum* spp. Mycotic keratitis • *Fusarium* spp. • *Aspergillus* spp. • *Candida* spp. Lymphocutaneous sporotrichosis • *Sporothrix schenckii*	Penicilliosis • *Talaromyces (Penicillium) marneffei* Paracoccidioidomycosis • *Paracoccidioides brasiliensis*	Trichosporonosis • *Trichosporon* spp. Aspergillus • *Aspergillus fumigatus* • *Aspergillus*, other spp. Mucormycosis • *Rhizopus* spp. • *Mucor* spp. Hyalohyphomycosis • *Acremonium* spp. • *Fusarium* spp. • *Paecilomyces* spp. • *Scedosporium* spp. Phaeohyphomycosis • *Alternaria* spp. • *Bipolaris* spp. • *Curvularia* spp. Pneumocystosis • *Pneumocystis jiroveci* Microsporidiosis

ROLE IN DISEASE

This section is a summary of the fungi associated with human disease. Again, I have restricted this to the most common fungal pathogens, recognizing that many of the molds are opportunistic pathogens that can cause disease in immunocompromised patients. Additionally, some fungi are restricted to residents of tropical areas of the world and would primarily be treated by physicians living in those communities. For those physicians, a more comprehensive book on tropical medicine would be appropriate.

	FUNGAL PATHOGEN		
Infection Site	Yeast and Yeastlike	Mold	Dimorphic Fungi
Blood	*Candida* *Cryptococcus* *Trichosporon* *Malassezia* *Rhodotorula*	*Fusarium* *Talaromyces*	*Blastomyces* *Histoplasma*

	FUNGAL PATHOGEN		
Infection Site	**Yeast and Yeastlike**	**Mold**	**Dimorphic Fungi**
Bone marrow		*Talaromyces*	*Histoplasma*
Central nervous system	*Cryptococcus* *Candida*	*Scedosporium* *Mucormycetes*	*Coccidioides* *Histoplasma*
Bone and joint	*Candida*	*Sporothrix* *Fusarium* *Aspergillus* *Talaromyces*	*Histoplasma* *Blastomyces* *Coccidioides*
Eye	*Candida* *Cryptococcus*	*Fusarium* *Aspergillus* *Mucormycetes*	
Urogenital system	*Candida* *Cryptococcus* *Trichosporon*		
Respiratory tract	*Cryptococcus* *Pneumocystis*	*Aspergillus* *Mucormycetes* *Fusarium* *Scedosporium*	*Blastomyces* *Histoplasma* *Coccidioides* Other endemic fungi
Skin and mucous membranes	*Candida* *Cryptococcus* *Trichosporon*	*Trichophyton* *Microsporum* *Epidermophyton* *Aspergillus* *Mucormycetes* *Fusarium* Dematiaceous molds *Sporothrix*	Endemic fungi
Multiple systemic sites	*Candida* *Cryptococcus* *Trichosporon*	Hyaline molds Dematiaceous molds	Endemic fungi

ANTIFUNGAL AGENTS

Management of fungal infections is complex because patients typically require prolonged treatment with a limited number of available drugs, many of which are toxic. Despite this, progress has been made in recent years with the development of the next antifungals and less toxic alternatives to older agents. This table is a list of the most commonly used antifungals for specific clinical indications. No effort has been made here to indicate the treatment of choice for specific diseases. That will be done in the following chapters.

Drug Class	Examples	Clinical Indications
Polyene	Amphotericin B Lipid-associated amphotericin B Nystatin	Candidiasis, cryptococcosis, aspergillosis, mucormycosis, dimorphic fungal infections Candidiasis (oral, topical)
Imidazole	Ketoconazole Clotrimazole Miconazole	Dermatophytosis (topical) Candidiasis (oral), dermatophytosis (topical) Dermatophytosis (topical)
Allylamines	Terbinafine	Dermatophytosis (topical), onychomycosis
Triazole	Itraconazole	Blastomycosis, coccidioidomycosis, paracoccidioidomycosis, histoplasmosis, sporotrichosis, dermatophytosis (topical), onychomycosis
	Fluconazole	Candidiasis, cryptococcal meningitis, coccidioidomycosis, onychomycosis
	Voriconazole	Candidiasis, aspergillosis, fusariosis, pseudallescheriasis
	Posaconazole	Candidiasis (oral pharyngeal)
Flucytosine	Flucytosine	Candidiasis, cryptococcosis, chromoblastomycosis
Echinocandin	Caspofungin Anidulafungin Micafungin	Candidiasis, aspergillosis Candidiasis Candidiasis
Sulfonamide	Trimethoprim-sulfamethoxazole	Pneumocystis
Aromatic diamidine	Pentamidine	Pneumocystis

Cutaneous and Subcutaneous Fungi

INTERESTING FACTS

- Ringworm is caused by fungi (dermatophytes) and not parasitic worms, and the cutaneous disease caused by dermatophytes does not resemble any parasitic infection
- *Microsporum canis* is a common dermatophyte in cats that can be spread among cats and dogs, as well as humans as an accidental host
- *Sporothrix* is a fungus found in sphagnum moss, organic rich soil, and rotting vegetation; infection is caused when nursery workers, farm laborers, gardeners, and others working with soil introduce the fungus into the subcutaneous tissues through cuts in the skin produced by thorns from roses, barberry bushes, and the like
- *Sporothrix* produces painless, nonhealing ulcers on the skin surface

There are a large number of fungi that are responsible for cutaneous and subcutaneous diseases. Rather than offer a comprehensive presentation of all diseases and pathogens, I want to focus on just a few clinical conditions: infections of the outermost layers of the skin caused by the dermatophytes (**dermatophytosis**), a specific subset of infections of the nails (**onychomycosis**), eye infections (**fungal keratitis**), and subcutaneous infections caused by *Sporothrix* (**lymphocutaneous sporotrichosis**). I will briefly mention other related fungal diseases as appropriate.

There are three primary genera of fungi responsible for infections of the keratinized outer layers of the skin, hair, and nails, as well as a number of minor genera—well, minor if you are not infected with these fungi. Let's get the minor fungi out of the way with a listing of the fungus, disease, and presentation.

Fungus	Disease	Presentation
Malassezia furfur	Tinea versicolor	Hypopigmented or hyperpigmented macules on upper trunk, arms, chest, shoulders, face, and neck
Hortaea werneckii	Tinea nigra	Solitary, irregular, brown to black macule usually on the palms or soles (resembles a melanoma in appearance)
Trichosporon spp.	White piedra	White to brown swelling along the shaft of hairs of the groin and axillae
Piedraia hortae	Black piedra	Small, dark nodules surrounding the shaft of scalp hairs

CLINICAL CASE

Tinea Versicolor

Holliday and Grider[1] reported a typical case of tinea versicolor in a 24-year-old woman. She presented with a 12-year history of a depigmenting rash over her neck, torso, and upper arms. It was most notable in the summer months, with spontaneous remission during the cooler seasons. Previous therapies with multiple topical antifungal agents had not regenerated the skin pigmentation. Scrapings of the skin and staining with periodic acid–Schiff stain revealed the presence of abundant fungi described as a "spaghetti and meatball" pattern. This is the classic description of Malassezia *in these lesions, with the presence of spherical and rodlike forms. It is likely that this diagnosis was previously suspected because she had been treated with antifungals, but recurrent infections are common and repigmentation may take months once the fungus is eliminated. Mild cases may be treated with 1% selenium sulfate (the active ingredient in dandruff shampoos) and more severe infections such as in this woman are treated with a course of oral fluconazole and topical ketoconazole.*

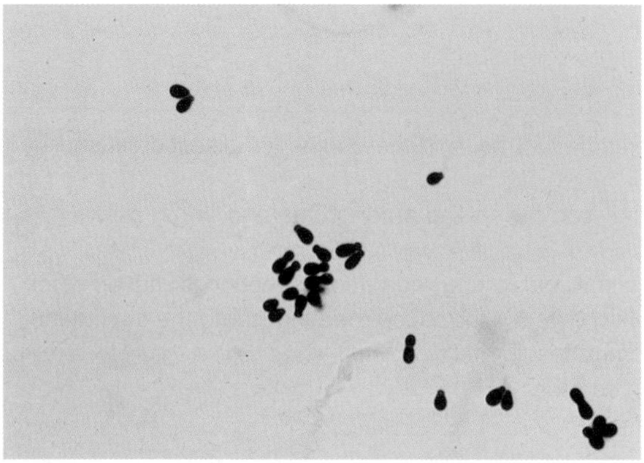

Gram stain of *Malassezia furfur* in skin scraping.

DERMATOPHYTOSIS

The three genera responsible for most cutaneous fungal infections are: *Trichophyton*, *Epidermophyton*, and *Microsporum*. All dermatophytes have the common ability to invade the skin, hair, or nails (not all species invade all these sites) and break down the outermost keratin layer. The fungi are grouped into the anatomic site where infection occurs:

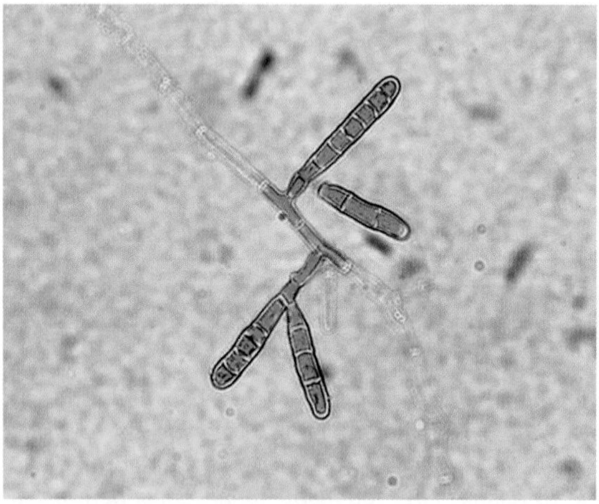

Culture of *Epidermophyton floccosum* showing smooth-walled macroconidia and absence of microconidia.

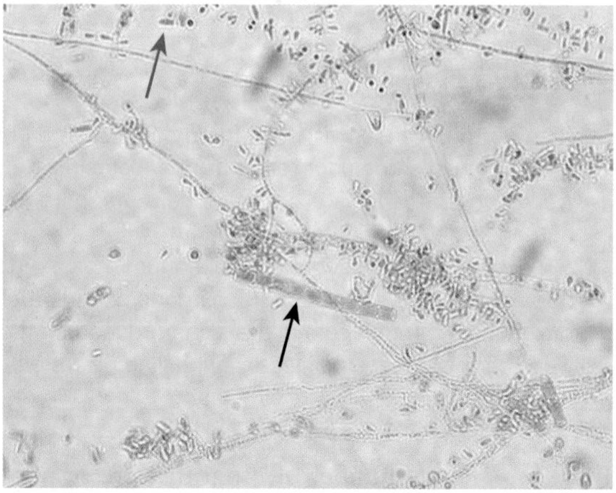

Culture of *Trichophyton rubrum*, showing multicelled macroconidia (*black arrow*) and microconidia (*red arrow*).

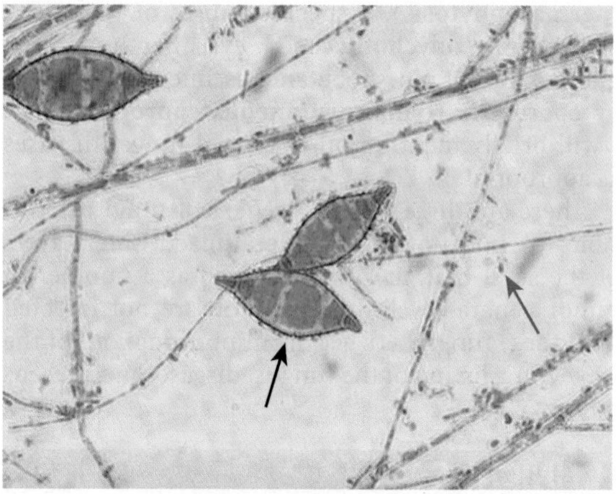

Culture of *Microsporum canis* showing rough-walled macroconidia (*black arrow*) and microconidia (*red arrow*).

Disease	Anatomic Site	Examples
Tinea capitis	Scalp, eyebrows, eyelashes	*Trichophyton tonsurans*
Tinea barbae	Beard	*Trichophyton rubrum, Trichophyton verrucosum*
Tinea corporis	Smooth or glabrous skin	*T. rubrum, Microsporum canis*
Tinea cruris	Groin	*T. rubrum, Epidermophyton floccosum*
Tinea pedis	Foot	*T. rubrum*
Tinea unguium	Nails	*T. rubrum*

Many species of dermatophytes are restricted to specific geographic areas of the world. Because the individual species may have very unique presentations, it is important to know the most common dermatophytes that you might encounter and their clinical presentation. That is beyond the scope of this text but the following summary is a good guideline for understanding these fungi.

Epidemiology	• Dermatophytes classified into three categories based on natural habitat: geophilic, zoophilic, and anthropophilic • Geophilic: live in soil and are an occasional pathogen of animals and humans • Zoophilic: infect animals but some species can be transmitted to humans • Anthropophilic: infect humans and may be transmitted person-to-person • Infections occur worldwide, especially in tropical and subtropical regions
Clinical Disease	• The clinical presentation is a function of the fungus, site of infection, and immune response of the host • Classic presentation on skin is the development of a ring of inflammation ("ringworm"); papules, pustules, or vesicles may develop • Nail infections are typically chronic with the nails becoming thickened, discolored, raised, friable, and deformed.
Diagnosis	• Demonstration of fungal hyphae by direct microscopy of skin, hair, or nail samples • Isolation of the organism in culture • Hair infections with some species can be diagnosed by a fluorescent yellow-green appearance when exposed to a Wood light
Treatment, Control, Prevention	• Localized infections that do not involve hair or nails may be treated effectively with topical antifungal agents (azoles, terbinafine, haloprogin) • All other infections require oral therapy (griseofulvin, itraconazole, fluconazole, terbinafine)

CLINICAL CASE

Dermatophytosis in an Immunocompromised Host

Squeo and associates[2] described a case of a 55-year-old renal transplant recipient with onychomycosis and chronic tinea pedis, who presented with tender nodules on his left medial heel. He then developed papules and nodules on his right foot and calf. A skin biopsy demonstrated periodic acid–Schiff-positive, thick-walled, round cells, 2 to 6 µm in diameter in the dermis. Skin biopsy culture grew Trichophyton rubrum. T. rubrum *has been described as an invasive pathogen in immunocompromised hosts. The clinical presentation, histopathology, and early fungal culture growth suggested* Blastomyces dermatitidis *in the differential diagnosis before the final identification of* T. rubrum.

CLINICAL CASE

Tinea Capitis in an Adult Woman

Martin and Elewski[3] *described an 87-year-old woman with a 2-year history of pruritic, painful, scaling scalp eruption and hair loss. Her previous treatment for this condition included numerous courses of systematic antibiotics and prednisone, without success. Of interest in her social history was that she had recently acquired several stray cats that she kept inside her home. On physical examination, there were numerous pustules throughout the scalp, with diffuse erythema, crusting, and scale extending to the neck. There was extremely sparse scalp hair and prominent posterior cervical lymphadenopathy. She had no nail pitting. A Wood light examination of the scalp produced negative findings. A skin biopsy specimen and fungal, bacterial, and viral cultures were obtained. Bacterial culture grew rare* Enterococcus species, *whereas viral cultures showed no growth. The scalp biopsy specimen revealed an endothrix dermatophyte infection. Fungal culture grew* Trichophyton tonsurans. *The patient was treated with griseofulvin and Selsun shampoo (active ingredient 1% selenium sulfide). When seen at a 2-week follow-up visit, the patient demonstrated new hair growth and a resolution of her pustular eruption. With the brisk clinical response and culture growth of* T. tonsurans, *treatment with griseofulvin was continued for 8 weeks. The scalp hair grew back normally without permanent alopecia. Adults with alopecia require an evaluation for tinea capitis, including fungal cultures.*

One additional comment should be made about nail infections. In addition to dermatophytes, there are a number of bacteria, as well as the yeast *Candida*, that can infect nails. Because treatment may differ for the specific pathogen, it is important to make the diagnosis by culture. One caution is damaged nail beds may be superficially colonized with fungi that are not responsible for the primary infection, so it is important to recover the fungus from multiple cultures or demonstrate the fungus specifically invading the nail tissues.

FUNGAL KERATITIS

This is a specific fungal infection that deserves mention. Fungal keratitis (infection of the cornea) is far less common than bacterial or viral infections, but threatens vision unless specifically diagnosed and treated. Although a number of molds can cause keratitis, the most common are *Fusarium* and *Aspergillus*. These and other molds are most commonly introduced following trauma to the eye. The yeast most commonly associated with keratitis is *Candida*. This yeast is acquired from the patient's normal population of organisms, and *Candida* infections are associated with prolonged ulceration, recent eye surgery, or corticosteroid use.

LYMPHOCUTANEOUS SPOROTRICHOSIS

Sporothrix schenckii is responsible for this lymphocutaneous disease that is characterized by the development of a skin ulcer at the primary site of inoculation of the fungus found in the soil, and then the development of subsequent ulcers along the lymphatics that drain the initial lesion. This is a dimorphic fungus, existing as yeast cells in the infected patient and a mold form in nature and when grown in laboratory culture. It is discussed in this chapter rather than the following chapter because the skin lesions are the primary presentation of disease. The clinical picture will develop slowly and can mimic infections caused by other organisms (e.g., mycobacteria and *Nocardia*) so a specific diagnosis is important for the proper treatment of the patient.

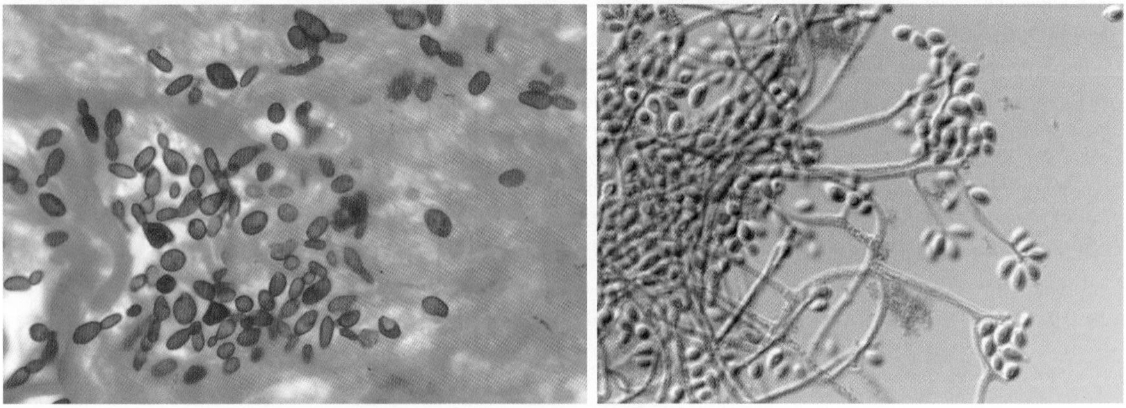

Sporothrix schenckii. (Left) Yeast cells in tissue biopsy; (Right) mold form in culture.

LYMPHOCUTANEOUS SPOROTRICHOSIS	
Epidemiology	• Worldwide distribution, especially in tropical and subtropical regions; present in North, Central, and South America • Infections associated with exposure to soil and plants, particularly rich organic soil • Trauma such as a minor cut while gardening (e.g., on rose thorn) is a common method for subcutaneous inoculation of the fungus
Clinical Disease	• Lymphocutaneous disease presents as an indolent papulonodular lesion that can ulcerate; secondary nodules and ulcerative lesions develop along the lymphatics draining the primary inoculation site • Dissemination can occur to the bones, lungs, and central nervous system although this is not common
Diagnosis	• Demonstration of the yeast form of the fungus in lesions is frequently difficult (relative few organisms may be present) but the culture of the lesions will be positive • Dimorphic fungus with cigar-shaped yeast cells in the lesions when observed and classic mold in the laboratory culture at 25–30°C; the mold has very thin hyphae and budding spores that resemble a flower ("flowerette"; a reminder of the source of the organism and association with gardening)
Treatment, Control, Prevention	• Itraconazole is the treatment of choice for the lymphocutaneous disease, with 3 to 6 months of treatment required • Disseminated disease may be treated with more prolonged itraconazole, or the use of amphotericin B followed by itraconazole

CLINICAL CASE

Sporotrichosis

Haddad and colleagues[4] described a case of lymphangitic sporotrichosis after injury with a fish spine. The patient was an 18-year-old male fisherman, resident in a rural town of São Paulo state in Brazil, who wounded his third left finger on the dorsal spines of a fish netted during his work. Subsequently, the area around the injury developed edema, ulceration, pain, and purulent secretion. The primary care physician interpreted the lesion as a pyogenic bacterial process and prescribed a 7-day course of oral tetracycline. No improvement was noted, and the therapy was charged to cephalexin, with similar results.

At examination 15 days after the accident, the patient presented with an oozing ulcer and nodules on the dorsum of the left hand and arm, forming an ascending nodular lymphangitic pattern. The diagnostic hypotheses considered were localized lymphangitic sporotrichosis, sporotrichoid leishmaniasis, and atypical mycobacteriosis (Mycobacterium marinum). *A histopathologic examination of material from the lesion revealed a chronic ulcerated granulomatous pattern of inflammation with intraepidermal microabscesses. No acid-fast bacilli or fungal elements were found. Culture of biopsy material on Sabouraud agar grew a mold characterized by thin septate hyphae, with conidia arranged in a rosette at the end of the conidiophores, consistent with* Sporothrix schenckii. *An intradermal reaction to the sporotrichin was positive as well. The patient was treated with oral potassium iodide, with clinical resolution at 2 months of therapy.*

The clinical presentation in this case was typical sporotrichosis; however, the source of the infection (fish spine) was unusual. Despite the greater incidence of infection by M. marinum *among fisherman and aquarists, sporotrichosis must be remembered when these workers show lesions in an ascending lymphangitic pattern after being injured by contact with fish.*

OTHER SUBCUTANEOUS INFECTIONS

Finally, as with cutaneous infections, there are a large collection of other fungi that cause subcutaneous infections. Most of these are observed in tropical areas and may be uncommonly seen outside the endemic regions. Still, it is important to be aware of these pathogens. Diagnosis is by observation of the fungus in the involved tissues and isolation in culture. Because these are slowly progressive infections, treatment must be used for months or years.

Disease	Examples of Pathogens	Comments
Eumycotic mycetoma	*Phaeoacremonium, Curvularia, Fusarium*; many other molds	Slowly developing infection particularly on lower limbs; characterized by chronic inflammation and fibrosis with progressive disfigurement
Chromoblastomycosis	*Fonsecaea, Cladosporium, Exophiala*; many other pigmented (dematiaceous) molds	As with mycetoma, a chronically progressive infection of lower limbs or exposed skin; characterized by "cauliflower-like" growth with satellite lesions; disfiguring; with secondary lesions and infections
Subcutaneous mucormycosis	*Conidiobolus, Basidiobolus* (nonseptate molds)	Subcutaneous introduction of the fungus to face or skin (shoulder, pelvis, thighs) that develops into a large subcutaneous mass
Subcutaneous phaeohyphomycosis	*Exophilia, Alternaria, Curvularia*; other dematiaceous molds	Usually single inflammatory cyst on the feet or legs; less commonly on the hands or other body surfaces; grows slowly over months to years

REFERENCES

1. Holliday A, Grider D. Images in clinical medicine. Tinea versicolor. *N Engl J Med.* 2016;374:e11.
2. Squeo RF, Beer R, Silvers D, Weitzman I, Grossman M. Invasive *Trichophyton rubrum* resembling blastomycosis infection in the immunocompromised host. *J Am Acad Dermatol.* 1998;39:379–380.
3. Martin ES, Elewski BE. Tinea capitis in adult women masquerading as bacterial pyoderma. *J Am Acad Dermatol.* 2003;49:S177–S179.
4. Haddad VJ, Miot HA, Bartoli LD, Cardoso Ade C, de Camargo RM. Localized lymphatic sporotrichosis after fish-induced injury (*Tilapia* sp.). *Med Mycol.* 2002;40:425–427.

20

Systemic Dimorphic Fungi

INTERESTING FACTS

- Dogs and cats, like humans, acquire blastomycosis by inhalation of spores present in acidic, moist soil, rich in organic material; transmission does not occur from domestic pet-to-pet, pet-to-human, or human-to-human
- Infections with *Blastomyces* and *Histoplasma* are associated with moist soil in river valleys; in contrast, *Coccidioides* is most commonly associated with dry soils in desert areas
- Although the source of *Blastomyces* and *Histoplasma* is well known, neither fungus is commonly isolated from organic soil
- All three dimorphic fungi produce an initial pulmonary disease that can be mistaken for tuberculosis or lung cancer

The fungi discussed in this chapter are associated with disseminated or systemic disease and characteristically exist in two morphologies: most commonly in a **yeast form** in human tissues (*Coccidioides* is the exception) and a multicellular **mold form** in nature. Disease with these fungi is initiated by exposure to the infectious mold form; specifically spores of the molds are inhaled, followed by development of mild to severe respiratory disease. Dissemination may occur to characteristic body sites (e.g., central nervous system [CNS], skin, bone marrow). Thus knowledge of the prevalent dimorphic fungi in specific geographic areas and the most common clinical presentation allows a rapid narrowing of the differential diagnosis. Three dimorphic fungi will be discussed in this chapter:

Dimorphic Fungus	Historic Perspective
Blastomyces dermatitidis	Blastomyces was first described by Thomas Gilchrist who named the fungus *B. dermatitidis*, recognizing the dermal presentation. The French biologist Philippe Van Tieghem recognized the disseminated form and named the disease **blastomycosis**. The disease is also referred to as **Gilchrist disease** after Thomas Gilchrist
Coccidioides immitis, Coccidioides posadasii	The first case of **coccidioidomycosis** was described by Alejandro Posadas (1892) in an Argentinean patient who had disseminated disease. The organism *C. immitis* and associated disease was first described by Rixford and Gilchrist (1896) from a patient observed in California. *C. immitis* infections are localized in California and *C. posadasii* is responsible for the majority of infections outside California.
Histoplasma capsulatum	**Histoplasmosis** was first described by Samuel Darling (1905), who reported the disease in a fatal case from Martinique. The name is derived from the observation that the yeast form of the fungus is found in the cytoplasm of reticuloendothelial cells. Disease is also referred to as **Darling disease**.

Two additional dimorphic fungi deserve brief mention: ***Paracoccidioides brasiliensis*** and ***Talaromyces (Penicillium) marneffei***. *P. brasiliensis* was originally described by Adolfo Lutz in 1908 in a Brazilian patient. In 1930 the current name was selected because the mold resembles *Coccidioides* and the majority of cases had been described in Brazil. Although the fungus resembles *Coccidioides*, disease is more like that caused by *Blastomyces*, hence the common name **South American Blastomycosis**. Disease is endemic throughout Latin America in areas with high humidity, rich vegetation, and moderate temperatures. **Paracoccidioidomycosis** may be subclinical, progressive with acute or chronic pulmonary disease, or disseminated disease involving the skin, lymph nodes, liver, spleen, CNS, and bones.

T. marneffei is an important cause of morbidity and mortality in HIV-infected and other immunosuppressed patients in Southeast Asia. The fungus was originally isolated in rats from Vietnam in 1952. It was believed to be a *Penicillium* species and was named in honor of Hubert Marneffe, Director of the Pasteur Institute in Indochina. It was renamed *T. marneffei* in 2015; however, the disease is still referred to as **penicilliosis**. Disease presents with fever, cough, and pulmonary infiltrates, and can progress to disseminated disease characterized by organomegaly, skin lesions, and hematologic disorders.

BLASTOMYCES DERMATITIDIS

B. dermatitidis is responsible for the disease **blastomycosis**. It is a dimorphic fungus that grows as a filamentous mold in moist, rich organic soil and as yeast cells in patients. Animals, particularly dogs, are also susceptible to disease with this organism.

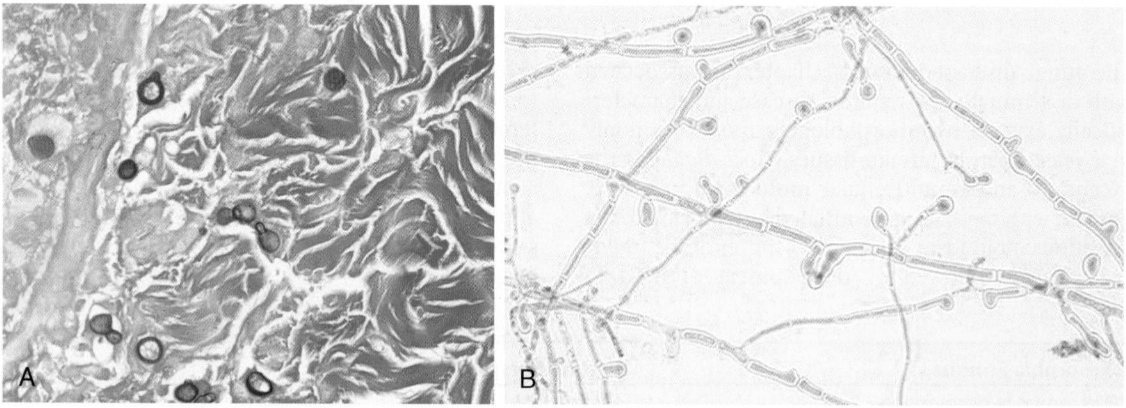

Blastomyces dermatitidis. (A) Yeast cells in biopsy tissue; (B) mold phase in culture with spores described as "lollipops" (infectious form found in nature).

BLASTOMYCES DERMATITIDIS	
Epidemiology	• Endemic in southeastern and south-central states, especially bordering the Ohio and Mississippi river basins; midwest states and Canadian provinces bordering the Great Lakes; and an area of New York and Canada along the St Lawrence River • Outbreaks of infections have been associated with occupational or recreational contact with soil and decaying organic matter • Infection is acquired by inhalation of infectious spores • Person-to-person spread does not occur
Clinical Disease	• Exposure may result in asymptomatic, transient colonization, or in disease • Disease is initiated with the development of pneumonia and may progress to dissemination to the skin and subcutaneous tissues (most common) as well as to bone, prostate, central nervous system, or other organs • Severity of disease is influenced by the magnitude of exposure and immune status of the patient

BLASTOMYCES DERMATITIDIS—cont'd	
Diagnosis	• Microscopic detection of characteristic yeast cells (typically large, single cells or pairs of cells with a thick wall) in tissue or draining skin lesions • Antigen detection in urine may be useful for diagnosis but is rarely performed • Antibody detection is not useful • Grows as a mold form (room temperature; 2–4 weeks) or yeast form (37°C; 3–5 days) in culture
Treatment, Control, Prevention	• Itraconazole is the drug of choice for mild to moderate pulmonary or non-CNS disease • Amphotericin B followed by itraconazole is the treatment for severe infection • Prevention and control of infections is not feasible because this fungus is endemic in the environment • Care should be used in handling laboratory cultures

CLINICAL CASE

Central Nervous System Blastomycosis

Buhari and colleagues[1] reported a case of CNS blastomycosis. The patient was a 56-year-old homeless man from Detroit who presented with a 2-week history of left hemiparesis, aphasia, and generalized headache. There was no history of rash, respiratory symptoms, or fever. His medical history was significant for a left craniotomy 30 years previously for intracranial hemorrhage caused by trauma. He lived in an abandoned building and was not taking any medicines. On examination he had expressive aphasia, new-onset left hemiparesis, and bilateral carotid bruits. The rest of the physical examination was unremarkable, as were routine serum chemistries and hematologic parameters. He was negative for antibodies to HIV. A chest radiograph was unremarkable. A contrast-enhanced computed tomography (CT) scan of the head demonstrated multiple ring-enhancing lesions in the right cerebrum, with surrounding vasogenic edema and midline shift; significant encephalomalacia and generalized atrophy were present in the left cerebral hemisphere. Serum and urine tests were negative for Cryptococcus *(serum) and* Histoplasma *(serum and urine) antigens. Tuberculin skin tests were nonreactive, and imaging studies of the sinuses, chest, and abdomen were unremarkable. A brain biopsy was performed, and histopathologic examination revealed granulomatous inflammation and budding yeasts consistent with* B. dermatitidis*. Subsequent culture confirmed the diagnosis of CNS blastomycosis. The patient was treated with dexamethasone and amphotericin B but developed hypertension and bradycardia, with subsequent cardiopulmonary arrest and death.*

This is an example of an unusual presentation of CNS blastomycosis without any other evidence of disseminated disease. The clinical syndrome of hypertension, bradycardia, and cardiopulmonary arrest suggest that the patient died of increased intracranial pressure, either as a complication of the infection or the diagnostic brain biopsy. Although Blastomyces *can disseminate to the brain as in this case, it is more typical that infection begins as a pulmonary infection and disseminates to the skin.* Cryptococcus *and* Histoplasma *are fungi that more commonly disseminate to the brain.*

COCCIDIOIDES IMMITIS AND *COCCIDIOIDES POSADASII*

C. immitis and *C. posadasii* are responsible for the disease **coccidioidomycosis**. The species are indistinguishable in appearance or pathogenicity, differentiated only by molecular methods. In contrast with the other dimorphic fungi, *Coccidioides* forms a spherule containing endospores in human tissues. A key to diagnosis is detection of these "bags of spores" in clinical specimens. The mold form of the fungus also has a characteristic morphology. Instead of forming spores along the sides or end of hyphae (mycelia), the growing mycelia are subdivided by septae (walls) into cells. Alternating cells will disintegrate, leaving mature barrel-shaped cells called **arthroconidia**. These arthroconidia are the infectious spores and are extremely resilient to harsh environmental conditions (typically this fungus is found in dry, hot climates). The spores can be carried hundreds of miles in wind currents to cause disease in distant populations.

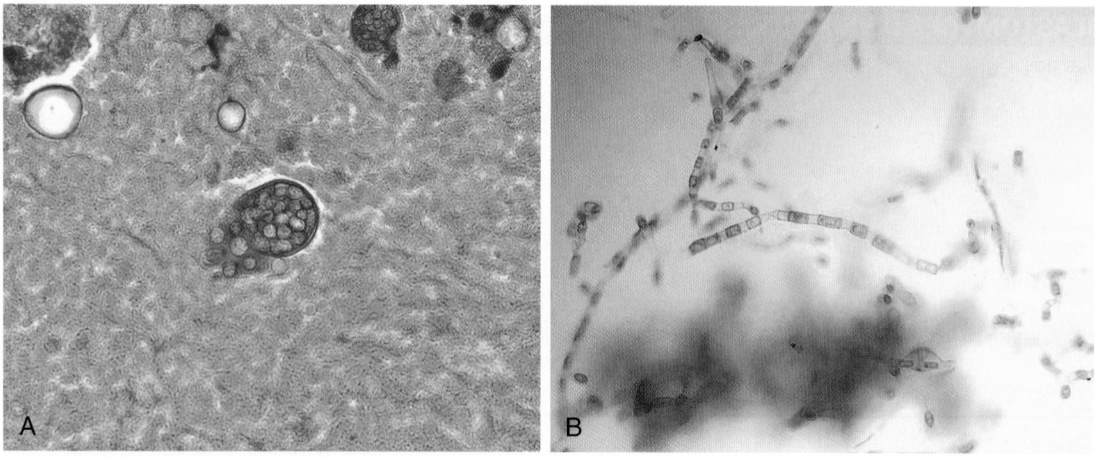

Coccidioides immitis. (A) Spherule observed in sputum; (B) mold phase in culture (infectious form found in nature).

COCCIDIOIDES IMMITIS **AND** ***COCCIDIOIDES POSADASII***	
Epidemiology	• Endemic to US southwest desert, northern Mexico, scattered areas of Central and South America • Spores can survive in nature for an extended period; germinate and grow as a mold following rain; then be disseminated in the wind during a windy, dry period • Exposure and asymptomatic or mild infections is very common in endemic areas • Infection caused by inhalation of infectious spores (arthroconidia) • Risk of disseminated disease highest in certain ethnic groups (Filipino, African American, Native American, Hispanic), women in third trimester of pregnancy, individuals with cellular immune deficiency, persons at extremes of age • Person-to-person spread does not occur • Laboratory infections handling the mold form of this organism are not uncommon so care must be exercised
Clinical Disease	• Infections can be asymptomatic or progress to disease • Pneumonia is most common clinical disease • Extrapulmonary dissemination is most commonly to the skin, joints and bones, and central nervous system (meningitis)
Diagnosis	• Histopathologic examination of tissues for endosporulating spherules • Spherules can also be observed in sputa or wound drainage • The mold form grows rapidly in culture and can be detected in as soon as 1–2 days; caution needed because sporulation can occur within a day or two so the mold form is highly infectious • Serology may be useful for diagnosis or prognostic evaluation
Treatment, Control, Prevention	• Most patients with primary infections do not require treatment • Those with severe disease or risk factors for progressive disease should be treated with amphotericin B followed by an oral azole as maintenance therapy • Azoles are used for chronic cavitary pulmonary disease or nonmeningeal disseminated disease • Meningeal coccidioidomycosis is treated with fluconazole, with other azoles as secondary choices • With the exception of careful handling of laboratory cultures, prevention and control of exposure is not feasible because the fungus is endemic in the regions

CLINICAL CASE

Coccidioidomycosis

Stafford and colleagues[2] describe a 31-year-old African-American US Army soldier who presented with fever, chills, night sweats, and a nonproductive cough of 4 weeks' duration. In addition, he had recently detected a painless right breast mass. His past medical history was unremarkable. He was stationed at Fort Irwin, California, where he was working as a telephone repairman. His physical exam was unremarkable except for a firm, nontender, 3-cm subcutaneous mass overlying the right breast. Multiple small (<1 cm) nontender lymph nodes were palpable in the axillae and groin. Laboratory studies revealed a white blood count of 11.9/μL, with 30% eosinophils. Serum chemistries were notable for an elevated alkaline phosphate level. Results of blood cultures, tests for serum Cryptococcus *antigen, urinary* Histoplasma *antigen, and HIV antibody were negative, as was a tuberculin skin test. A chest radiograph showed bilateral interstitial micronodules in a military pattern, as well as a right-sided paratracheal fullness. A CT scan of the chest confirmed the presence of diffuse 1- to 2-mm micronodules in all lobes. The CT scan also showed a lobular parenchymal mass lesion in the right middle lobe and a right chest wall mass. A fine-needle aspirate of the right breast mass revealed spherules filled with endospores, consistent with coccidioidomycosis. Culture of the material grew* C. immitis. *A serology panel for* C. immitis *was positive and revealed immunoglobulin G complement fixation titers at a dilution of greater than 1:256. Cerebrospinal fluid analysis was normal, but a bone scan revealed multiple regions of increased osteoblastic activity involving the left scapula, right anterior fifth rib, and midthoracic vertebral regions. Treatment was initiated with amphotericin B, but increasing neck pain prompted further imaging, which demonstrated a lytic lesion of the C1 vertebral body and a paravertebral mass. Despite antifungal therapy, progressive enlargement of the mass necessitated surgical debridement. The patient was continued on amphotericin B lipid formulation, with plans for long-term, perhaps lifelong, antifungal therapy.*

This is an example of the serious problems posed by coccidioidomycosis. Clues leading to diagnosis of disseminated coccidioidomycosis in this patient included an infectious prodrome, peripheral eosinophilia, hilar lymphadenopathy, characterization of pattern of organ involvement (lungs, bones, soft tissues), residence in an endemic area, and African-American ethnicity (higher risk group of dissemination).

HISTOPLASMA CAPSULATUM

Histoplasmosis is caused by two variants of *H. capsulatum*: *H. capsulatum* var. *capsulatum* is responsible for pulmonary and disseminated disease in the eastern half of the United States and most of Latin America, and *H. capsulatum* var. *duboisii* causes predominantly skin and bone lesions in tropical areas of Africa. The mold form of the fungi is indistinguishable but the variants are separated by the different morphology of the yeast cells. The yeast forms of both variants are only observed as intracellular pathogens.

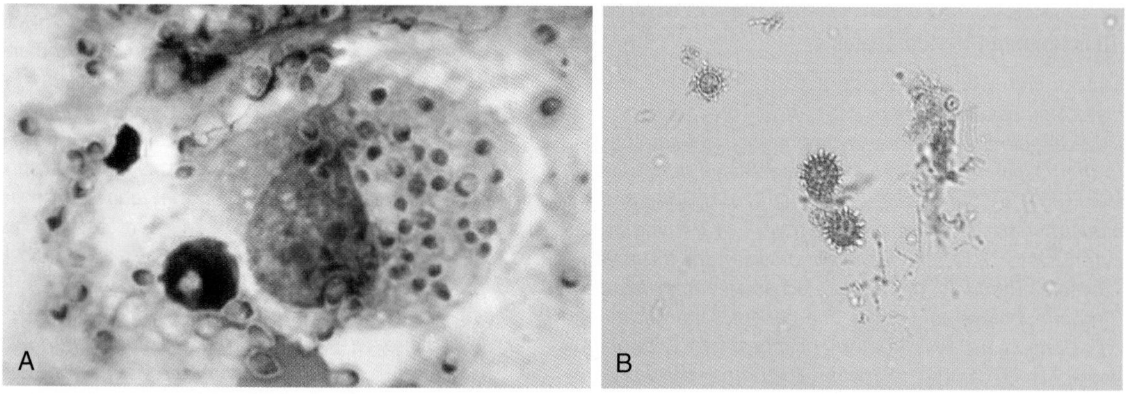

Histoplasma capsulatum. (A) Giemsa stain of intracellular yeast forms; (B) infectious mold form found in nature.

HISTOPLASMA CAPSULATUM	
Epidemiology	• *H. capsulatum* var. *capsulatum* is localized to Ohio and Mississippi river valleys and throughout Mexico and Central and South America • *H. capsulatum* var. *duboisii* is confined to tropical Africa (e.g., Gabon, Uganda, Kenya) • Found in soil with high nitrogen content such as areas contaminated with bird or bat droppings • Outbreaks of disease associated with exposure to bird roosts, caves, and decaying buildings or urban renewal projects involving excavation and demolition • Infection acquired by inhalation of infectious spores • Person-to-person spread does not occur • Immunocompromised patients and children most susceptible to develop symptomatic disease • Reactivation of disease and dissemination common among immunosuppressed individuals (e.g., AIDS patients)
Clinical Disease	• Severity of symptoms and course of disease depend on extent of exposure and immune status of infected individual • Most infections are asymptomatic or mild, self-limited flulike disease • Acute pulmonary disease caused by *H. capsulatum* var. *capsulatum* is characterized by high fever, headache, nonproductive cough, and chest pain; symptoms most commonly resolve within 10 days but can progress to disseminated disease, involving multiple organ systems • Pulmonary disease is rare in African histoplasmosis caused by *H. capsulatum* var *duboisii*; disease is characterized by regional lymphadenopathy with lesions of skin and bone; a more fulminant progressive disease can occur in AIDS patients
Diagnosis	• Direct microscopy and culture of respiratory material confirms the diagnosis of histoplasmosis • Serology is useful for all but AIDS patients • Detection of *Histoplasma* antigen in urine or serum is useful for extrapulmonary disease
Treatment, Control, Prevention	• Mild or moderate pulmonary histoplasmosis can be treated symptomatically or with itraconazole • Moderate to severe disease is treated with amphotericin B followed by itraconazole • Exposure in endemic areas is difficult to avoid but areas where birds may have roosted should be avoided, particularly for immunocompromised patients • Care should be exercised in handling laboratory cultures

CLINICAL CASE

Disseminated Histoplasmosis

Mariani and Morris[3] describe a case of disseminated histoplasmosis in a patient with AIDS. The patient was a 42-year-old El Salvadoran woman who was admitted to the hospital for evaluation of progressive dermatitis involving the right nostril, cheek, and lip, despite antibiotic therapy. She was positive for HIV (CD4 lymphocyte count 21/μL) and had lived in Miami for the past 18 years. The lesion first appeared on the right nostril 3 months before admission. The patient sought medical attention and was treated unsuccessfully with oral antibiotics. Over the following 2 months, the lesion increased in size, involving the right nares and malar region, and was accompanied by fever, malaise, and a 50-lb weight loss. A necrotic area developed on the superior aspect of the right nostril, extending to the upper lip. A presumptive diagnosis of leishmaniasis was entertained, based in part on the patient's country of origin and possible exposure to a sandfly bite.

Laboratory studies revealed anemia and lymphopenia. A chest radiograph was normal, and a CT scan of the head showed a soft-tissue mass in the right nasal cavity. Histopathologic evaluation of a skin biopsy showed chronic inflammation, with intracytoplasmic budding yeasts. Culture of the biopsy grew H. capsulatum*, and the results of a urine* Histoplasma *antigen test were positive. The patient was treated with amphotericin B followed by itraconazole with good results.*

This case underscores the ability of H. capsulatum *to remain clinically latent for many years, only to reactivate upon immunosuppression of the host. Cutaneous manifestations of histoplasmosis are usually a consequence of progression from primary (latent) to disseminated disease. Histoplasmosis is not endemic to southern Florida but is endemic to much of Latin America, where the patient had lived before moving to Miami. A high index of suspicion and conformation with skin biopsies, cultures, and testing for urinary antigen are crucial for timely and appropriate treatment of disseminated histoplasmosis.*

REFERENCES

1. Buhari. *Infect Med.* 2007;24(suppl 8):12–14.
2. Stafford CM, Lim ML, Lamb C, Amundson DE, Bradshaw DA. Case in point: fever and a chest wall mass in a young man. *Infect Med.* 2007;24(suppl 8):23–25.
3. Mariani, Morris. *Infect Med.* 2007;24(suppl 8):17–19.

21

Opportunistic Fungi

INTERESTING FACTS

- *Candida albicans* is the most common yeast that causes opportunistic fungal diseases
- *Aspergillus fumigatus* is the most common mold that causes opportunistic fungal diseases
- *Cryptococcus neoformans* is the most common cause of fungal meningitis
- *Pneumocystis jiroveci* is the most common opportunistic pathogen in AIDS patients

There are many examples of opportunistic fungi but this chapter will be restricted to examples of the most commonly encountered human pathogens. Most of the opportunistic fungi are filamentous molds commonly found in the environment and produce disease in humans following inhalation of spores or following trauma (**exogenous infections**). In general, infections are primarily restricted to individuals with a compromised immune system or some other underlying disease (e.g., diabetes). There are three important exceptions to the rule that opportunistic fungi are molds. *Cryptococcus* is a yeast that exists in nature and is acquired by inhalation of the yeast cells and not spores. *Candida* is a yeast that colonizes humans and produces **endogenous infections**; that is, the yeast moves from normally colonized mucosal surfaces to the blood or other normally sterile sites. *Pneumocystis*, formerly classified as a parasite, is another yeastlike fungus that colonizes humans but produces disease in immunocompromised patients.

The three genera of fungi that will be the focus of this chapter are *Candida*, *Cryptococcus*, and *Aspergillus*. Other fungi of interest will be mentioned briefly at the end of the chapter.

CANDIDA ALBICANS AND RELATED SPECIES

More than 20 species of *Candida* have been associated with human disease, but most infections are caused by relatively few species:

***Candida* Species**	**Most Common Diseases**
Candida albicans	Mucosal infections (thrush, vaginitis), cutaneous and nail infections, cardiovascular infections (fungemia, endocarditis, intravenous line–related or intravenous drug abuse–related sepsis), deep tissue infections
Candida glabrata	Urinary tract infections; many other less common infections
Candida parapsilosis	Catheter-related fungemia, particularly in children receiving lipid-rich hyperalimentation
Candida tropicalis	Fungemia in patients with hematologic malignancies
Candida krusei	Fungemia

Candida species are the most common cause of all fungal diseases, infecting healthy individuals (e.g., cutaneous and nail infections, vaginitis) as well as life-threatening infections in immunocompromised patients. Diagnosis is generally not a problem because these yeasts will grow in 1 to 3 days in culture and identification can be easily accomplished for the most common species. One potential diagnostic problem is relatively few yeasts circulate in the blood of patients with disseminated infections, so documentation of fungemia may be difficult. Therapeutic management of infected patients has been complicated in recent years by the increased observation of azole-resistance in certain *Candida* species (e.g., ***Candida krusei, Candida glabrata***). The following is a summary for *Candida* species:

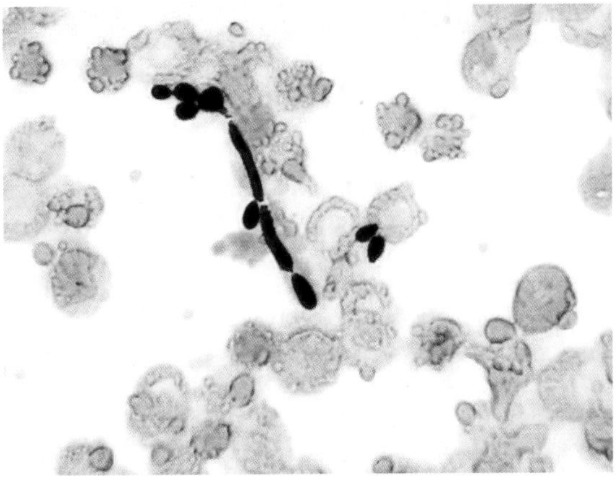

Candida albicans in blood culture.

CANDIDA ALBICANS **AND RELATED SPECIES**	
Epidemiology	• Opportunistic yeasts • Most infections caused by *C. albicans* • Colonize humans and other warm-blooded animals • Primary site of colonization is gastrointestinal tract, although present in mouth, vagina, and on warm, moist skin surfaces • Most infections are endogenous; exogenous infections occur in the hospital (e.g., contaminated intravascular line) • Risk factors for blood infections with *Candida* include hematologic malignancies and neutropenia, HIV infections, prior exposure to broad-spectrum antibacterials, recent abdominal surgery or trauma, prematurity in infants, elderly patients • Use of azoles for antifungal prophylaxis in hematologic malignancy patients and recipients of stem cell transplantation increase the risk for infections caused by *Candida glabrata* and *Candida krusei*
Clinical Disease	• Cause infections ranging from superficial mucosal and cutaneous disease to hematogenously disseminated, often fatal, infections
Diagnosis	• Observation of yeasts by microscopy and culture • Use of antigen tests to detect fungal antigens or nucleic acid amplification tests to detect presence of *Candida* in normally sterile specimens • Care must be used to interpret microscopy and culture because *Candida* normally colonizes the skin and mucosal surfaces; abnormal predominance of yeast in these body sites is consistent with disease
Treatment, Control, Prevention	• Mucosal and cutaneous infections can be treated with itraconazole, fluconazole, miconazole, many other agents; invasive infections, particularly in immunocompromised patients, must be treated more aggressively using azoles, echinocandins, or amphotericin B • *C. glabrata* and *C. krusei* have decreased susceptibility to azoles (e.g., fluconazole) so treatment with an echinocandin (e.g., anidulafungin, caspofungin, micafungin) or amphotericin B may be required • Antifungal prophylaxis for high-risk patients has reduced the incidence of disease

CLINICAL CASE

Candidemia

Posteraro and associates[1] describe a case of recurrent fungemia in a 35-year-old woman. The patient was seen at 5 weeks' gestation after intrauterine insemination. She presented with fever, tachycardia, and hypotension. The white blood cell count was 23,500/µL with 78% neutrophils. She experienced a spontaneous abortion. Severe chorioamnionitis was diagnosed, placental and fetal tissues were cultured, and blood cultures and vaginal swabs were obtained. The patient was treated with broad-spectrum antibacterial agents. Five days later, no clinical improvement was seen. The cultured blood and placental samples grew the yeast C. glabrata*, which was also isolated from the patient's vaginal cultures. On the basis of fluconazole minimal inhibitory concentrations, which indicated that the organism was susceptible, the patient was placed on fluconazole. Four weeks later, she experienced complete resolution of her symptoms, with eradication of the fungus from her bloodstream. Antifungal treatment was discontinued, and the patient was sent home where she did well. Six months later she was readmitted to the hospital with fever, chills, and fatigue. The white blood cell count was elevated at 21,500/µL with 73% neutrophils. Consecutive blood cultures were again positive for* C. glabrata*, which was also found in cultures of vaginal fluid. All isolates were found to be resistant to fluconazole. On the basis of these findings the patient was treated with amphotericin B. Within 1 week that patient's clinical condition was improved. After 1 month of amphotericin B treatment, blood cultures were sterile, and she was discharged from the hospital. Three years later she remained free of any evidence of infection.*

This was an unusual case in that the patient was not immunocompromised yet experienced recurrent candidemia with C. glabrata*. The use of fluconazole as initial therapy, although apparently successful, induced up-regulation of drug efflux pumps in the organism and allowed later isolates to become resistant to fluconazole and other azoles.*

CRYPTOCOCCUS NEOFORMANS

Cryptococci are spherical yeasts that are surrounded by a large, prominent **polysaccharide capsule** (an important diagnostic feature). *C. neoformans* is found worldwide in soil, particularly soil enriched with pigeon droppings. A related species, *Cryptococcus gatti*, is in a more geographically restricted region of the US Pacific northwest. Infection with both species is acquired by inhalation of the yeast cells followed by an initial mild or asymptomatic process in the lungs. The fungi have a predisposition to disseminate to the central nervous system in susceptible patients. Indeed, *Cryptococcus* is the most common fungal pathogen responsible for **meningitis**. Although both species can cause disease in immunocompetent patients, *C. neoformans* is most commonly observed as an opportunistic pathogen in patients with underlying defects in cellular immunity, such as HIV-infected patients and solid organ transplants. The incidence of cryptococcosis has decreased in recent years with the use of prophylactic antifungal agents (e.g., fluconazole) in high-risk patients. Diagnosis of disease is generally made by observation of encapsulated yeast in spinal fluid or detection of the **capsular polysaccharide** by a specific antigen test (positive for both cryptococcal species). Occasionally yeasts are detected in the blood of infected patients, but blood culture alone is an unreliable diagnostic test because relatively few organisms may be circulating in the blood and culture will require 3 to 7 days before growth is detected.

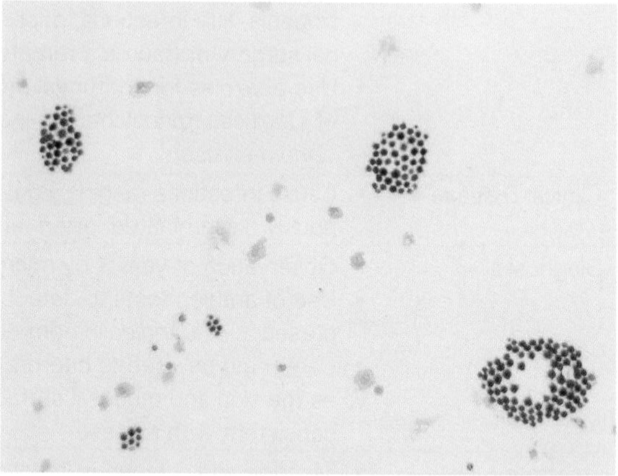

Cryptococcus neoformans in cerebrospinal fluid. Note the clusters of individual cells separated by clear spaces occupied by the unstained surrounding envelope.

CRYPTOCOCCUS NEOFORMANS	
Epidemiology	• Worldwide distribution, commonly in soil contaminated with avian excreta; *Cryptococcus gatti* more restricted to tropical and subtropical regions (associated with eucalyptus and fir trees) • Infections typically acquired by inhalation • Prevalence of infections less common with the use of prophylactic antifungals such as fluconazole in immunocompromised patients
Clinical Disease	• Infections initially develop in **lungs** although dissemination in the blood, particularly to the central nervous system, is common • **Meningitis** is usually the presenting disease
Diagnosis	• Definitive diagnosis by culture of the organism in blood, sputum, or cerebrospinal fluid (CSF) (most reliable source) • Microscopic examination of CSF may demonstrate characteristic budding cells (**India ink** is used as a contrasting dye to detect the presence of a clear capsule surrounding the yeast cell) • Use of antigen tests to detect the polysaccharide capsular material; this is more reliable than stains for CSF (white blood cells may be misidentified as *Cryptococcus* by an inexperienced microscopist)
Treatment, Control, Prevention	• Meningitis uniformly fatal if untreated • Amphotericin B and fluconazole used initially, followed by maintenance use of fluconazole or itraconazole; antigen test can be used to monitor response to therapy • Prophylactic use of antifungals recommended for high-risk patients

CLINICAL CASE

Cryptococcosis

Pappas and colleagues[2] *describe a case of cryptococcosis in a heart transplant recipient. The 56-year-old patient, who underwent heart transplant surgery 3 years earlier, presented with new-onset cellulitis of his left leg and a mild headache of 2 weeks' duration. The patient was on chronic immunosuppressive therapy with cyclosporine, azathioprine, and prednisone and was admitted for intravenous antibiotics. Despite 5 days of intravenous nafcillin, the patient failed to improve, and a skin biopsy of the cellulitic area was obtained for histopathologic studies and culture. Laboratory results revealed the presence of a yeast consistent with* C. neoformans. *A lumbar puncture was also performed, and an examination of the cerebrospinal fluid (CSF) disclosed cloudy fluid and an elevated opening pressure of 420 mm H_2O. Microscopic examination revealed encapsulated budding yeast forms. Cryptococcal antigen titers of CSF and blood were markedly elevated. Blood, CSF, and skin biopsy cultures grew* C. neoformans. *Systematic antifungal therapy with amphotericin B and flucytosine was initiated. Unfortunately the patient suffered progressive mental status decline despite aggressive management of intracranial pressure and maximal doses of antifungals. He experienced slow, progressive decline, leading to death 13 days after initiation of antifungal therapy. CSF cultures obtained 2 days before death remained positive for* C. neoformans.

The patient in this case was highly immunocompromised and presented with cellulitis and headache. Such presentations should arouse suspicion of atypical pathogens such as C. neoformans. *Given the high mortality associated with cryptococcal infection, rapid and accurate diagnosis is important. Unfortunately, despite these efforts and the use of aggressive therapy, many such patients succumb to infection.*

MISCELLANEOUS YEASTLIKE FUNGI

The following is a summary of other medically important, single-cell fungi that can produce disseminated disease:

Fungus	Diseases and Comments
Malassezia	Catheter-related sepsis, particularly in infants receiving lipid infusions (some species require **lipids** for growth); treatment by removal of line and discontinuation of the lipid infusions
Trichosporon	Catheter-related sepsis in neutropenic patients; **high mortality** because susceptibility to most antifungals including amphotericin B is variable
Rhodotorula	Catheter-related sepsis in immunocompromised patients; amphotericin B and fluconazole with good activity
Microsporidia	Many genera; disease dependent on infecting species; most common diseases following ingestion include chronic diarrhea, hepatitis, or peritonitis in AIDS patients; treatment with albendazole
Pneumocystis	**Most common opportunistic pathogen in AIDS patients**; respiratory tract is the main portal of entry and pneumonia the most common presentation, although dissemination occurs less commonly; treatment and prophylaxis of high-risk patients is with trimethoprim-sulfamethoxazole

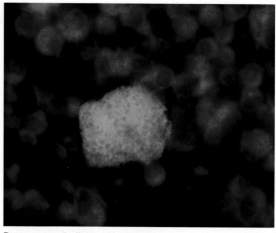

Pneumocystis jiroveci in bronchoalveolar lavage stained with immunofluorescent antibodies.

ASPERGILLUS FUMIGATUS

Aspergillus is the most common mold that causes opportunistic infections. A large number of species has been described, but the number of species associated with human disease is relatively limited, with *A. fumigatus* by far the most common. Aspergilli are environment fungi whose spores are inhaled, producing a wide range of diseases including allergic hypersensitivity reactions, primary pulmonary disease, or highly aggressive disseminated disease. A preliminary diagnosis of infection is made by observation of the fungus in tissue (typical appearance is branching, septate [divided into compartments], nonpigmented [hyaline] hyphae) and confirmed by growth of the mold in 2 to 5 days in culture. Identification of the individual species is by the morphologic appearance of the mold growing in culture (color of the colonies, arrangement of spores on the fruiting structures attached to the hyphae). The spores are not observed in patient tissues.

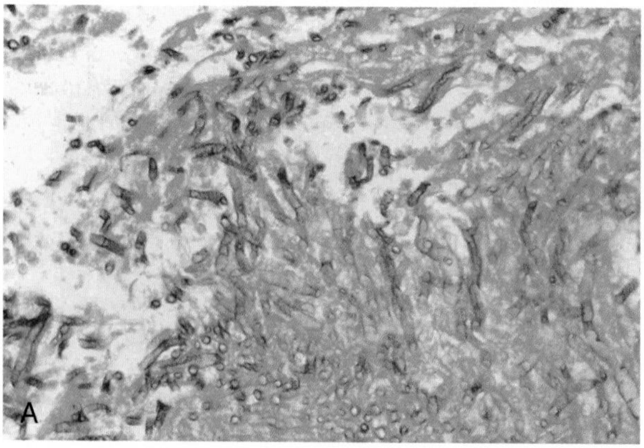

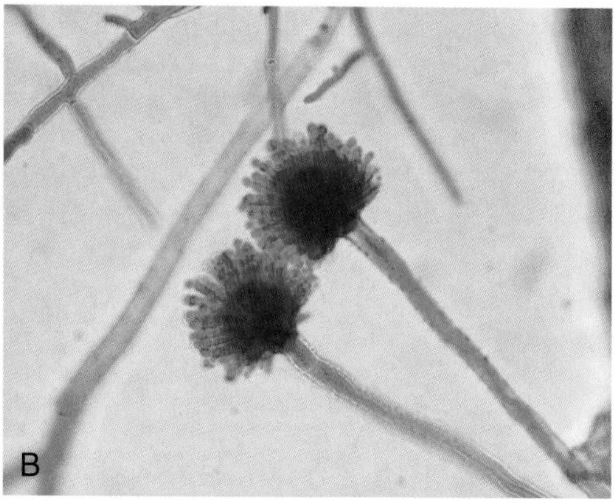

Aspergillus fumigatus. (A) Mold form in lung tissue; (B) mold form with fruiting conidia structure in culture.

ASPERGILLUS FUMIGATUS	
Epidemiology	• Worldwide distribution with spores ubiquitous in air, soil, and decaying vegetation • Within the hospital environment, *Aspergillus* may be found in air, showerheads, water storage tanks, potted plants, and in areas of construction and remodeling • Infections most commonly acquired by inhalation • Most infections caused by *A. fumigatus* (most common), *Aspergillus flavus*, *Aspergillus niger*, and *Aspergillus terreus*
Clinical Disease	• Disease is a function of the host immune response and, less so, the *Aspergillus* species or strain • Exposure to fungal spores may result in a hypersensitive reaction (**allergic aspergillosis**) or **invasive disease** • Invasive disease marked by **angioinvasion** (invasion of blood vessels) and tissue destruction • Hematogenous dissemination to the brain (most common), heart, kidneys, gastrointestinal tract, liver, spleen
Diagnosis	• Diagnosis is by observation of the mold in tissue and isolation in culture; isolation in asymptomatic patients may represent insignificant colonization so additional cultures and demonstration of tissue involvement is required • Antigen tests can be used to complement culture • Nucleic acid amplification tests are controversial because environmental contamination of reagents is common
Treatment, Control, Prevention	• Treatment of chronic pulmonary aspergillosis may involve steroids as well as long-term antifungal therapy, usually with an azole agent • Therapy for invasive aspergillosis usually involves administration of voriconazole or amphotericin B; efforts to decrease immunosuppression are generally necessary • Prophylaxis of high-risk neutropenic patients usually with itraconazole, posaconazole, or voriconazole • Exposure is difficult to control because the mold is present in the environment; however, high-risk patients should avoid areas of remodeling, construction, and excavation

CLINICAL CASE

Invasive Aspergillosis

Guha and associates[3] describe a case of invasive aspergillosis in a renal transplant recipient. The patient was a 34-year-old woman who presented with 2-day history of weakness, dizziness, left calf pain, and black tarry stools. She denied chest pain, cough, or shortness of breath. Her past medical history was significant for diabetes leading to renal failure, for which she received a cadaveric renal transplant in 2002. Three weeks before presentation, acute graft rejection developed. She was placed on an immunosuppressive regimen of alemtuzumab, tacrolimus, sirolimus, and prednisone. On admission, she was tachycardic, hypertensive, and febrile. Physical examination revealed a tender venous cord palpable in the popliteal fossa. An initial chest radiograph showed no abnormalities. Laboratory studies showed anemia and azotemia. The white cell blood count was 4800/μL with 80% neutrophils. The patient was given four units of packed red blood cells, and empirical treatment with gatifloxacin. On hospital day 6, vesicular rash developed on the buttocks and left calf, cultures of which were positive for herpes simplex virus, and she was placed on acyclovir. The patient's clinical condition stabilized except for her renal function, and intermittent hemodialysis was started on hospital day 8. On hospital day 12, the patient exhibited decreased responsiveness, became obtunded, and was intubated for respiratory distress. A chest radiograph showed diffuse bilateral lung nodules. Culture of bronchoalveolar lavage fluid was positive for Aspergillus *species, and viral inclusion bodies suggestive of cytomegalovirus were seen. Her immunosuppression was decreased, and liposomal amphotericin B was started. The patient experienced an acute myocardial infarction and became comatose. Multiple acute infarcts in the frontal lobe and cerebellum were seen on a magnetic resonance imaging scan of the brain. The patient's condition continued to deteriorate, and multiple skin nodules developed on her arm and trunk. Biopsy specimens of the skin nodules grew* Aspergillus flavus *on culture. The patient subsequently died on hospital day 23. At autopsy,* A. flavus *was detected in multiple organs, including heart, lung, adrenal gland, thyroid, kidney, and liver.*

This case serves as an extreme example of disseminated aspergillosis in an immunocompromised host.

MISCELLANEOUS OPPORTUNISTIC MOLDS

The following is a summary of other medically important, multicellular molds that can produce disseminated disease:

Fungus	Diseases and Comments
Mucorales (e.g., *Rhizopus, Mucor, Rhizomucor*)	Genera of nonseptate, nonpigmented molds that cause invasive disease in immunocompromised patients, particularly **diabetes** patients, patients with **metabolic acidosis**, and those with hematologic malignances
Fusarium, Scedosporium, Paecilomyces	Septated, nonpigmented molds that cause disseminated infections in immunocompromised patients; one of the few molds that are isolated in blood cultures
Alternaria, Bipolaris, Curvularia	Septated, pigmented molds that cause either localized subcutaneous disease following trauma or disseminate to multiple organs in immunocompromised patients

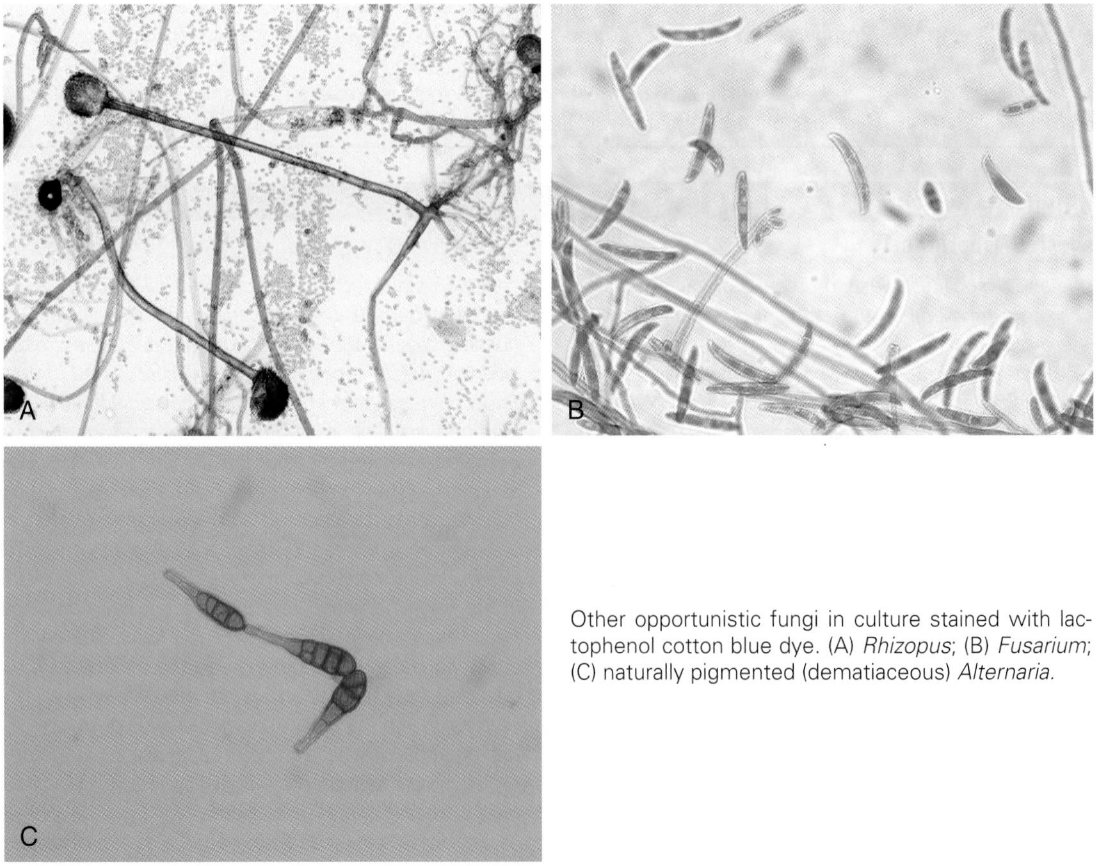

Other opportunistic fungi in culture stained with lactophenol cotton blue dye. (A) *Rhizopus*; (B) *Fusarium*; (C) naturally pigmented (dematiaceous) *Alternaria*.

CLINICAL CASE

Fusariosis

Badley and associates[4] describe a 38-year-old man, undergoing chemotherapy for recently diagnosed acute myeloid leukemia, who developed neutropenia and fever. He was placed on broad-spectrum antibacterial agents but remained febrile for 96 hours. A left internal jugular catheter was in place. Blood and urine cultures showed no growth. To combat a potential fungal infection, voriconazole was added to the therapeutic regimen. After 1 week of treatment, the patient was still febrile and neutropenic, and his antifungal therapy was changed to caspofungin. Four days later, the patient developed a mildly painful rash. Initially the rash developed on the upper extremities and consisted of papular, erythematous, plaquelike lesions with centers that became necrotic. Blood cultures and skin biopsy specimens were sent to the laboratory for analysis. The laboratory report indicated that the blood cultures were positive for "yeast", based on the presence of budding cells and pseudohyphae. *The skin biopsy showed "mold" consistent with* Aspergillus. *However, serum galactomannan testing was negative. All cultures grew* Fusarium solani. *The patient's caspofungin was discontinued, and he was switched to a lipid preparation of amphotericin B and voriconazole. Despite the antifungal therapy, the lesions increased in number over the next 2 weeks and spread throughout the extremities, trunk, and face. The neutropenia and fever persisted, and he died approximately 3 weeks after the initial diagnosis.*

The combination of skin lesions and positive blood cultures are typical findings in fusariosis. Although "yeast" were reported from the blood cultures, closer examination revealed the microconidia and hyphae of Fusarium. *Likewise, the appearance of septate hyphae in the skin biopsy could represent a number of different hyaline molds, including* Fusarium.

REFERENCES

1. Posteraro B, Tumbarello M, La Sorda M, et al. Azole resistance of *Candida glabrata* in a case of recurrent fungemia. *J. Clin Microbiol.* 2006;44:3046–3047.
2. Pappas. www.FrontlineFungus.org.
3. Guha. *Infect Med.* 2007;24(suppl 8):8–11.
4. Badley. www.FrontlineFungus.org.

22 Introduction to Parasites

OVERVIEW

Parasites are the most complex of all microbes. All parasites are classified as eukaryotic, some are unicellular and others are multicellular, some are as small as 4 to 5 μm in diameter and others are up to 10 meters in length, and some are amorphous with minimal features whereas others have characteristic structures, such as a head, body, and legs. Historically, parasitic infections were viewed as exotic diseases acquired only in remote regions of the world, but the reality is that some of the more common parasitic infections can be acquired in most communities in developed countries, and global transportation can bring diseases restricted to remote regions of the world to anyone's doorsteps. The epidemiology of these diseases is equally challenging, with some parasites spread from person to person while others require a complex series of hosts for development into infectious forms. The difficulties confronting students are not only an understanding of the spectrum of diseases caused by parasites but also an appreciation of the epidemiology of these infections, which is vital for developing a differential diagnosis and an approach to the control and prevention of parasitic infections. With literally hundreds of parasites associated with human disease, the student needs some help in organizing the most relevant information. In this chapter and subsequent ones, I will concentrate on only the most common parasites associated with human disease, recognizing that avirulent parasites, particularly those classified in the kingdom Protozoa, can colonize humans and create confusion when detected in clinical specimens. In this chapter, I first provide a classification structure for the parasites and then a view of the parasites from the perspective of the diseases they cause. I also provide an overview of the antiparasitic agents that can be used to treat these infections. In the subsequent chapters, I provide a more detailed view of the biology, epidemiology, clinical disease, diagnosis, and treatment of these organisms.

CLASSIFICATION

The parasites of humans are classified in three kingdoms: Protozoa, Stramenopila, and Animalia. **Protozoa** are simple, unicellular parasites that are microscopic in size. Stramenopila include a number of unicellular plantlike organisms (e.g., algae) and one organism, *Blastocystis*, is commonly observed in fecal specimens but is of uncertain clinical significance (actually, of controversial significance). The kingdom of Stramenopila will not be discussed further. The last kingdom, Animalia, includes all eukaryotic organisms that are not Protozoa, Stramenopila, or Fungi. For our purposes here, this kingdom includes the "**worms**" and the "**bugs**".

Kingdom	General Class	Organism	Disease
Protozoa	Ameba	*Entamoeba histolytica*	Amebiasis (amebic dysentery)
		Acanthamoeba spp.	Keratitis, encephalitis
		Naegleria fowleri	Meningoencephalitis
	Flagellate	*Giardia duodenalis*	Giardiasis (diarrheal disease)
		Trichomonas vaginalis	Trichomoniasis (vaginitis)
		Leishmania spp.	Leishmaniasis (cutaneous or visceral disease)
		Trypanosoma brucei	African sleeping sickness
		Trypanosoma cruzi	Chagas disease
	Sporozoan	*Cryptosporidium* spp.	Diarrheal disease
		Cyclospora cayetanensis	Diarrheal disease
		Cystoisospora belli	Diarrheal disease
		Toxoplasma gondii	Toxoplasmosis (disseminated disease)
		Plasmodium spp.	Malaria
		Babesia spp.	Babesiosis (malaria-like disease)
Animalia	Nematodes (roundworms)	*Enterobius vermicularis*	Enterobiasis (perianal itching)
		Trichuris trichiura	Trichuriasis (diarrheal disease)
		Ascaris lumbricoides	Ascariasis (intestinal disease)
		Strongyloides stercoralis	Strongyloidiasis (intestinal disease)
		Necator americanus	Hookworm (intestinal disease)
		Ancylostoma duodenale	Hookworm (intestinal disease)
		Brugia malayi	Filiariasis or elephantiasis
		Wuchereria bancrofti	Filiariasis or elephantiasis
		Loa loa	Disseminated disease
		Onchocerca volvulus	Onchocerciasis (disseminated disease with blindness)
		Trichinella spiralis	Trichinosis (disseminated disease)
		Toxocara canis	Visceral larva migrans
		Ancylostoma braziliense	Cutaneous larva migrans
	Trematodes (flatworms)	*Fasciolopsis buski*	Intestinal disease
		Fasciola hepatica	Hepatic disease
		Opisthorchis sinensis (also known as *Clonorchis sinensis*)	Hepatic disease
		Paragonimus westermani	Pulmonary disease
		Schistosoma spp.	Schistosomiasis (disseminated disease)
	Cestodes (tapeworms)	*Taenia saginata*	Intestinal disease
		Taenia solium	Intestinal disease; cysticercosis (disseminated)
		Diphyllobothrium latum	Intestinal disease
		Hymenolepis spp.	Intestinal disease
		Dipylidium caninum	Intestinal disease
		Echinococcus granulosus	Echinococcosis (disseminated disease)
	Arthropods	Mosquito	Vector for many diseases
		Tick	Vector for many diseases
		Flea	Vector for many diseases
		Lice	Vector for many diseases
		Mite	Vector for many diseases
		Fly	Vector for many diseases

ROLE IN DISEASE

In this section, I present a summary of the parasites that are associated with human disease from the perspective of the clinical presentation. This is the view of the physician when presented with an ill patient; however, it is critical that he or she know the most likely parasites responsible for the clinical symptoms. The goal of this section and subsequent chapters is to give the physician the tools to develop this differential diagnosis.

	PARASITE			
Disease	**Protozoa**	**Nematode**	**Trematode**	**Cestode**
Systemic				
Dissemination and multiorgan involvement	*Plasmodium falciparum, Toxoplasma, Leishmania*	*Toxocara, Strongyloides, Trichinella*		
Iron deficiency		*Necator, Ancylostoma*		
Vitamin B_{12} deficiency				*Diphyllobothrium*
Blood				
Malaria	*Plasmodium*			
Babesiosis	*Babesia*			
Filariasis		*Brugia, Loa, Wuchereria*		
Lymphatics				
Lymphedema		*Brugia, Loa, Wuchereria*		
Lymphadenopathy	*Toxoplasma, Trypanosoma*			
Bone Marrow				
Leishmaniasis	*Leishmania*			
Central Nervous System				
Meningoencephalitis	*Naegleria, Trypanosoma, Toxoplasma*			
Granulomatous encephalitis	*Acanthamoeba*			
Mass lesion, brain abscess	*Toxoplasma, Acanthamoeba*		*Schistosoma japonicum*	*Taenia solium*
Eosinophilic meningitis	*Plasmodium falciparum*	*Toxocara*		
Cerebral paragonimiasis			*Paragonimus*	
Eye				
Keratitis	*Acanthamoeba*	*Oncocerca*		
Chorioretinitis, conjunctivitis	*Toxoplasma*	*Loa, Oncocerca*		
Ocular cysticercosis				*Taenia solium*
Toxocariasis		*Toxocara*		
Intestinal Tract				
Anal puritis	*Enterobius*			
Colitis	*Entamoeba histolytica*			
Toxic megacolon	*Trypanosoma cruzi*			

	PARASITE			
Disease	**Protozoa**	**Nematode**	**Trematode**	**Cestode**
Rectal prolapse		*Trichuris*		
Abdominal pain, diarrhea, dysentery	*Entamoeba histolytica, Giardia, Cryptosporidium, Cyclospora, Cystoisospora*	*Strongyloides, Trichuris, Necator, Ancyclostoma*	*Schistosoma mansoni*	Taenia, Diphyllobothrium, Hymenolepsis, Dipylidium
Obstruction, perforation		*Ascaris, Fasciolopsis*		
Genitourinary Tract				
Vaginitis, urethritis	*Trichomonas*	*Enterobius*		
Cystitis, hematuria	*Plasmodium*		*Schistosoma haematobium*	
Renal failure	*Plasmodium, Leishmania*			
Liver, Spleen				
Abscess	*Entamoeba histolytica*		*Fasciola*	
Hepatitis	*Toxoplasma*			
Biliary obstruction		*Ascaris*	*Opisthorchis, Fasciola*	
Cirrhosis	*Leishmania*	*Toxocara*	*Schistosoma*	
Mass lesion				*Taenia solium, Echinococcus*
Heart				
Myocarditis	*Toxoplasma, Trypanosoma cruzi*			
Lung				
Abscess	*Entaemoeba histolytica*		*Paragonimus*	
Nodule, mass				*Echinococcus*
Pneumonitis	*Toxoplasma*	*Ascaris, Ancylostoma, Strongyloides, Toxocara*	*Paragonimus*	
Muscle				
Generalized myositis		*Trichinella, Toxocara*		
Myocarditis	*Trypanosoma cruzi*	*Trichinella, Toxocara*		
Skin and Subcutaneous Tissue				
Ulcerative lesion	*Leishmania*			
Nodule, swelling	*Trypanosoma cruzi, Acanthamoeba*	*Oncocerca, Loa, Toxocara*		
Rash, vesicles	*Toxoplasma*	*Ancylostoma*	*Schistosoma*	

ANTIPARASITIC AGENTS

Treatment of parasitic infections poses a potential problem. Because both parasites and humans are eukaryotic, many antiparasitic agents also act on human metabolic pathways; that is, these agents can pose a risk of toxicity. Differential toxicity is achieved by preferential uptake, metabolic alteration of the drug by the parasite, or differences in susceptibility between host and parasite. Agents used for the treatment of **protozoan infections** generally target nucleic acid synthesis, protein synthesis, or specific metabolic pathways that are unique for the rapidly proliferating parasites. In contrast, agents used for treatment of the **helminth infections** target unique metabolic pathways in the nonproliferating adult worms. Because the student may not be familiar with the antiparasitic agents, I will first present a listing of the different classes of agents and then summarize the specific agents used to treat each parasite. The following is a summary of the major antiparasitic agents and clinical indications.

Drug Class	Examples	Clinical Indications
Antiprotozoal Agents		
Heavy metals	Melarsoprol, sodium stibogluconate, meglumine antimoniate	Trypanosomiasis, leishmaniasis
Aminoquinoline analogs	Chloroquine, mefloquine, quinine, primaquine, halofantrine, lumefantrine	Malaria prophylaxis and therapy
Folic acid antagonists	Sulfonamides, pyrimethamine, trimethoprim	Toxoplasmosis, malaria, cyclosporiasis
Inhibitors of protein synthesis	Clindamycin, spiramycin, paromomycin, tetracycline, doxycycline	Malaria, babesiosis, amebiasis, cryptosporidiosis, leishmaniasis
Diamidines	Pentamidine	Leishmaniasis, trypanosomiasis
Nitromidazoles	Metronidazole, benznidazole, tinidazole	Amebiasis, giardiasis, trichomoniasis, trypanosomiasis
Nitrofurans	Nifurtimox	Trypanosomiasis
Phosphocholine analog	Miltefosine	Leishmaniasis
Sulfated naphthylamine	Suramin	Trypanosomiasis
Thiazolides	Nitazoxanide	Cryptosporidiosis, giardiasis
Antihelminth Agents		
Benzimidazoles	Mebendazole, thiabendazole, albendazole	Broad-spectrum antihelminthic for nematodes and cestodes
Tetrahydropyrimidine	Pyrantel pamoate	Ascariasis, pinworm, hookworm
Piperazine	Piperazine, diethylcarbamazine	Ascaris and pinworm infections
Avermectins	Ivermectin	Filarial infections, strongyloidiasis, ascariasis, scabies
Prazinoisoquinoline	Praziquantel	Broad-spectrum antihelminthic for cestodes and trematodes
Phenol	Niclosamide	Infesting tapeworm
Quinolone	Bithionol, oxamniquine	Paragonimiasis, schistosomiasis
Organophosphate	Metrifonate	Schistosomiasis
Sulfated naphthylamidine	Suramin	Onchocerciasis

The following table is a list of primary and secondary treatments for the most common parasites. Please note that for many of the groups of parasites, the same antiparasitic agents are used for treatment.

Parasite	Primary Antiparasitic Agents	Secondary Antiparasitic Agents
Intestinal Protozoa		
Entamoeba histolytica	Metronidazole + paromomycin	Iodoquinol; tinidazole + paromomycin
Cryptosporidium spp.	Nitazoxanide	Paromomycin + azithromycin
Cystoisospora belli	Trimethoprim-sulfamethoxazole	Ciprofloxacin; pyrimethamine
Cyclospora cayetanensis	Trimethoprim-sulfamethoxazole	Ciprofloxacin
Giardia duodenalis	Metronidazole; nitazoxanide	Furazolidone; paromomycin; quinacrine

Parasite	Primary Antiparasitic Agents	Secondary Antiparasitic Agents
Urogenital Protozoa		
Trichomonas vaginalis	Metronidazole	
Blood and Tissue Protozoa		
Acanthamoeba spp.	Miltefosine	
Naegleria fowleri	Miltefosine; amphotericin B	
Plasmodium spp.	Chloroquine; refer to current Centers for Disease Control and Prevention recommendations	
Babesia microti	Clindamycin + quinine; atovaquone + azithromycin	
Toxoplasma gondii	Pyrimethamine + sulfadiazine	
Leishmania spp.	Sodium stibogluconate; meglumine antimonite; miltefosine	Pentamidine; amphotericin B
Trypanosoma brucei	Suramin; pentamidine; malarsoprol (for central nervous system disease)	
Trypanosoma cruzi	Benznidazole; nifurtimox	
Intestinal Nematodes		
Ascaris lumbricoides	Albendazole	Mebendazole; pyrantel pamoate
Enterobius vermicularis	Mebendazole	Albendazole; pyrantel pamoate
Ancylostoma duodenale	Albendazole; mebendazole; pyrantel pamoate	
Necator americanus	Albendazole; mebendazole; pyrantel pamoate	
Strongyloides stercoralis	Ivermectin	Albendazole; mebendazole
Trichuris trichiura	Albendazole; mebendazole	
Blood Nematodes		
Brugia malayi	Diethylcarbamazine	Albendazole
Wuchereria bancrofti	Diethylcarbamazine	Albendazole
Loa loa	Diethylcarbamazine	
Onchocerca volvulus	Ivermectin	
Tissue Nematodes		
Trichinella spiralis	Mebendazole (adult worms only)	
Intestinal Trematodes		
Fasciolopsis buski	Praziquantel	Niclosamide
Tissue Trematodes		
Fasciola hepatica	Triclabendazole	Bithionol
Opisthorchis sinensis	Praziquantel	Albendazole
Paragonimus westermani	Praziquantel	Triclabendazole
Blood Trematodes		
Schistosoma mansoni	Praziquantel	Oxamniquine
Schistosoma japonica	Praziquantel	
Schistosoma haematobium	Praziquantel	

Continued

Parasite	Primary Antiparasitic Agents	Secondary Antiparasitic Agents
Intestinal Cestodes		
Taenia spp.	Praziquantel	Niclosamide
Diphyllobothrium latum	Praziquantel	Niclosamide
Hymenolepis spp.	Praziquantel	Niclosamide
Dipylidium caninum	Praziquantel	Niclosamide
Tissue Cestodes		
Echinococcus spp.	Albendazole	Mebendazole; praziquantel

23

Protozoa

INTERESTING FACTS

- *Entamoeba histolytica* is the most common ameba responsible for diarrheal disease
- *Cryptosporidium* is the most common cause of water-borne outbreaks of enterocolitis
- *Giardia duodenalis* is the most common flagellate responsible for diarrheal disease
- *Trichomonas vaginalis* is the most common parasite responsible for vaginitis
- *Acanthamoeba* is the most common parasite responsible for keratitis
- *Plasmodium* is the most important blood-borne parasite in the world

Protozoa are simple, unicellular parasites that are microscopic in size. Classification of protozoa is complex but the easiest way to organize these parasites is by where they produce disease. It is also useful to understand the reservoirs and vectors of these parasites.

Group	Parasite	Reservoir	Vector
Intestinal amoeba	*Entamoeba histolytica*	Humans	—
Coccidia	*Cyclospora cayetanensis*	Humans	—
	Cryptosporidium spp.	Humans	—
	Cystoisospora belli	Humans	—
Flagellates	*Giardia duodenalis*	Humans, beavers, muskrats	—
	Trichomonas vaginalis	Humans	—
Free-living amoeba	*Naegleria* spp.	Environment	
	Acanthamoeba spp.	Environment	
Blood and Tissue Protozoa	*Plasmodium* spp.	Humans	Mosquito
	Babesia microti	Rodents	Tick
	Toxoplasma gondii	Cat	—
	Leishmania spp.	Rodents, dogs	Sandfly
	Trypanosoma brucei	Domestic animals, humans, cattle, sheep, wild game	Tsetse fly
	Trypanosoma cruzi	Wild animals	Reduviid bug

The protozoa listed in this chapter are certainly not a comprehensive list of all protozoa or even all protozoa associated with human disease; however, the most important species are included in this chapter.

INTESTINAL AMOEBA

The intestinal protozoa can be subdivided into the amebae, coccidia, and flagellates. *E. histolytica* represents the intestinal amebae and must be differentiated from a number of nonpathogenic amebae that can also be found in the intestines (this is done by their morphologic appearance and is not discussed further in this chapter). Although not common in the United States, infections can be acquired when traveling to countries with poor hygienic standards.

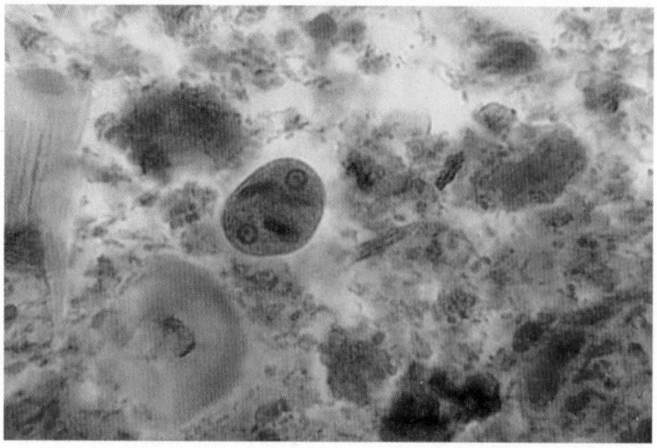

Trichrome stain of *Entamoeba histolytica* cyst with two nuclei and an elongated chromatoidal bar in the cytoplasm.

ENTAMOEBA HISTOLYTICA	
Epidemiology	• Worldwide distribution • Most prevalent in tropical and subtropical regions with poor hygiene • Many asymptomatic carriers serve as reservoirs for disease • Two forms of parasites: infectious cysts and noninfectious, replicating trophozoites • Trophozoites replicate in the lumen of the colon • Transmission through contaminated water and food or through oral-anal sexual practices
Clinical Disease	• **Asymptomatic carriage** • **Intestinal amebiasis**: localized infection of the colon presenting with abdominal pain, cramping, and diarrhea • **Extraintestinal amebiasis**: dissemination to liver with abscess formation is most common
Diagnosis	• Intestinal amebiasis most commonly diagnosed by microscopic detection of trophozoites and cysts in stool specimens • Nucleic acid amplification tests (NAATs) available for detection of *E. histolytica* in stool specimens • Parasites may not be observed in stool specimens for patients with extraintestinal infections; serology is the most reliable diagnostic method for these patients
Treatment, Prevention, Control	• Acute infections treated with metronidazole plus paromomycin; alternative iodoquinol (asymptomatic carriage) or tinidazole plus paromomycin • Prevention and control through implementation of appropriate sanitation standards and use of chlorination and filtration of water where necessary

CLINICAL CASE

HIV and Amebic Liver Abscess

Liu and colleagues[1] described a 45-year-old homosexual man who developed intestinal and hepatic amebiasis. The patient initially presented with intermittent fever followed by right upper quadrant pain and diarrhea. On admission to the hospital, he was afebrile with an elevated white blood cell count and abnormal liver function tests. Stool examinations were positive for occult blood and white blood cells. He underwent colonoscopy, and multiple discrete ulcers were detected in the rectum and colon. The diagnosis of amebic colitis was confirmed by the demonstration of numerous trophozoites on histopathologic examination of colon biopsy specimens. Ultrasound examination of the abdomen revealed a large heterogeneous mass within the liver, consistent with an abscess. Percutaneous drainage of the abscess obtained chocolate-like pus, and examination of a biopsy from the margin of the abscess revealed only a necrotic material, without evidence of amebae. Polymerase chain reaction (PCR) amplification of amebic 16S ribosomal RNA from the aspirate was positive, indicating infection with E. histolytica. *The patient was treated with metronidazole followed by iodoquinol to eradicate the luminal amebae. Subsequent history revealed he traveled to Thailand 2 months before the onset of the present illness. HIV serology was positive as well. The patient improved rapidly on antiamebic therapy and was discharged on antiretroviral therapy.*

Although amebic cysts are frequently detected in the stools of homosexual men, previous studies in Western countries suggested that almost all isolates belong to the nonpathogenic species Entamoeba dispar, *and invasive amebiasis was considered rare in HIV-positive individuals. This case illustrates that invasive amebiasis, such as amebic liver abscess and colitis, can accompany HIV infection. The possible association of invasive amebiasis with HIV infection should be considered for patients living in or with a history of travel to areas where* E. histolytica *is endemic.*

COCCIDIA

Three **coccidia** are discussed in this chapter: *Cyclospora*, *Cryptosporidium*, and *Cystoisospora*. *Cyclospora* infections in the United States are typically associated with food-related outbreaks such as with raw fruits or vegetables shipped from countries with poor hygienic conditions. *Cryptosporidium* and *Cystoisospora* were initially implicated in intestinal disease in HIV-infected individuals, but are now recognized as pathogens of immunocompetent and immunocompromised individuals. *Cryptosporidium* in particular is associated with large outbreaks when drinking water or recreational waters are contaminated. Many species of *Cryptosporidium* infect a variety of animals, but *Cryptosporidium hominis* and *Cryptosporidium parvum* are most commonly associated with human infections.

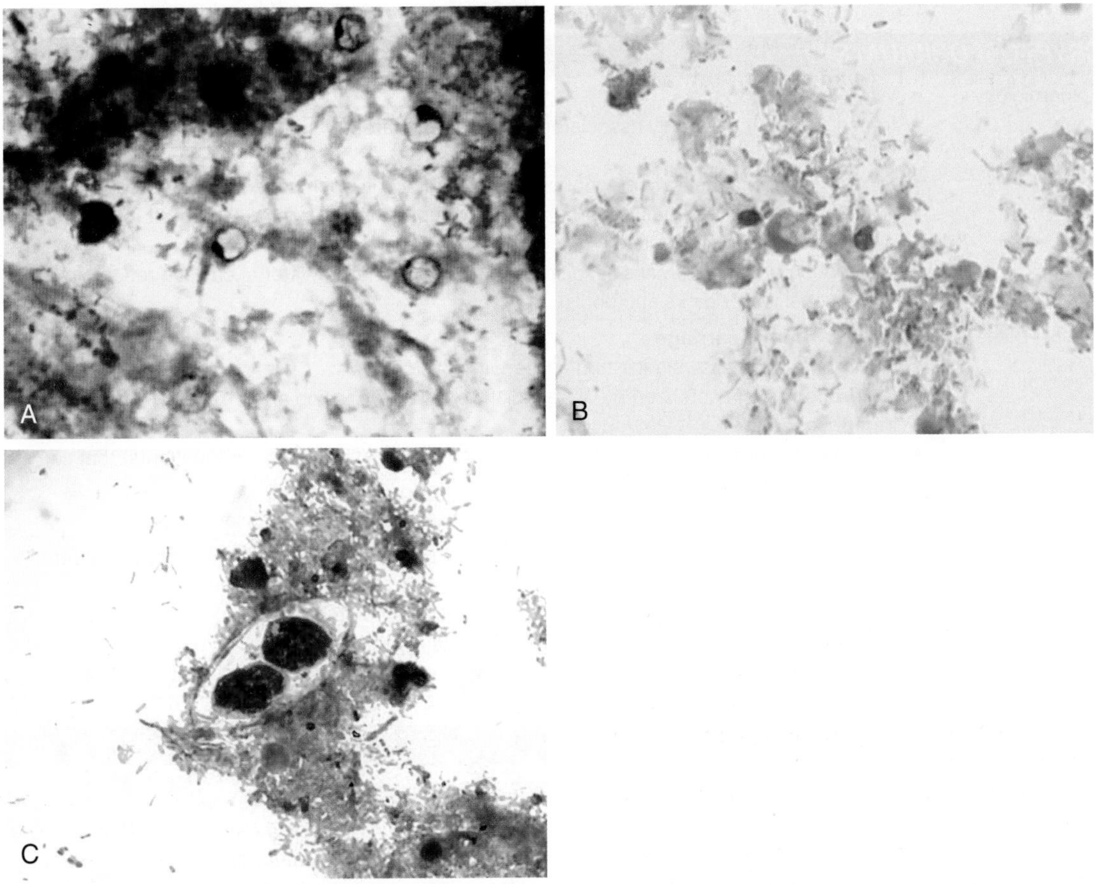

Acid-fast stains of (A) *Cyclospora*, (B) *Cryptosporidium*, and (C) *Cystoisospora*.

CYCLOSPORA CAYETANENSIS	
Epidemiology	• Worldwide distribution • Most prevalent in tropical and subtropical regions with poor hygiene • Infection from ingestion of contaminated food (e.g., raw fruits and vegetables) or water; person-to-person transmission not observed • Outbreaks most commonly occur in spring and summer months • Small (8–10 μm), spherical, noninfectious oocysts are passed in stool; in the external environment they develop two internal sporocysts, each of which contain two sporozoites • When the oocyst is ingested, the sporozoites are liberated and enter the epithelial cells of the **small intestine** where they establish disease
Clinical Disease	• **Asymptomatic carriage** • **Mild to severe diarrheal disease** with nausea, anorexia, abdominal cramping, and watery diarrhea; self-limiting disease in immunocompetent patients although symptoms may persist for weeks • **Chronic infection** can occur, particularly in HIV-infected patients
Diagnosis	• Infection most commonly diagnosed by microscopic detection of oocysts in stool specimens
Treatment, Prevention, Control	• Drug of choice is trimethoprim-sulfamethoxazole; alternative ciprofloxacin • Maintain personal hygiene and high sanitary conditions • Treatment of water with chlorine or iodine is generally not effective because the oocysts are relatively resistant

CRYPTOSPORIDIUM SPP.	
Epidemiology	• Worldwide distribution • Infection most commonly associated with contaminated water or fecal-oral, oral-anal transmission • Small (4–6 μm), spherical, infectious oocysts containing sporozoites are excreted in feces • Ingested sporozoites attach to brush border of epithelial cells lining the **small intestine** where they establish disease • Well-documented outbreaks associated with contaminated water such as in reservoirs or recreational water parks and pools
Clinical Disease	• **Asymptomatic carriage** • Symptomatic disease similar to disease with *Cyclospora* • **Enterocolitis** characterized by watery diarrhea with remission after 10 days in immunocompetent patients • More **severe enterocolitis** in immunocompromised patients (e.g., HIV patients) that can evolve into chronic disease
Diagnosis	• Detection of oocysts in stool specimens by microscopy, immunoassay, or NAATs
Treatment, Prevention, Control	• Nitazoxanide is used to treat immunocompetent patients but no effective treatment for immunocompromised patients; alternative paromomycin plus azithromycin • Prevention of disease is difficult because widespread distribution in animals and inadvertent contamination of water supplies and recreational waters • Maintain personal hygiene and high sanitary conditions; avoid oral-anal sexual practices

CLINICAL CASE

Cryptosporidiosis

Quiroz and colleagues[2] described an outbreak of cryptosporidiosis that was linked to a food handler. In the fall of 1998 an outbreak of gastroenteritis among university students was reported to the Department of Health. Preliminary findings suggested that the illness was associated with eating at one of the campus cafeterias; four employees of this cafeteria had a similar illness. The outbreak was thought to be caused by a viral agent until C. parvum *was detected in the stool specimens of several cafeteria employees. In a case control study of 88 case patients and 67 control patients, eating in 1 or 2 cafeterias was associated with diarrheal illness.* C. parvum *was detected in stool samples of 16 (70%) of 23 ill students and 2 of 4 ill employees. One ill food handler with laboratory-confirmed cryptosporidiosis prepared raw produce on the days surrounding the outbreak. All 25* C. parvum *isolates submitted for DNA analysis, including 3 from the ill food handler, were genotype 1. This outbreak illustrates the potential for cryptosporidiosis to cause food-borne illness. Epidemiologic and molecular evidence indicate that an ill food handler was the likely outbreak source.*

CYSTOISOSPORA BELLI	
Epidemiology	• Worldwide distribution • Most prevalent in tropical and subtropical regions with poor hygiene • Infection from ingestion of contaminated food or water, or oral-anal sexual contact • Large, oblong, noninfectious oocysts are passed in stool; in the external environment they develop two internal sporocysts, each of which contain four sporozoites • When the oocyst is ingested, the sporozoites are liberated and enter the epithelial cells of the **small intestine** where they establish disease
Clinical Disease	• **Asymptomatic carriage** • **Mild to severe diarrheal disease,** similar to giardiasis • **Chronic infection** can occur, particularly in HIV-infected patients
Diagnosis	• Infection most commonly diagnosed by microscopic detection of oocysts in stool specimens
Treatment, Prevention, Control	• Drug of choice is trimethoprim-sulfamethoxazole; alternative ciprofloxacin or pyrimethamine • Maintain personal hygiene and high sanitary conditions; avoid oral-anal sexual practices

FLAGELLATES

Two flagellates (so named because their flagella, or hairlike structures, are a key morphologic feature for their identification) are discussed in this chapter: the intestinal protozoa *G. duodenalis* and the urogenital protozoa *T. vaginalis.*

In contrast with most of the other parasites discussed in this chapter, *G. duodenalis* (also called *Giardia lamblia* and *Giardia intestinalis*) is widely disseminated in the United States. Wild animals are an important reservoir for this parasite and their feces can contaminate many streams and lakes as well as drinking water such as from wells.

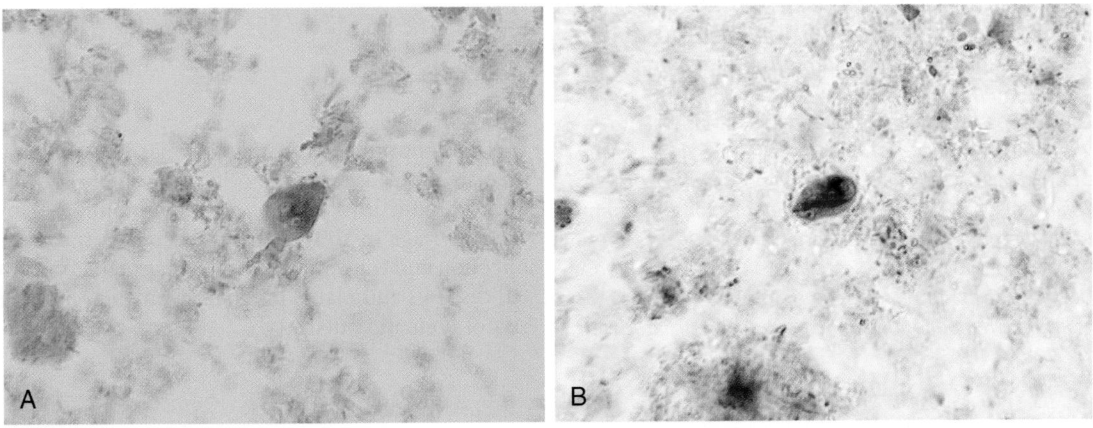

Trichrome stain of *Giardia duodenalis* (A) trophozoite and (B) cyst.

GIARDIA DUODENALIS	
Epidemiology	• Worldwide distribution • Animals such as beavers and muskrats serve as the natural reservoir • Asymptomatic human carriers also serve as a reservoir • Two forms of parasite: infectious cysts and noninfectious, replicating trophozoites • Human infections most commonly from ingestion of cyst-contaminated water or food products • Person-to-person spread through fecal-oral contamination • Outbreaks reported in day-care facilities, nurseries, and long-term care institutions
Clinical Disease	• **Asymptomatic carriage** • Infection (**giardiasis**) of **small intestine** with symptoms ranging from diarrhea to malabsorption syndrome • Incubation period on average 10 days; onset sudden with foul-smelling watery diarrhea, abdominal cramps, flatulence • Symptoms persist for 1–2 weeks although chronic disease may develop
Diagnosis	• Intestinal giardiasis most commonly diagnosed by microscopic detection of trophozoites and cysts in stool specimens • NAATs now available for detection of *G. duodenalis* in stool specimens • Immunoassays and fluorescent antibody tests are available but less sensitive than NAATs
Treatment, Prevention, Control	• Drug of choice is metronidazole or nitazoxanide; alternatives furazolidone; paromomycin; quinacrine • Avoid contaminated water and food • Chlorine treatment alone is insufficient because the cysts are relatively resistant; water should be boiled or filtered

CLINICAL CASE

Drug-Resistant Giardiasis

Abboud and colleagues[3] described a case of metronidazole- and abendazole-resistant giardiasis that was successfully treated with nitazoxanide. The patient was a 32-year-old homosexual man with AIDS, who was admitted to the hospital because of intractable diarrhea. Examination of stool revealed the presence of numerous cysts of G. duodenalis (G. lamblia). *The patient was unsuccessfully treated five times with metronidazole and albendazole without improvement of diarrhea or cyst shedding. Although combined antiretroviral therapy was also administered, it was ineffective, and viral genotypic analysis found mutations associated with high resistance to most antiretroviral drugs. The patient was subsequently treated for giardiasis with nitazoxanide, which resulted in resolution of the diarrhea and negative results of tests for stool cyst shedding. Resistance of the infecting strain of* G. duodenalis *to both metronidazole and albendazole was confirmed by* in vivo *and* in vitro *studies. Nitazoxanide may be considered as a useful alternative therapy for resistant giardiasis.*

The importance of *T. vaginalis* has been underappreciated because the majority of women and men infected with this parasite are asymptomatic. However, carriage of this organism increases the risk of infection and transmission of other sexually transmitted diseases and places pregnant women at increased risk of premature delivery.

TRICHOMONAS VAGINALIS	
Epidemiology	• Worldwide distribution • Trophozoite is the only form; colonizes urethra and vagina in women and urethra in men • Person-to-person transmission through sexual intercourse
Clinical Disease	• Most infected individuals are **asymptomatic** • **Vaginitis** and **urethritis**: inflammation of the epithelial lining with associated itching, burning, painful urination, vaginal discharge in women, and urethral discharge • Without treatment, infections can persist for months or years
Diagnosis	• Detection of parasite by microscopic examination, culture, or NAAT of discharge • NAAT is the most sensitive test and preferred for detection of asymptomatic and symptomatic infected individuals
Treatment, Prevention, Control	• Metronidazole is the drug of choice • To avoid reinfection, both sexual partners must be treated • Safe sexual practices must be maintained

FREE-LIVING AMOEBA

Two free-living amebae are discussed in this chapter: *Naegleria* and *Acanthamoeba*. Both are important human pathogens capable of causing overwhelming and rapidly fatal disease, but fortunately are relatively uncommon.

NAEGLERIA SPP.	
Epidemiology	• Worldwide distribution • Common in soil and freshwater lakes and rivers • Infections are most common after exposure to trophozoites in contaminated waters in the warm summer months • Parasite enters the body through the nose and migrates to the brain; infections are not caused by ingestion of contaminated waters
Clinical Disease	• **Primary amebic meningoencephalitis**: rapidly progressive and fatal destruction of brain tissue
Diagnosis	• Because of the rapid progression of disease, diagnosis by history of exposure and clinical symptoms is confirmed postmortem • Detection of parasite by microscopic examination of cerebrospinal fluid or brain tissue • NAATs available only in reference laboratories
Treatment, Prevention, Control	• Treatment is generally ineffective because of the rapid progression of disease, although the experimental drug miltefosine is available through the Centers for Disease Control and Prevention (CDC); alternative amphotericin B • Prevention is difficult because of the widespread distribution of the parasite

ACANTHAMOEBA SPP.	
Epidemiology	• Worldwide distribution • Common in soil and freshwater lakes and rivers; in tap water and bottle water; can contaminate dialysis fluids and contact lens cleaners • Infections of the eye most commonly associated with improperly cleaned contact lenses used by patients with mild preexisting trauma to the cornea (e.g., scratched or irritated cornea)
Clinical Disease	• **Keratitis**: symptoms can range from irritation, redness, and mild eye pain to rapid destruction of the cornea • **Granulomatous amebic encephalitis**: disease primarily in immunocompromised patients with a longer incubation period and slower progression than that observed with *Naegleria* infections

Continued

ACANTHAMOEBA SPP.—cont'd	
Diagnosis	• Culture of eye scrapings is a sensitive and rapid method to diagnose amebic keratitis (specimens are inoculated onto an agar plate covered with a film of gram-negative bacteria; the trail of migrating amebae is easily visualized after overnight incubation) • Detection of the parasite by microscopic examination of the brain tissue is the test of choice for amebic encephalitis
Treatment, Prevention, Control	• Treatment is generally ineffective although the experimental drug miltefosine is available through the CDC • Eye infections are avoided by using sterile cleaning solutions for contact lenses and avoiding the use of lenses if the eye is irritated

BLOOD AND TISSUE PROTOZOA

Two protozoa are important blood-borne parasites: *Plasmodium* and *Babesia*. In contrast with the protozoa discussed previously, all the blood and tissue protozoa require important vectors for transmission of disease: the *Anopheles* mosquito for malaria (*Plasmodium*) and the tick for babesiosis (*Babesia*).

Five species of *Plasmodium* are responsible for malaria in humans: *Plasmodium falciparum*, *Plasmodium vivax*, *Plasmodium ovale*, *Plasmodium malariae*, and *Plasmodium knowlesi*, with the first two species the most common. In 2013 the World Health Organization estimated that there were almost 200 million cases of malaria and 500,000 deaths, primarily children in Africa. Approximately 1500 cases of malaria occur in the United States each year, mainly in travelers and immigrants from endemic areas, although transmission in the United States is well documented.

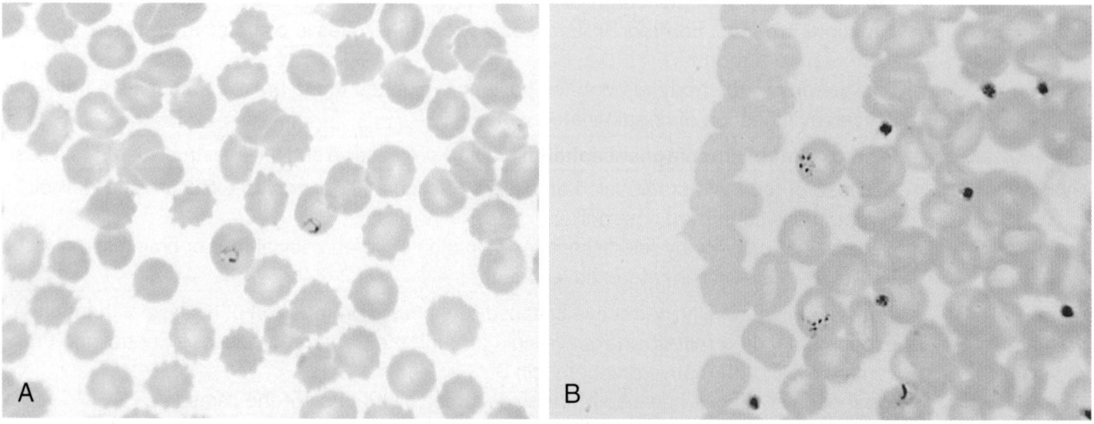

Giemsa stain of peripheral blood with infection with (A) *Plasmodium falciparum* and (B) *Babesia microti*.

PLASMODIUM SPP.	
Epidemiology	• Tropical and subtropical regions of Africa, India, Southeast Asia, Russia, China • Individual species can be geographically restricted • Plasmodium species share a similar lifecycle • Human infection initiated by the bite of the *Anopheles* **mosquito** which transmits infectious sporozoites into the blood; sporozoites are carried to the liver cells where replication occurs; when the hepatocytes rupture, infectious merozoites are released into the blood and the merozoites attach, penetrate, and replicate in erythrocytes • Mosquitos are infected when they ingest sexually mature forms of the parasite—gametocytes

PLASMODIUM SPP.—cont'd	
Clinical Disease	• The clinical presentation of **malaria** is a function of the individual species of *Plasmodium* (e.g., *Plasmodium falciparum* produces the most severe symptoms) and preexisting exposure (milder disease can occur in patients with partial immunity) • Onset of disease can be acute following a period of replication in the liver cells; symptoms include chills, fever, and myalgias and can progress to nausea, vomiting, and diarrhea; symptoms can be periodic (a day of acute symptoms followed by a few days of mild symptoms) corresponding to synchronized infection and rupture of erythrocytes • *Plasmodium vivax* and *Plasmodium ovale* can establish a **dormant liver phase** that can be activated months or years after the primary infection, producing symptoms of an acute infection
Diagnosis	• Detection of the parasite in infected erythrocytes by microscopy (Giemsa stain) • Detection of characteristic forms in infected cells is used to differentiate the individual species • NAAT is the most sensitive method for detection and identification of parasites but these tests are not currently widely available • Immunoassays are available; these tests are rapid but not as sensitive as microscopy
Treatment, Prevention, Control	• Treatment is complicated because resistance to the most commonly used drug, chloroquine, is widespread; the CDC (or similar organization) guidelines should be followed for treatment of infections with known or suspected resistant strains • Risk of infection can be reduced through the use of protective clothing, mosquito repellants on exposed skin, and prophylactic antibiotics when traveling in endemic regions • Vaccines for prevention of infections are under investigation

CLINICAL CASE

Malaria

Mohin and Gupta[4] described a case of severe malaria caused by P. vivax. *The patent was a 59-year-old man who presented with a 1-day history of high-grade fever after recently returning from Guyana in South America. He did not take any medications before, during, or after the trip. He noted that his symptoms were similar to those of a malaria infection 5 years previously, also acquired in Guyana. A peripheral blood smear as a part of the initial workup showed numerous red blood cells with schizonts consistent with* Plasmodium *infection, with more than 5% parasitemia. Several blood tests, including a DNA PCR, were sent for parasite species determination. The patient was started on quinine and doxycycline oral therapy because of the concerns regarding chloroquine-resistant malaria. During the next 4 days the patient developed more severe thrombocytopenia and nonoliguric renal failure, acute respiratory failure, and circulatory failure, despite a decrease in parasitemia to less than 0.5%. He received intravenous quinidine and an exchange transfusion to treat* P. falciparum *infection, suspected at the time because of the severity of his symptoms. The next day, however, the PCR results of the blood revealed the parasite was* P. vivax *and not* P. falciparum. *The patient gradually improved and was treated with primaquine to prevent relapse.*

This case shows that although it is unusual, severe respiratory and circulatory compromise may complicate P. vivax *malaria.* P. vivax *should be considered if the patient's condition deteriorates despite the presence of relatively low parasite levels. As opposed to* P. falciparum, P. vivax *infections carry the additional risk of relapse, which warrants appropriate and adequate treatment. This case also emphasizes the importance of chemoprophylaxis and personal protective measures for anyone planning a trip to a malaria-infested region.*

Many species of *Babesia* cause human disease worldwide, but the focus in this chapter is the most common species in the United States responsible for disease, with almost 2000 cases reported annually.

BABESIA MICROTI	
Epidemiology	• Northeastern and upper Midwestern states in the United States • Wild rodents (e.g., white footed mouse) are the primary reservoir • *Ixodes* (deer) **ticks** are the vector of disease and either become infected by feeding on an infected rodent or transovarianly; humans are accidental hosts • Most infections result from the nymph stage of the tick so a history of a tick bite may not be elicited (nymphs are very tiny [size of poppy seed]) • Most infections are during the spring and summer months • During the blood meal, infectious sporozoites are released into the human blood stream and enter into erythrocytes where the parasites replicate
Clinical Disease	• **Babesiosis** is characterized by the onset of malaise, fever, headache, chills, sweating, and fatigue; more severe disease occurs in immunocompromised patients
Diagnosis	• Detection of the parasite in infected erythrocytes by microscopy (Giemsa stain) • NAATs are available primarily in reference laboratories
Treatment, Prevention, Control	• Atovaquone plus azithromycin is used for mild disease; clindamycin plus quinine, and exchange transfusion is used for severe disease • Infections are prevented by use of protective clothing and insect repellents; prompt removal of ticks (although they may not be noticed) because they must feed for several hours to transmit disease

Three genera of tissue protozoa are discussed here: *Toxoplasma* which is found worldwide including in the United States, and *Leishmania* and *Trypanosoma* which have a more restricted geographic distribution.

Unfortunately, we do not have to travel very far to be exposed to this parasite—it is as close as the pet cat. The parasitic lifecycle is maintained in cats, which shed *T. gondii* oocysts that mature into infectious forms in a few days. The infectious forms are consumed by rodents, which in turn are consumed by cats. Humans are the unfortunate accidental hosts.

TOXOPLASMA GONDII	
Epidemiology	• Worldwide distribution • Domestic **cats** serve as the reservoir • Parasite replicates in the intestinal epithelial cells; noninfectious oocysts are passed in cat feces; the oocysts mature over 2–3 days forming two sporocysts, each containing four sporozoites • Human infections develop following exposure to infectious oocysts following handling cat feces or ingestion of **oocysts** in improperly cooked meat from infected animals (e.g., pork, lamb); transplacental transmission can also occur
Clinical Disease	• **Asymptomatic infection** • Symptoms of **toxoplasmosis** are dependent on the immune status of the host (disease most severe for the fetus *in utero* and in immunocompromised patients) and the tissues involved (e.g., lung, heart, lymphoid organs, and central nervous system) • Disease characterized by tissue destruction with abscess formation and formation of cysts • Encephalopathy, meningoencephalitis, and cerebral mass lesion can develop in immunocompromised patients
Diagnosis	• Most infections diagnosed by serology or microscopic detection of cysts in infected tissue • NAATs available in reference laboratories
Treatment, Prevention, Control	• Mild infections can be managed symptomatically; severe or disseminated infections treated with pyrimethamine plus sulfadiazine; treatment may be lifelong • Pregnant women and immunocompromised patients should avoid exposure to cat feces or consumption of under-cooked meat

CLINICAL CASE

Toxoplasmosis

Vincent and colleagues[5] described a 67-year-old woman with a 3-year history of Hodgkin disease, who received chemotherapy followed by autologous stem-cell transplantation. Shortly afterward she became febrile and neutropenic, and treatment with broad-spectrum antibiotics was started. The results of blood and urine cultures were negative. After resolution of neutropenia (1 month posttransplantation), confusion and lethargy developed. Imaging studies of the brain revealed micro-infarcts in both hemispheres and the midbrain. Findings from a lumbar puncture were unrevealing. Based on the suspicion of toxoplasmosis, pyrimethamine and sulfadiazine were added to the patient's regimen. When toxic epidermal necrolysis developed, the sulfadiazine was discontinued and clindamycin was begun. Multiorgan failure ensued, and the patient died 1 week later. At autopsy, cyst forms with bradyzoites were detected in the woman's brain and heart. Histopathologic findings and immunohistochemical staining confirmed a diagnosis of disseminated toxoplasmosis.

Disseminated toxoplasmosis is rare, especially after autologous stem-cell transplantation. The likely cause of reactivation and dissemination of Toxoplasma in this patient was the cell-mediated immunosuppression associated with Hodgkin disease and its treatment. In addition to the brain, the heart, liver, and lungs are frequently involved in cases of disseminated toxoplasmosis.

The taxonomy of *Leishmania* is in a state of flux and the names of the individual species are not critical for understanding the diseases they produce.

LEISHMANIA SPP.

Epidemiology	• Individual species restricted to specific geographies • Parasites found in Southern Europe and tropical and subtropical regions including Africa, Asia, Middle East, Latin America • Reservoir hosts include rodents and dogs; transmission from host-to-humans or human-to-human is through the bite of a **sandfly** (smaller than a mosquito) • **Promastigote** stage of the parasite is in the saliva of an infected sandfly; after injection, the promastigote transforms into the **amastigote** stage and invades the human reticuloendothelial cells where they multiply; rupture of the cells and further replication produces localized or disseminated disease • Sandflies become infected when they ingest a blood meal with amastigotes; these transform to infectious promastigotes in the fly midgut and migrate to the salivary gland during a blood meal • Clinical manifestations are a function of the species of parasite and immune status of patient
Clinical Disease	• **Cutaneous leishmaniasis**: a localized ulcer at the site of the bite • **Mucocutaneous leishmaniasis**: progression of disease with destruction of adjacent mucous membranes • **Disseminated or visceral leishmaniasis**: self-limited mild disease; fulminant disease with multiorgan destruction (e.g., liver, spleen, kidneys); or chronic process
Diagnosis	• Clinical diagnosis in endemic region confirmed by demonstration of amastigotes in tissue by microscopy, immunoassay, or NAATs
Treatment, Prevention, Control	• Treatment of choice for all forms of leishmaniasis is sodium stibogluconate, meglumine antimonite, or miltefosine; alternatives pentamidine or amphotericin B • Prevention by control of vector and treatment of infected humans

Two species of *Trypanosoma*, *Trypanosoma brucei* and *Trypanosoma cruzi*, produce very different diseases in different regions of the world, so they are presented separately. Additionally, *T. brucei* is subdivided into subspecies that are geographically restricted to regions of Africa and produce variants on the disease most commonly called **African Sleeping Sickness** due to the parasites' effects on the central nervous system.

TRYPANOSOMA BRUCEI

Epidemiology	• ***T. brucei gambiense*** in tropical West and Central Africa (Democratic Republic of Congo, Angola, Sudan, Central African Republic, Chad, northern Uganda) • ***T. brucei rhodensiense*** in East Africa (Tanzania, Uganda, Malawi, Zambia) • Animal reservoir for *T. b. gambiense* is most likely domestic animals and humans; reservoirs for *T. b. rhodensiense* are cattle, sheep, and wild game • Transmission by **tsetse flies** (*Glossina*) • An infected tsetse fly injects **trypomastigotes** into skin tissue during a blood meal; these mature and are transported by blood to other body fluids (cerebrospinal fluid, lymph) where replication continues • Tsetse flies become infected when they ingest bloodstream trypomastigotes that will multiply in the fly midgut; this form transforms into the **epimastigote** and migrates to the salivary glands where replication continues
Clinical Disease	• **African sleeping sickness**: *T. b. gambiense* disease develops after an incubation period of days to a few weeks; an ulcer may develop at the site of the bite; fever, myalgia, arthralgia, and lymph node enlargement; chronic disease progresses to central nervous system, involvement with lethargy, tremors, meningoencephalitis, mental retardation, and eventual death • *T. b. rhodensiense* disease has a more acute progression with death occurring in the first year in untreated patients
Diagnosis	• Detection of trypomastigotes in blood and spinal fluid is the diagnostic test of choice • Immunoassays and NAATs are insensitive
Treatment, Prevention, Control	• Suramin or pentamidine is used to treat acute infections; if central nervous system involvement is suspected, malarsoprol is the drug of choice • Control by reducing the human reservoir and insect control, although this is difficult in resource-limited countries

TRYPANOSOMA CRUZI

Epidemiology	• Mexico, Central America, and South America • Reservoir is a variety of wild animals and the vector for transmission is the **reduviid bug** (kissing bug) • Vector nests in homes, particularly with mud walls and thatched roofs • Human infections can also be transmitted congenitally, in contaminated blood products and following organ transplantation • Transmission occurs during a blood meal when **trypomastigotes** in the bug feces contaminate the bite wound; the parasites invade cells at the bite wound, transform into the **amastigote** stage, and replicate; the amastigote stage transforms in the trypomastigote stage and exits the cell to either reinfect other cells or be ingested by a feeding bug • In the reduviid bug, the trypomastigotes are transformed into epimastigotes and replicate in the midgut, which in turn are transformed into trypomastigotes in the hindgut
Clinical Disease	• **Asymptomatic disease** • **Acute Chagas disease**: characterized by erythema and induration at the site of the bug bite; followed by fever, chills, malaise, myalgia, and fatigue • **Chronic Chagas disease**: progression to chronic stage characterized by hepatosplenomegaly, myocarditis, and enlargement of the esophagus and colon; central nervous system involvement with meningoencephalitis may also occur
Diagnosis	• Detection of trypomastigotes in blood in the early stages of disease or amastigotes in infected tissues • Serology and NAATs are insensitive
Treatment, Prevention, Control	• All infected patients should be treated; the drugs of choice are benznidazole and nifurtimox, although these are less effective for chronic disease • Bug control through use of insecticides and quality home construction will reduce exposure

CLINICAL CASE

Trypanosomiasis

Herwaldt and colleagues[6] described a case in which the mother of an 18-month-old boy in Tennessee found a triatomine (reduviid) bug in his crib, which she saved because it resembled a bug shown on a television program about insects that prey on mammals. An entomologist identified the bug as Triatoma sanguisuga, *a vector of Chagas disease. The bug was found to be engorged with blood and infected with* T. cruzi. *The child had been intermittently febrile for the preceding 2 to 3 weeks but was otherwise healthy except for pharyngeal edema and multiple insect bites of unknown type on his legs. Whole-blood specimens obtained from the child were negative by buffy coat examination and hemoculture, but positive for* T. cruzi *by PCR and DNA hybridization, suggesting that he had low-level parasitemia. Specimens obtained after treatment with benznidazole were negative. He did not develop anti–*T. cruzi *antibody; 19 relatives and neighbors were also negative. Two of three raccoons trapped in the vicinity had positive hemocultures for* T. cruzi. *The child's case of* T. cruzi *infection—the fifth reported US autochthonous case—would have been missed without his mother's attentiveness and the availability of sensitive molecular techniques. Given that infected triatomine bugs and mammalian hosts exist in the southern United States, it is not surprising that humans could become infected with* T. cruzi. *Furthermore, given the nonspecific clinical manifestations of the infection, it is likely that other cases have been overlooked.*

REFERENCES

1. Liu C, Hung C, Chen M, Lai Y, Chen P, Huang S, Chen D. Amebic liver abscess and human immunodeficiency virus infection: a report of three cases. *J Clin Gastroenterol.* 2001;33:64–68.
2. Quiroz E, Bern C, MacArthur J, Xiao L, Fletcher M, Arrowood M, Shay D, Levy M, Glass R, Lal A. An outbreak of cryptosporidiosis linked to a foodhandler. *J Infect Dis.* 2000;181:695–700.
3. Abboud P, Lemée V, Gargala G, Brasseur P, Ballet J, Borsa-Lebas F, Caron F, Favennec L. Successful treatment of metronidazole- and albendazole-resistant giardiasis with nitazoxanide in a patient with acquired immunodeficiency syndrome. *Clin Infect Dis.* 2001;32:1792–1794.
4. Mohin G, Gupta A. A rare case of multiorgan failure associated with *Plasmodium vivax* malaria. *Infect Dis Clin Pract.* 2007;15:209–212.
5. Vincent. *Infect Med.* 2006;23:300.
6. Herwaldt B, Grijalva M, Newsome A, McGhee C, Powell M, Nemec D, Steurer F, Eberhard M. Use of polymerase chain reaction to diagnose the fifth reported US case of autochthonous transmission of *Trypanosoma cruzi*, in Tennessee 1998. *J Infect Dis.* 2000; 181:395–399.

24

Nematodes

INTERESTING FACTS

- *Enterobius* (pinworm) infections are the most common nematode infection in the United States
- An estimated 1 billion people worldwide are infected with *Trichuris* (whipworms); likewise, 1 billion people are infected with *Ascaris* (roundworms) and hookworms
- Elephantiasis (enlargement of arms, legs, and genitals due to blockage of the lymphatics) is caused by three blood roundworms: *Wuchereria bancrofti, Brugia malayi*, and *Brugia timori*
- Trichinosis is uncommon in the United States since the introduction of regulations for pork production, with most cases associated with consumption of undercooked wild game, e.g., bear meat

The helminths or "worms" are subdivided into three groups: nematodes ("roundworms"), trematodes ("flatworms"), and cestodes ("tapeworms"). Roundworms are presented in this chapter, and the flatworms and tapeworms in the following two chapters. It is easiest to remember roundworms based on where they are found in human infections.

Intestinal Nematodes	*Enterobius vermicularis* ("pinworm")
	Trichuris trichiura ("whipworm")
	Ascaris lumbricoides ("roundworm")
	Strongyloides stercoralis ("threadworm")
	Necator americanus and *Ancylostoma duodenale* ("hookworm")
Blood Nematodes	*Brugia malayi* ("Malayan filariasis" or "elephantiasis")
	Wuchereria bancrofti ("Bancroft filariasis" or "elephantiasis")
	Loa loa ("African eye worm")
	Onchocerca volvulus (onchocerciasis or "river blindness")
Tissue Nematodes	*Trichinella spiralis* ("trichinosis")
	Toxocara canis ("visceral larva migrans")
	Ancylostoma braziliense ("cutaneous larva migrans")

INTESTINAL NEMATODES

These nematodes share a number of important features. They have a simple lifecycle with **humans as their only hosts**, and infections are the result of ingestion of infectious eggs containing larvae (*Enterobius*, *Trichuris*, *Ascaris*) or exposure to larvae (*Strongyloides*, *Necator*, *Ancylostoma*) present in the soil that invade through exposed skin (i.e., bare feet). Because their lifecycles involve shedding of eggs or (with *Strongyloides*) larvae in feces, these are diseases in communities with poor sanitary conditions. The exception to this is infection with *Enterobius* where the adult worms deposit eggs on the anal folds at night and the eggs are infectious within a few hours. Enterobius infections are readily spread person-to-person so they are common in most communities. With the exception of *Enterobius*, asymptomatic infections with intestinal nematodes are common in residents of communities where the worms are endemic, while acute symptomatic disease is more common in previously unexposed visitors. Diagnosis is made by detecting characteristic eggs or larvae in fecal specimens, again with the exception of *Enterobius* where the eggs are deposited on the skin surrounding the anus and are not found in feces. Treatment for all these infections is the same, as are preventive measures. The following are some important general facts about the intestinal nematodes:

Intestinal Nematode	Route of Infection	Migration Through Lungs (Pneumonitis)	Diagnosis	Primary Treatment
Enterobius vermicularis	Ingestion of eggs	No	Eggs in anal folds	Albendazole, mebendazole
Trichuris trichiura	Ingestion of eggs	No	Eggs in stool	Albendazole, mebendazole
Ascaris lumbricoides	Larvae penetrate skin	Yes	Eggs in stool	Albendazole, mebendazole
Necator americanus	Larvae penetrate skin	Yes	Eggs in stool	Albendazole, mebendazole
Ancylostoma duodenale	Larvae penetrate skin	Yes	Eggs in stool	Albendazole, mebendazole
Strongyloides stercoralis	Larvae penetrate skin	Yes	Larvae in stool	Ivermectin

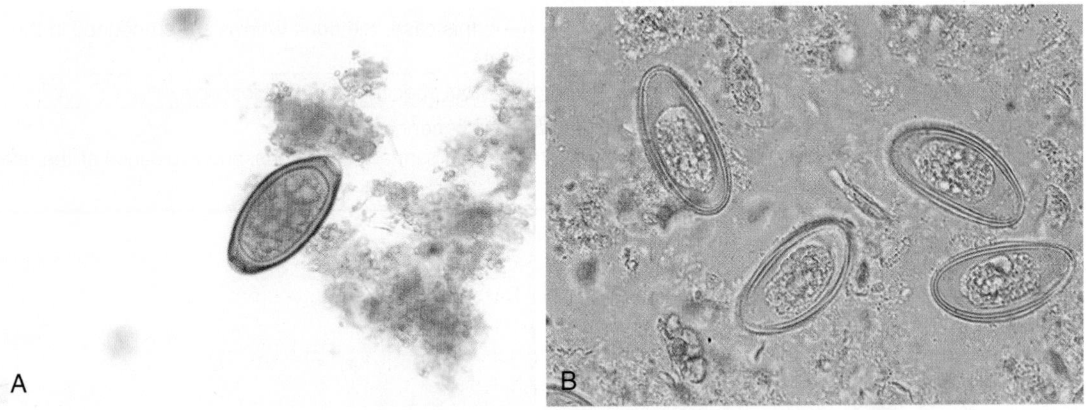

Eggs of (A) *Trichuris* in stool and (B) Enterobius in anal fold.

ENTEROBIUS VERMICULARIS	
Epidemiology	• Worldwide distribution • Humans are the only host for pinworm infections; no animal reservoir or insect vector • Infection through ingestion of eggs • Adults mature in 3–4 weeks and female worms migrate to the anus to discharge their eggs; the embryonated eggs develop to the infective stage in 4–6 hours • Infections most common in children, members of a household with children, and residents of institutionalized care facilities • Highly infectious for humans; pets and other animals are not susceptible to this parasite
Clinical Disease	• **Enterobiasis** characterized by irritation of the anal fold by the migrating adult worms when they deposit their eggs leading to severe itching and loss of sleep

Continued

ENTEROBIUS VERMICULARIS—cont'd	
Diagnosis	• Detection and identification of worm eggs at the anus; eggs are collected on a sticky paddle and examined by microscopy; occasionally small adult worms will also be observed • Eggs are not typically observed in stool specimens
Treatment, Prevention, Control	• The drug of choice is mebendazole, alternatives are albendazole or pyrantel pamoate; treatment consists of a single dose followed by another dose 2 weeks later • The entire household should be treated to reduce the risk of reinfections

TRICHURIS TRICHIURA	
Epidemiology	• Worldwide, particularly in tropical regions where sanitation is poor • Humans are the only hosts for whipworm infections; no animal reservoir or insect vector • Human infection by ingestion of embryonated egg, primarily from food products grown in soil contaminated with human feces • Eggs hatch in the small intestine, releasing the larval form that migrates to the **colon** where it develops into an adult worm; egg production begins after about 2 months; eggs are passed in the stool and require 2–4 weeks in soil to develop into infective forms
Clinical Disease	• **Asymptomatic infection** is the most common condition in endemic areas • Symptomatic **trichuriasis** may present with abdominal pain, bloody diarrhea, weakness, and weight loss; severe infections with rectal prolapse due to straining during defecation, and anemia and eosinophilia (characteristic findings in parasitic infections characterized by tissue invasion—in this case, the adult worms are embedded in the mucosal layer of the large intestine)
Diagnosis	• Detection of characteristic eggs in stool specimens by microscopy
Treatment, Prevention, Control	• The drug of choice is albendazole or mebendazole • Good personal hygiene, maintenance of sanitary conditions, and avoidance of the use of human feces as fertilizer

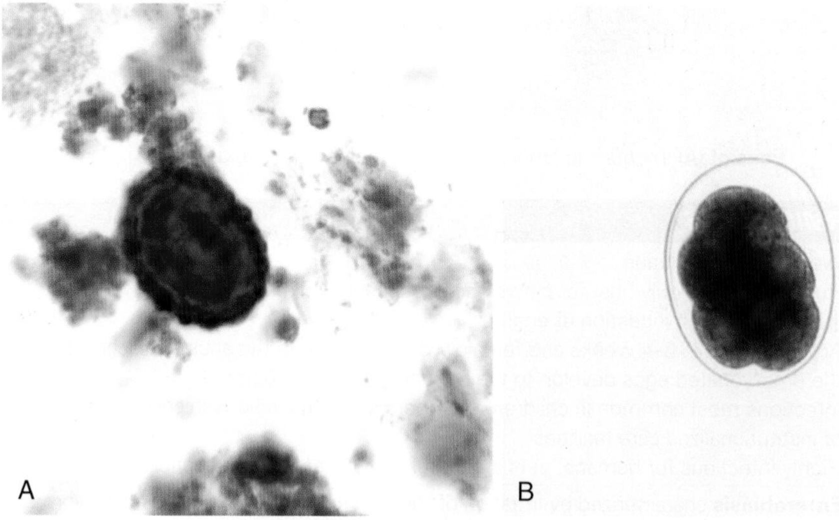

Eggs of (A) *Ascaris* and (B) hookworm in stool.

ASCARIS LUMBRICOIDES	
Epidemiology	• Worldwide distribution, particularly in tropical regions where sanitation is poor • Humans are the only hosts for roundworm infections; no animal reservoir or insect vector • Human infection by ingestion of embryonated egg, primarily from food products grown in soils contaminated with human feces • Eggs hatch in the **small intestine**, releasing the larval form that invades the intestinal mucosa and is carried by the circulatory system to the lungs, where larvae mature for approximately 2 weeks; they then penetrate the alveolar walls, ascend to the throat and are swallowed; the larvae mature into adult worms in the small intestine and initiate egg production approximately 3 months after the eggs were initially ingested
Clinical Disease	• **Asymptomatic infection** is the most common condition in endemic areas • Migration of the larvae through the lungs can produce an irritation (**pneumonitis**) with cough and eosinophilia • Symptomatic **ascariasis** can be mild abdominal discomfort (light infections) or intestinal obstruction (heavy infections with these very large adult worms)
Diagnosis	• Detection of characteristic eggs in stool specimens by microscopy • Passage of an adult worm can be alarming because of the size (20–35 cm) but is diagnostic because it is the largest of the intestinal helminths
Treatment, Prevention, Control	• The drug of choice is albendazole; alternatives are mebendazole or pyrantel pamoate • Good personal hygiene, maintenance of sanitary conditions, and avoidance of the use of human feces as fertilizer

CLINICAL CASE

Hepatic Ascariasis

Hurtado and colleagues[1] described a case of a 36-year-old woman who presented with recurrent right upper quadrant (RUQ) abdominal pain. One year earlier, she also presented with RUQ abdominal pain, abnormal liver function tests, and positive serology for hepatitis C. An abdominal ultrasonography examination showed biliary dilation and endoscopic retrograde cholangiopancreatography (ERCP) showed multiple stones in the common bile duct, left hepatic duct and left intrahepatic duct. The majority of the stones were removed. Examination of the bile-duct aspirate was negative for ova and parasites. One month before the more recent admission, the patient experienced recurrent RUQ pain and jaundice. Repeat ERCP again showed multiple stones in the common and left main hepatic ducts; partial removal was accomplished. One month later, the patient was admitted with severe epigastric pain and fever. The patient was born in Vietnam and had immigrated to the United States when she was in her early 20s. She had no history of recent travel. An abdominal computed tomography (CT) scan contrast showed abnormal perfusion of the left hepatic lobe and dilation of the left biliary radicles with multiple filing defects. ERCP showed partial obstruction of the left main hepatic duct, a few small stones, and purulent bile. Magnetic resonance imaging showed diffuse enhancement of the left lobe and left portal vein, suggestive of inflammation. Cultures of blood grew Klebsiella pneumoniae, *and examination of a stool sample revealed a few* Strongyloides stercoralis *rhabditiform larvae. Biliary stents were placed, and the patient was treated with levofloxacin. Two weeks later the patient was admitted to the hospital, where a partial hepatectomy was performed for treatment of recurrent pyogenic cholangitis. Gross examination of the left hepatic lobe showed ectatic bile ducts containing bile-stained calculi. Microscopic examination of the calculous material revealed collections of parasite eggs and a degenerated and fragmented nematode.* Klebsiella *spp. were identified in cultures by the microbiology laboratory. The findings were consistent with recurrent pyogenic cholangiohepatitis with infection by* Ascaris lumbricoides *and* Klebsiella *spp. In addition to antibiotics for the bacterial infection, the patient was treated with ivermectin for the* Strongyloides *infection and albendazole for the* Ascaris *organisms.*

NECATOR AMERICANUS AND ANCYLOSTOMA DUODENALE	
Epidemiology	• Worldwide although the individual parasites differ geographically • *N. americanus* distribution in the United States more limited with improved hygienic conditions • Present in warm, moist climates where the soil is contaminated with human feces • Humans are the only hosts for hookworm infections; no animal reservoir or insect vectors • Human infections occur when infectious larvae (**filariform larvae**) present in the soil penetrate exposed skin, migrate in the blood to the lungs, penetrate into the pulmonary alveoli, ascend to the pharynx and are swallowed; in the **small intestine** the larvae mature to adult worms, attach to the intestinal wall, and initiate egg production; eggs are passed in the stool and when in contact with the soil, release their immature larvae (**rhabditiform larvae**) which mature into the infectious filariform larvae in approximately 2 weeks
Clinical Disease	• **Asymptomatic infection** is the most common condition in endemic areas • Migration of the larvae through the lungs can produce an irritation (**pneumonitis**) with cough and eosinophilia • **Hookworm infections** can produce symptoms of nausea, vomiting, and diarrhea, as well as anemia from the feeding adult worms
Diagnosis	• Detection of characteristic eggs in stool specimens by microscopy • The eggs of both hookworms cannot be differentiated
Treatment, Prevention, Control	• The drugs of choice are albendazole, mebendazole, or pyrantel pamoate • Good personal hygiene, maintenance of sanitary conditions, and avoidance of contamination of soil with human feces

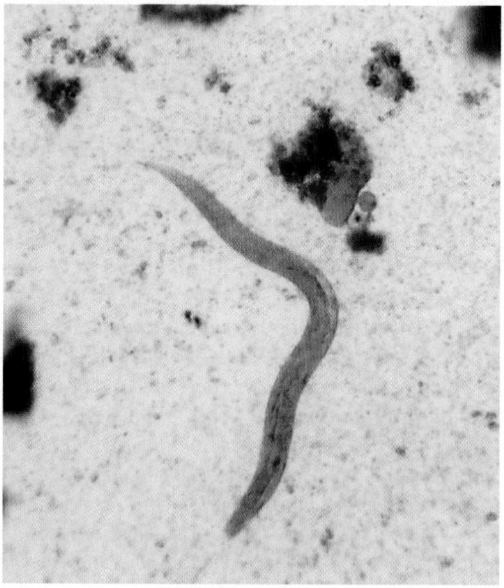

Strongyloides larva in stool.

STRONGYLOIDES STERCORALIS

Epidemiology	• Worldwide distribution, particularly in tropical regions where sanitation is poor • Estimated between 30 and 100 million persons are infected worldwide • Humans are the only hosts for threadworm infections; no animal reservoir or insect vectors • Lifecycle is very similar to hookworms; infectious filariform larvae present in the soil penetrate through exposed skin and migrate to the small intestine either directly or through the lungs; the worms mature into adults, attach to the wall of the **small intestine**, and produce eggs • In contrast with hookworms, the rhabditiform larvae in the eggs are released into the lumen of the intestine and that is the form detected in stool specimens • Rhabditiform larvae mature to filariform larvae in the soil; alternatively, rhabditiform larvae can mature to filariform larvae in patients with heavy worm burdens and reinfect the patient (autoinfection) without undergoing a stage of external development • Infections can persist for many years
Clinical Disease	• **Asymptomatic infection** is the most common condition in endemic areas • Migration of the larvae through the lungs can produce an irritation (**pneumonitis**) with cough and eosinophilia • Symptomatic **strongyloidiasis** can produce symptoms of epigastric pain and tenderness, vomiting, diarrhea, and malabsorption • Severe, chronic infections can develop in immunocompromised patients
Diagnosis	• Detection of larvae in stool specimens by microscopy; multiple specimens may need to be examined because shedding may be infrequent • Larvae can also be detected by spreading a stool specimen in the center of an agar plate; after overnight incubation, larvae can be detected by a trail of bacteria on the agar surface as the larvae migrates to the periphery of the plate
Treatment, Prevention, Control	• The drug of choice is ivermectin; alternatives are albendazole or mebendazole • Good personal hygiene, maintenance of sanitary conditions, and avoidance of contamination of soil with human feces

CLINICAL CASE

Strongyloides Hyperinfection

Gorman and colleagues2 described a case of necrotizing myositis complicated by diffuse alveolar hemorrhage and sepsis after corticosteroid therapy. The patient was a 46-year-old Cambodian man with a history of Raynaud phenomenon. He presented to the rheumatology clinic with worsening symptoms of Raynaud syndrome and diffuse muscle aches. He was employed as a truck driver and had emigrated from Cambodia 30 years earlier. Pertinent laboratory studies showed markedly elevated creatine kinase and aldolase levels. Pulmonary function studies showed decreased forced vital capacity, forced expiratory volume, and carbon monoxide diffusing capacity. A high-resolution CT scan of the chest showed mid ground-glass changes in both lung bases and interlobular septate thickenings. Muscle biopsy showed myocyte necrosis and random atrophy but no inflammatory cells. Bronchoscopy was unremarkable, and all cultures were negative. The patient was started on prednisone for presumed necrotizing myopathy secondary to undifferentiated connective tissue disease. He was admitted to the hospital 1 month later with profound muscle weakness and dyspnea, which improved with the administration of methylprednisolone and intravenous immunoglobulin. Three weeks later the patient was readmitted with fever, nausea, vomiting, abdominal pain, and diffuse joint pain. A CT scan of the abdomen suggested small bowel intussusception and colitis, but his symptoms improved without treatment. Another high-resolution CT scan of the chest showed early honeycombing and worsening interstitial infiltrates. The patient was scheduled for a lung biopsy; however, while awaiting the biopsy he suffered an abrupt fulminant deterioration with hemoptysis and hypoxemic respiratory failure that required intubation and mechanical verification. A chest radiograph showed new, diffuse, bilateral infiltrates. The patient developed an acute abdomen accompanied by purpura on the lower trunk. An abdominal CT showed pancolitis. Refractory septic shock caused by Escherichia coli *bacteremia and lactic acidosis ensued. Bronchoscopy showed diffuse alveolar hemorrhage, and numerous larvae of* S. stercoralis *were demonstrated on staining of an aspirate of*

CLINICAL CASE—cont'd

Strongyloides Hyperinfection

*endotracheal secretions. Serology was positive for anti-*Strongyloides *antibodies. Despite treatment with ivermectin, albendazole, cefepime, vancomycin, vasopressors, steroids, and dialysis, the patient died. This case of* Strongyloides *hyperinfection syndrome emphasizes the importance of screening and treating persons at risk for latent* S. stercoralis *infection (endemic in tropical and subtropical areas) before the initiation of immunosuppressive therapy. Contact precautions should be taken in patients with hyperinfection syndrome because of the risk of infection to health care workers and visitors upon exposure to infectious larvae in the patient's stool and secretions.*

BLOOD NEMATODES

The blood nematodes are grouped together because dissemination of **microfilariae** in the blood is an important feature of human disease. These nematodes have a more complex lifecycle with an **insect vector** important for transmission of all four parasites, but **humans are the only hosts**. Like the intestinal nematodes, there is **no animal reservoir** so control and elimination of disease is focused on rapid diagnosis and treatment of human disease, with insect control playing a secondary role. These diseases are also much more restricted in their geographic distributions, which offers a realistic opportunity to focus public health efforts on elimination of these diseases. However, it must be realized that a significant proportion of the population in endemic regions is infected asymptomatically. Disease is associated with migration of microfilariae in the blood and tissues and, with *Brugia* and *Wuchereria*, the obstruction of lymphatic flow with subsequent enlargement of distal tissues ("elephantiasis"). Diagnosis of disease is by detecting microfilariae in the blood of individuals (*Brugia*, *Wuchereria*, and *Loa*) or in the skin of patients infected with *Onchocerca*. The microfilariae have a characteristic morphology which allows differentiation of individual species. The following are some important general facts about the blood nematodes:

Blood Nematode	Vector	Location of Adult Worm	Diagnosis	Treatment (Microfilariae)
Brugia malayi	Mosquito	Lymphatics, lymph nodes	Microfilariae in blood	Diethylcarbamazine
Wuchereria bancrofti	Mosquito	Lymphatics, lymph nodes	Microfilariae in blood	Diethylcarbamazine
Loa loa	Deerfly	Subcutaneous tissues	Microfilariae in blood	Diethylcarbamazine
Onchocerca volvulus	Blackfly	Subcutaneous tissues	Microfilariae in skin	Ivermectin

BRUGIA MALAYI* AND *WUCHERERIA BANCROFTI	
Epidemiology	• Broad geographic distribution in tropical and subtropical areas of Africa, Mediterranean coast, India, Southeast Asia, Japan, parts of the Caribbean, and South America • An estimated 120 million people are infected worldwide • Infectious larvae transmitted to humans by **mosquito** bite; larvae migrate to **lymphatics and lymph nodes** where they develop into adult worms; female worm produces microfilariae which circulate in the blood and can infect a biting mosquito; after 1–2 weeks in the mosquito, the microfilariae develop into infectious filariform larvae
Clinical Disease	• Early symptoms of **filariasis** are fever, lymphangitis and lymphadenitis with chills, and recurrent fevers • Progressive infection with lymph node swelling leading to obstruction by adult worms with subsequent enlargement of distal tissues (**elephantiasis**)
Diagnosis	• Demonstration of microfilariae in the peripheral blood by microscopy
Treatment, Prevention, Control	• Diethylcarbamazine is the drug of choice for treating microfilariae but is not effective against the adult worms; alternative is albendazole • Mosquito control and use of protective clothing and insect repellents reduce the risk of exposure • Treatment of patients reduces the risk of human-to-mosquito-to-human transmission

LOA LOA	
Epidemiology	• West and Central African countries where as many as 80% of the residents in the rain forests in some countries report a history of infection • Human infection (**loiasis** or **African eye worm** infection) from the bite of the **deerfly** in the genus *Chrysops* • Deerflies most active in the day during the rainy season • Infectious larvae are transmitted to humans by the bite of the infected fly; larvae develop into adults in the subcutaneous tissues and produce microfilariae; during the day (corresponding to the feeding patterns of the fly) the microfilariae are in the patient's blood; flies ingest the microfilariae during their blood meal and these will migrate to the thoracic muscles of the fly where they develop into infectious larvae; larvae then migrate to the fly's proboscis from where they can then be transmitted during the next meal
Clinical Disease	• **Asymptomatic infection** is the most common condition in endemic areas • Symptomatic **loiasis** most commonly presents with itching over the entire body, muscle and joint pains, and tiredness • **Calabar swellings**: localized, nontender swellings that occur most commonly on the extremities; associated with itching • **Eye worm**: migration of an adult worm across the surface of the eye, associated with eye pain, itching, and light sensitivity; permanent damage to the eye does not occur
Diagnosis	• Diagnosis by clinical signs (Calabar swellings with associated pruritis; observation of adult worm in the eye) confirmed by the presence of microfilariae in the blood during daytime hours
Treatment, Prevention, Control	• Diethylcarbamazine is the drug of choice for treating microfilariae and adult worms, but may result in severe allergic reaction • Protection from fly bites and use of insect repellents • Prompt treatment of infected individuals

ONCHOCERCA VOLVULUS	
Epidemiology	• Distribution in sub-Saharan Africa, Yemen, Brazil, and Venezuela • Human infection (**onchocerciasis** or "**river blindness**") from the bite of the **blackfly** in the genus *Simulium* • Blackflies are active around streams and rivers • Multiple bites are generally necessary for transmission so infections are rare in short-term visitors • Infectious larvae are transmitted to humans by the bite of the infected fly; larvae develop into adults in the subcutaneous connective tissues and produce microfilariae; microfilariae are primarily in the skin and lymphatics of connective tissues, but also occasionally in the blood, urine, and sputum; flies ingest the microfilariae during their blood meal and these will migrate to the thoracic muscles of the fly where they develop into infectious larvae; larvae then migrate to the fly's proboscis from where they can then be transmitted during the next meal
Clinical Disease	• **Onchocerciasis** characterized by involvement of the skin, subcutaneous tissue, lymph nodes, and eyes; acute and chronic inflammation in response to microfilariae as they migrate through the skin; infection of the cornea leads to conjunctivitis progressing to sclerosing keratitis and eventual **blindness** • **Skin nodules** with loss of elasticity and depigmentation; pruritis, hyperkeratosis, and thickening
Diagnosis	• Demonstration of microfilariae in the skin; skin surface shaved with a razor, placed in saline, and after a few hours examined for microfilariae
Treatment, Prevention, Control	• Surgical removal of encapsulated nodules with adult worms; single dose of ivermectin to reduce the microfilariae but does not kill the adult worms • Humans are the reservoir of infections so control of human infections will control disease; mass chemotherapy of populations in endemic regions with ivermectin reduces the burden of disease and reduces the risk of transmission • Control of the insect vector is difficult

CLINICAL CASE

Onchocerciasis

Choudhary and Choudhary[3] *described the case of a 21-year-old man who emigrated from Sudan to the United States 1 year before presenting with a maculopapular rash that was associated with severe pruritus. The rash and pruritus had been present for the past 3 to 4 years. In the past, the patient had undergone multiple treatments for this condition, including corticosteroids, without relief. The patient denied any systemic symptoms but did complain of blurred vision. On physical examination, his skin was somewhat thickened over different parts of the body, and he had scattered maculopapular lesions with increased pigmentation; some lesions had keloid nodules as well as wrinkling. There was no lymphadenopathy. The remainder of his evaluation was unremarkable. Because of the presence of intense pruritus unresponsive to treatment, blurred vision, and the prevalence of onchocerciasis in his native country, skin snips were taken from the scapular area. Microfilariae of* Onchocerca volvulus *were revealed on microscopic examination. Ivermectin was prescribed, to which the patient's condition responded. Onchocerciasis, although not common in the United States, should be considered in immigrants and expatriates with suggestive symptoms if they came from areas in which the disease is endemic.*

TISSUE NEMATODES

Tissue nematodes differ from the other roundworms in that humans are dead-end, accidental hosts and animal reservoirs are important for these diseases. In these infections the complete lifecycle occurs within the host so transmission to humans is by accidental exposure to infectious larvae in meat (*Trichinella*) or eggs (*Toxocara*, dog roundworm; *Ancylostoma braziliense*, dog hookworm). In infections with *Toxocara* and *A. braziliense* the eggs are not passed in feces to complete their lifecycle in the environment; instead, the eggs hatch and the larvae wander in tissues producing their disease. With *Trichinella* infections, the larvae move through tissues and become encysted, primarily in muscles. Because *Trichinella* infections are the most common, these are summarized here.

TRICHINELLA SPIRALIS	
Epidemiology	• Worldwide distribution • Human disease produced when eating raw or undercooked meat from an infected animal with encysted larvae in striated muscle • Transmission most commonly associated with ingestion of undercooked pork although many carnivorous animals are infected • The larvae leave the meat in the small intestine, develop into adults within 2 days, and initiate production of larvae within 3 months; larvae migrate to **striated muscles** and encyst • The lifecycle of *T. spiralis* in pigs and other animals is identical to human disease
Clinical Disease	• Acute, early symptoms of **trichinosis** are fever, lymphangitis, and lymphadenitis with chills, recurrent febrile attacks, and eosinophilia • Symptoms in progressive disease related to the host inflammatory response to migrating microfilariae, obstruction of lymphatics by the worms with subsequent enlargement of tissues (e.g., **filarial elephantiasis**) and muscle pain
Diagnosis	• Clinical symptoms and a history of consumption of improperly cooked pork or bear meat, confirmed by serology or observation of encysted larvae in a muscle biopsy
Treatment, Prevention, Control	• Symptomatic because there are no effective treatments for larvae in tissues; mebendazole is used to treat adult worms • Disease in the United States has been significantly reduced by implementation of controls in the domestic pork industry; however, pigs raised on farms with exposure to rodents are at significant risk of acquiring infections • Pork and bear meat should be cooked thoroughly; microwave, smoking, or drying meat does not kill all larvae

REFERENCES

1. Hurtado RM, Sahani DV, Kradin RL. Case records of the Massachusetts General Hospital. Case 9-2006. A 35-year-old woman with recurrent right-upper-quadrant pain. *N Engl J Med*. 2006;354:1295-1301.
2. Gorman S, Duncan R, Dellaripa P. Recognizing Strongyloides hyperinfection. *Infect Med*. 2006;23:480–484.
3. Choudhary IA, Choudhary SA. Resistant pruritus and rash in an immigrant. *Infect Med*. 2005;22:187–189.

25

Trematodes

INTERESTING FACTS

- Although humans can be a host for fluke infections, person-to-person spread does not occur because intermediate hosts are required
- Human fluke infections are acquired by consumption of raw aquatic plants (*Fasciolopsis buski, Fasciola hepatica*) or undercooked freshwater fish (*Opisthorchis sinensis* [also known as *Clonorchis sinensis*]) or crustaceans (*Paragonimus westermani*)
- Adult Chinese liver flukes (*O. sinensis*) may persist in the human gall bladder for up to 50 years, so infection is frequently seen in Asian refugees many years after they have left the endemic region
- In contrast with other fluke infections, human disease with *Schistosoma* follows direct skin penetration with the parasite (cercariae stage) rather than consumption of an undercooked food product

The trematodes (also called **flatworms** or **flukes**, based on the shape of the adult worms) are more geographically restricted compared to other parasites. This is because of the complexity of their lifecycle. All of these parasites have a **primary host** where adult worms are found and an **intermediate host** where larval forms mature. In each example in this chapter, the intermediate host is a snail. In the cases of the intestinal and tissue trematodes, there is a second intermediate host (this does not exist with the blood trematodes).

Site of Infection	Flatworm	Primary Host	First Intermediate Host	Second Intermediate Host	Treatment
Intestinal Trematode	*Fasciolopsis buski* ("giant liver fluke")	Pigs, dogs, rabbits; **humans are accidental hosts**	Snail	Aquatic plants (e.g., water chestnuts)	Praziquantel
Tissue Trematodes	*Fasciola hepatica* ("sheep liver fluke")	Herbivores (sheep, cattle); **humans are accidental hosts**	Snail	Aquatic plants (e.g., watercress)	Triclabendazole
	Opisthorchis sinensis ("Chinese liver fluke")	Dogs, cats, fish-eating mammals; **humans are accidental hosts**	Snail	Freshwater fish	Praziquantel
	Paragonimus westermani ("oriental lung fluke")	Wild boars, pigs, monkeys; **humans are accidental hosts**	Snail	Freshwater crustaceans (e.g., crabs, crayfish)	Praziquantel

Site of Infection	Flatworm	Primary Host	First Intermediate Host	Second Intermediate Host	Treatment
Blood Trematodes	*Schistosoma mansoni* ("intestinal bilharziasis")	Primates, rodents, marsupials; **humans are accidental hosts**	Snail	None	Praziquantel
	Schistosoma japonica ("oriental blood fluke")	Cats, dogs, cattle, horses, pigs; **humans are accidental hosts**	Snail	None	Praziquantel
	Schistosoma haematobium ("urinary bilharziasis")	Monkeys, baboons, chimpanzees; **humans are accidental hosts**	Snail	None	Praziquantel

INTESTINAL TREMATODE

A number of intestinal flukes exist in different regions of Southeast Asia and China, with *F. buski* the largest and most common. Epidemiology, disease, and treatment of these flukes are similar, so *F. buski* is presented as a model for these infections.

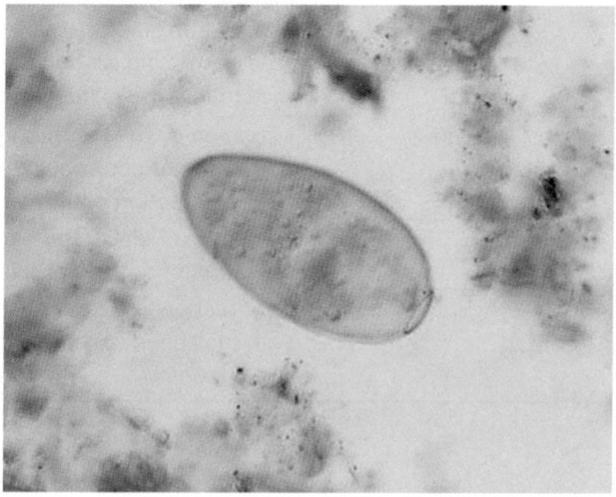

Egg of *Fasciolopsis*.

FASCIOLOPSIS BUSKI	
Epidemiology	• Present in China, Vietnam, Thailand, Indonesia, Malaysia, and India • Reservoir hosts are pigs, dogs, and rabbits; humans are accidental hosts • Human exposure to encysted larvae (**metacercariae**) when the husks from aquatic vegetables (e.g., **water chestnuts**) are peeled with the teeth; larvae are swallowed and develop into immature flukes in the duodenum; attach to mucosa of the small intestine and develop into adults; eggs are produced and passed in feces • Free-swimming larvae (**miracidia**) hatch from the eggs, penetrate snails, and undergo maturation; final stage (**cercariae**) released from snails and encyst on aquatic vegetation
Clinical Disease	• Attachment of adult worms to the small intestine produces inflammation, ulceration, and hemorrhage; abdominal discomfort and diarrhea; **malabsorption syndrome** • Marked eosinophilia
Diagnosis	• Detection of characteristic eggs in feces; adult flukes are rarely observed in feces
Treatment, Prevention, Control	• The drug of choice is praziquantel; niclosamide is an alternative • Implementation of proper sanitation and control of human feces reduces the incidence of infections

TISSUE TREMATODES

The tissue trematodes have a very similar lifecycle to *F. buski* except the adult worm does not reside in the intestines. The adult forms of two worms reside in the gall bladder (*F. hepatica* and *O. sinensis*) and their characteristic eggs are found in the feces, while the third worm (*P. westermani*) lives in the lungs and the eggs are expectorated in sputum (if swallowed they would be found in stool specimens).

FASCIOLA HEPATICA	
Epidemiology	• Worldwide distribution in sheep- and cattle-raising areas, including former Soviet Union, Japan, Egypt, and many Latin American countries • Reservoir hosts are herbivores, particularly sheep and cattle; humans are accidental hosts • Human exposure to ingestion of **watercress** with encysted metacercariae; flukes migrate through the duodenal wall to the liver and then to the **gallbladder** where they mature into adults; eggs are produced and passed in the feces • Free-swimming larvae (miracidia) hatch from the eggs, penetrate snails, and undergo maturation; final stage (cercariae) released from snails and encyst on aquatic vegetation
Clinical Disease	• Migration of worms through the liver produces inflammation, tenderness, and hepatomegaly; right upper quadrant pain, fever, and eosinophilia • Severe infection with biliary obstruction, hepatitis, and cirrhosis
Diagnosis	• Detection of characteristic eggs in the feces; eggs indistinguishable from *F. buski* so detection of eggs in gallbladder confirms diagnosis of *F. hepatica* infection
Treatment, Prevention, Control	• Poor response to praziquantel (reason important to differentiate from *F. buski*); treat with triclabendazole; alternative is bithionol • Avoid ingestion of watercress and uncooked aquatic vegetation in endemic areas

CLINICAL CASE

Fascioliasis

Echenique-Elizondo and colleagues[1] described a case of acute pancreatitis caused by the liver fluke F. hepatica. *The patient was a 31-year-old female who was admitted to the hospital because of a sudden onset of nausea and upper abdominal pain. She was otherwise healthy and gave a negative history of drug abuse, alcohol ingestion, gallstone disease, abdominal trauma, or surgery. On physical examination, she was markedly tender in the epigastric region and had hypoactive bowel sounds. Serum chemistries showed elevated pancreatic enzymes (amylase, lipase, pancreatic phospholipase A2, and elastase). Her white blood cell count was elevated, as were tests for alkaline phosphatase and bilirubin. Serum blood urea nitrogen, creatinine, lactate dehydrogenase, and calcium were normal. Abdominal ultrasonography and computed tomographic scan showed diffuse enlargement of the pancreas, and a cholangiogram demonstrated dilation and numerous filing defects in the common bile duct. An endoscopic sphincterotomy was performed, with extraction of numerous large flukes that were identified as* F. hepatica. *The patient was treated with a single oral dose of triclabendazole (10 mg/kg). Follow-up demonstrated normal blood chemistries and no evidence of disease 2 years postprocedure.*

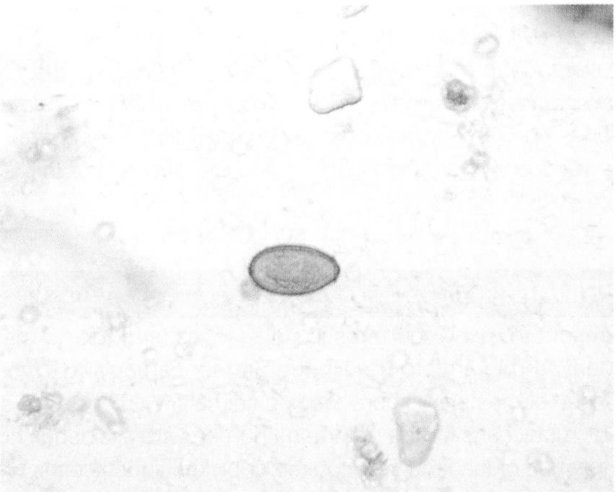

Egg of *Opisthorchis*.

OPISTHORCHIS SINENSIS	
Epidemiology	• Present in China, Japan, Korea, and Vietnam • Reservoir hosts are dogs, cats, and fish-eating mammals; humans are accidental hosts • Human exposure to ingestion of **uncooked freshwater fish** with encysted metacercariae; flukes migrate through the duodenal wall to the liver and then to the **gallbladder** where they mature to adults; eggs are produced and passed in feces • In contrast with *F. hepatica*, the eggs are ingested by snails and undergo maturation; final stage (cercariae) released from snails and penetrate under the scales of freshwater fish where they develop into metacercariae
Clinical Disease	• Usually asymptomatic or mild • Severe infections of the gallbladder results in fever, diarrhea, epigastric pain, hepatomegaly, anorexia, and jaundice; eosinophilia; biliary obstruction • Chronic infection can result in adenocarcinoma of bile ducts
Diagnosis	• Detection of characteristic small eggs in feces
Treatment, Prevention, Control	• The drug of choice is praziquantel; alternative is albendazole • Avoid eating uncooked freshwater fish; implement proper sanitation policies including disposal of human, dog, and cat feces in sites that avoid contamination of water

CLINICAL CASE

Cholangitis Caused by *Opisthorchis Sinensis*

Stunell and colleagues[2] described a 34-year-old Asian woman who presented to a local emergency department with a 2-day history of right upper quadrant abdominal pain, fever, and rigors. She had emigrated from Asia to Ireland 18 months earlier and gave a history of intermittent upper abdominal pain occurring over a 3-year period. On examination, she appeared acutely ill and was clammy to the touch. She was febrile, tachycardic, and had mild scleral icterus. Her abdomen was tender, with guarding in the upper right quadrant. Routine hematologic and biochemical studies revealed a marked leukocytosis and obstructive liver function tests. Contrast-enhanced computed tomography of the abdomen demonstrated evidence of multiple ovoid opacities within dilated intrahepatic bile ducts in the right lobe of the liver. The remainder of the liver parenchyma appeared normal. Upon stabilization of the patient, an endoscopic retrograde cholangiopancreatography was performed for biliary decompression. This demonstrated intrahepatic and extrahepatic bile duct dilation, with multiple filing defects and strictures. A stool sample sent for

Continued

analysis confirmed the presence of ova and adult flukes of O. sinensis. *The patient recovered with medical management (praziquantel) and had negative stool samples 30 days after treatment. This case, as well as the previous clinical case, demonstrates the various complications of liver fluke infestation. Of note, praziquantel is the drug of choice for treating the Oriental liver fluke* (O. sinensis), *whereas triclabendazole is used to treat fascioliasis, thus emphasizing the importance of an epidemiologic history and identification of the fluke.*

PARAGONIMUS WESTERMANI	
Epidemiology	• Present in many countries in Asia, Africa, and Latin America • Many immigrants to the United States, particularly from Indonesia, are infected • Reservoir hosts are shore-feeding animals (wild boars, pigs, monkeys) that ingest infected crustaceans (**crabs, crayfish**); humans are accidental hosts with infections following ingestion of inadequately cooked or pickled crustaceans with encysted metacercariae • In humans the metacercariae hatch in the stomach, migrate through the intestinal wall to the abdominal cavity, through the diaphragm, to the pleural cavity; adult worms in lungs produce eggs that appear in sputum or are swallowed and found in feces • Embryonated eggs passed by the reservoir hosts hatch releasing miracidia that penetrate snails; after maturation in the snail, cercariae are released, invade crustaceans, and develop in metacercariae that encyst in the tissues
Clinical Disease	• Symptoms correspond to migration of larvae through tissues and are associated with fever, chills, and high eosinophilia • Adult worms stimulate an inflammatory response with fever, cough, and increased sputum production • Progressive infections lead to cavitary lung disease and fibrosis of lung tissues
Diagnosis	• Detection of characteristic eggs in sputum or pleural effusion
Treatment, Prevention, Control	• Drug of choice is praziquantel; alternative is triclabendazole • Avoid consumption of uncooked or pickled crabs and crayfish, as well as meat from animals in the endemic regions • Proper sanitation and control of the disposal of human feces are essential

CLINICAL CASE

Paragonimiasis

Singh and colleagues[3] described a case of pleuropulmonary paragonimiasis mimicking pulmonary tuberculosis. The patient was a 21-year-old man who was admitted to the hospital for progressive dyspnea, with a 1-month history of headache, fever, cough with scant hemoptysis, fatigue, pleuritic pain, anorexia, and weight loss. He had a history of antituberculous therapy for 6 months without clinical improvement. Two months before admission, after ingesting three raw crabs, he had a 3-day episode of watery diarrhea. On hospital admission the patient was cachectic and afebrile. There was bilateral dullness to percussion and absent breath sounds in the lower two-thirds of the chest. He was found to be anemic and had clubbing without lymphadenopathy, cyanosis, or jaundice. A chest radiograph showed bilateral pleural effusions that were also confirmed by computed tomography. Ultrasound-guided thoracentesis of the right lung yielded about 200 mL of yellowish fluid. The fluid was exudative and contained 2700 white blood cells/mL, 91% of which were eosinophils. Gram stain of the fluid was negative, as was culture for bacteria and fungi. Sputum smears revealed operculated yellowish eggs consistent with Paragonimus westermani *infection. The patient was treated with a 3-day course of praziquantel and responded well. Of note, the right-sided plural effusion did not recur after the thoracentesis and praziquantel treatment. This case emphasizes the importance of making an etiologic diagnosis of a pleuropulmonary process to differentiate paragonimiasis from tuberculosis in regions where both are endemic infectious diseases.*

BLOOD TREMATODES

Schistosomes differ from the other flukes in that male and female worms exist and they are intravascular parasites—the adult worms are not found in the intestines, tissues, or cavities. As with the other flukes, snails are an important intermediate host, but the free-swimming cercariae that are released from the snails directly penetrate human skin rather than establishing residence on a secondary host. Disease is related to where the adults establish residence in the circulatory system and release their eggs.

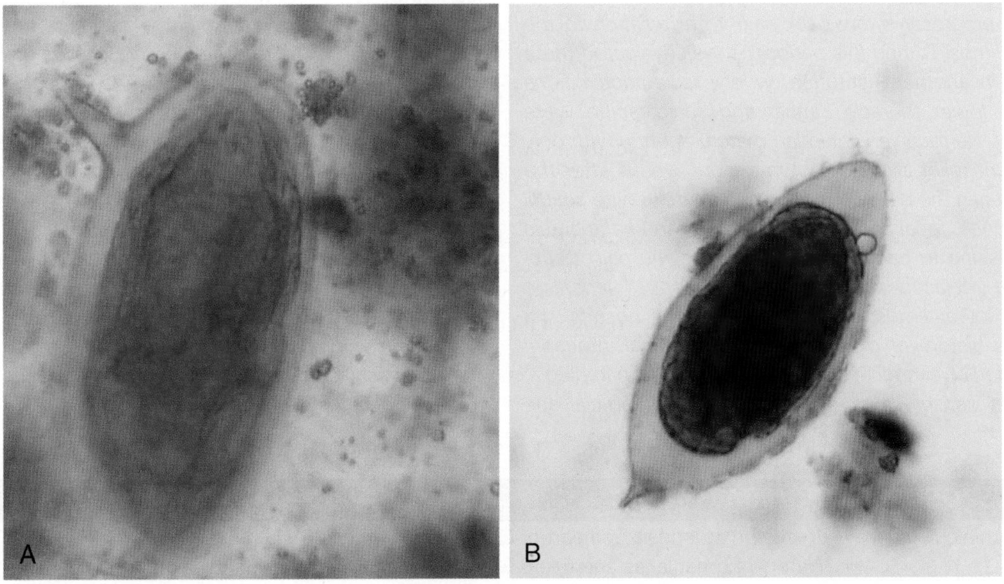

(A) *Schistosoma mansoni* (note lateral spine) and (B) *Schistosoma haematobium* (note terminal spine).

SCHISTOSOMA MANSONI	
Epidemiology	• *S. mansoni* is the most widespread schistosome; endemic in southern and sub-Saharan Africa, the Nile River valley in Sudan and Egypt, South America including Brazil, Suriname, and Venezuela, and the Caribbean West Indies • Waters of great lakes and rivers where host snail is present and sanitation is poor • Reservoir host include primates, marsupials, and rodents; snails are intermediate hosts • Residents (and tourists), particularly children, at risk when swimming or bathing in waters contaminated with free-swimming cercariae • After skin penetration, the parasites enter the circulatory system and migrate to portal blood in the liver and mature to adults; paired adult male and female worms migrate to the inferior mesenteric vein near the lower colon, laying eggs that circulate to the liver and are shed in stools
Clinical Disease	• Penetration through the skin results in itching, allergic reaction, and dermatitis • Migration through the lungs and liver results in cough and hepatitis, respectively • Egg laying by adult worms produces fever, malaise, abdominal pain, and liver tenderness; inflammation and thickening of the bowel wall is related to inflammatory response to deposited eggs with abdominal pain, diarrhea, and bloody stools • Chronic infections with hepatosplenomegaly
Diagnosis	• Detection of characteristic eggs in feces
Treatment, Prevention, Control	• The drug of choice is praziquantel; alternative is oxamniquine; treatment terminates egg production but does not alleviate the host response to deposited eggs • Implementation of proper sanitation and control of human feces reduces the incidence of infections

CLINICAL CASE

Schistosomiasis

Ferrari[4] described a case of neuroschistosomiasis caused by Schistosoma mansoni *in an 18-year-old Brazilian man. The patient was admitted to the hospital because of the recent onset of paraplegia. He was in good health until 33 days before admission, when he noted the onset of progressive low back pain with radiation to the lower limbs. During this period, he was evaluated three times in another institution, where radiographic films of the lower thoracic lumbar and sacral spine were normal. He received antiinflammatory agents, with only transient relief in his symptoms. Four weeks after the pain began the disease progressed acutely, with sexual impotence, fecal and urinary retention, and paraparesis progressing to paraplegia. At this time the pain disappeared, replaced by a marked impairment of sensation in the lower limbs. On admission to the hospital, he gave a history of exposure to schistosomal infection. Neurologic examination revealed flaccid paraplegia, marked sensory loss, and absence of superficial and deep reflexes at and below the level T11. The cerebrospinal fluid contained 84 white blood cells/mL (98% lymphocytes, 2% eosinophils) and 1 red blood cell, 82 mg/dL total protein, and 61 mg/dL glucose. Myelography, computed tomography-myelography, and magnetic resonance imaging showed a slight widening of the conus. The diagnosis of neuroschistosomiasis was confirmed by the demonstration of viable and dead eggs of* S. mansoni *on rectal mucosal biopsy. The concentration of cerebrospinal fluid immunoglobulin G against soluble egg antigen of* S. mansoni *quantitated by enzyme-linked immunosorbent assay was 1.53 μg/mL. He was treated with prednisone and praziquantel. Despite therapy, his condition remained unaltered at follow-up 7 months later.* S. mansoni *is the most frequently reported cause of schistosomal myeloradiculopathy worldwide. Schistosomal myeloradiculopathy is among the most severe forms of schistosomiasis, and prognosis depends largely on early diagnosis and treatment.*

SCHISTOSOMA JAPONICA	
Epidemiology	• Present in Indonesia and part of China and Southeast Asia • Waters of great lakes and rivers where host snail is present and sanitation is poor • Reservoir hosts include cats, dogs, cattle, horses, and pigs • Residents (and tourists), particularly children, at risk when swimming or bathing in waters contaminated with free-swimming cercariae • After skin penetration, the parasites enter the circulatory system and migrate to portal blood in the liver and mature to adults; paired adult male and female worms migrate to the superior mesenteric vein near the small intestine and the inferior mesenteric vein, laying eggs that circulate to liver and are shed in stools
Clinical Disease	• Similar to *S. mansoni* infections; however, smaller eggs and higher egg production can lead to more severe disease and dissemination to other organs including the brain
Diagnosis	• Detection of characteristic eggs in feces
Treatment, Prevention, Control	• Drug of choice is praziquantel • Implementation of proper sanitation and control of human feces reduces the incidence of infections

SCHISTOSOMA HAEMATOBIUM	
Epidemiology	• Present throughout Africa; also in Cyprus, southern Portugal, and India • Waters of great lakes and rivers where host snail is present and sanitation is poor • Reservoir hosts include monkeys, baboons, and chimpanzees • Residents (and tourists), particularly children, at risk when swimming or bathing in waters contaminated with free-swimming cercariae • After skin penetration, the parasites enter the circulatory system and migrate to vesical, prostatic, and uterine plexuses of the venous circulation and mature into adults; large eggs are produced and deposited in the bladder wall as well as uterine and prostatic tissues

SCHISTOSOMA HAEMATOBIUM—cont'd	
Clinical Disease	• Early stages of disease as with other schistosomes with dermatitis, allergic reactions, fever, and malaise • Disease progresses to urinary symptoms including hematuria, dysuria, and urinary frequency • Chronic infections associated with bladder carcinoma
Diagnosis	• Detection of characteristic eggs in urine; eggs not found in the feces
Treatment, Prevention, Control	• Drug of choice is praziquantel

REFERENCES

1. Echenique-Elizondo M, Amondarain J, Lirón de Robles C. Fascioliasis: an exceptional cause of acute pancreatitis. *JOP*. 2005;6:36–39.
2. Stunell H, Buckley O, Geoghegan T, Torreggiani WC. Recurrent pyogenic cholangitis due to chronic infestation with *Clonorchis sinensis* (2006: 8b). *Eur Radiol.* 2006;16:2612–2614.
3. Singh TN, Kananbala S, Devi KS. Pleuropulmonary paragonimiasis mimicking pulmonary tuberculosis—a report of three cases. *Indian J Med Microbiol.* 2005;23:131–134.
4. Ferrari TC. Spinal cord schistosomiasis. a report of 2 cases and review emphasizing clinical aspects. *Medicine (Baltimore).* 1999;78:176–190.

26

Cestodes

INTERESTING FACTS

- Tapeworm infections in the United States are relatively uncommon, with the most common infections caused by *Hymenolepis nana* (mouse tapeworm), and *Diphyllobothrium latum* (fish tapeworm)
- Adult tapeworms can range in size from a few centimeters (*H. nana*) to more than 10 m long (*D. latum* and *Taenia saginata*)
- Adult tapeworms consist of a head and long, segmented body or proglottids, with the head the smallest unit and the most distal proglottids the largest
- *Echinococcus* eggs deposited in the soil can remain infectious for up to 1 year
- Human infections with *Echinococcus multilocularis* can remain asymptomatic for 5 to 15 years but untreated infections are progressive and fatal

Cestodes are flat, ribbon-like worms (the reason they are called "**tapeworms**") that have a head (**scolex**) with suckers and hooks for attachment to the intestinal wall and a long segmented body (**proglottids**). The worms are hermaphroditic, so as they develop the segments closest to the head are immature and the most distal proglottids are gravid (filled with eggs). These gravid proglottids break off from the worm and are shed in the feces. The morphologic features of the proglottids and eggs are the diagnostic clues that are used to distinguish these worms. The size of these worms is impressive, with *T. saginata* and *D. latum* up to 30 feet long and *H. nana* and *Dipylidium caninum* only a few inches long. The lifecycles of tapeworms generally involve at least two hosts, with the adult worms developing in the primary host and the larval forms developing in the intermediate host. Human disease is primarily restricted to intestinal symptoms, except for infection where humans are accidental secondary hosts.

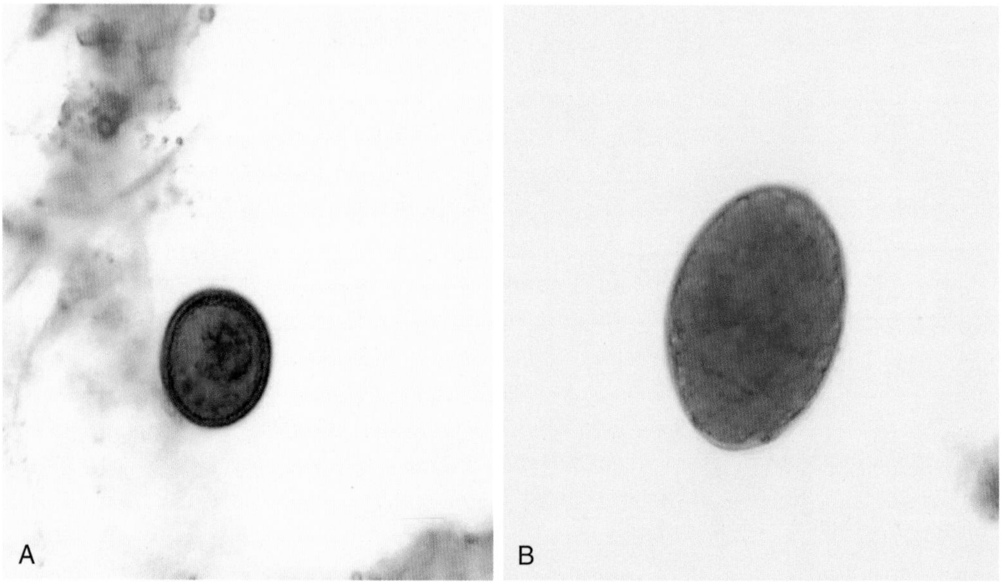

Eggs of (A) *Taenia* and (B) *Diphyllobothrium*.

Site of Infection	Tapeworm	Primary Host	Intermediate Host	Treatment
Intestinal Cestodes	*Taenia saginata* ("beef tapeworm")	Humans	Cattle	Praziquantel, niclosamide
	Taenia solium ("pork tapeworm")	Humans	Pigs	Praziquantel, niclosamide
	Diphyllobothrium latum ("fish tapeworm")	Humans	Copepods (1st stage), fish (2nd stage)	Praziquantel, niclosamide
	Hymenolepis nana ("dwarf tapeworm")	Mice; **humans are accidental hosts**	Beetles	Praziquantel, niclosamide
	Hymenolepis diminuta ("rat tapeworm")	Rats; **humans are accidental hosts**	Beetles	Praziquantel, niclosamide
	Dipylidium caninum ("dog tapeworm")	Dogs, cats; **humans are accidental hosts**	Fleas	Praziquantel, niclosamide
Tissue Cestodes	*Taenia solium* ("cysticercosis")	Humans	**Humans are accidental hosts**	Praziquantel, niclosamide
	Echinococcus granulosus ("unilocular cystic hydatid disease")	Dogs	Sheep, cattle, goats, pigs; **humans are accidental hosts**	Albendazole
	Echinococcus multilocularis ("alveolar hydatid disease")	Wolves, foxes, dogs (uncommon)	Rodents; **humans are accidental hosts**	Albendazole

INTESTINAL CESTODES

TAENIA SAGINATA AND *TAENIA SOLIUM*	
Epidemiology	• *T. saginata* in Eastern Europe, Eastern Africa, Latin America • *T. solium* in Eastern Europe, India, Asia, sub-Saharan Africa, Latin America, and the United States • Animals (cattle, *T. saginata*; pigs, *T. solium*) infected when eggs or proglottids (tapeworm segments with mature eggs) are ingested; eggs hatch in intestine releasing onchospheres (larvae) that migrate to muscles where they develop into cysticerci; human infection develops following ingestion of raw or undercooked **beef or pork** • In the human intestine, the cysticerci develop into adult worms • Adult worms release proglottids filled with eggs that are released in feces; can survive in the environment for days to months
Clinical Disease	• **Asymptomatic** or **mild** with abdominal pain, loss of appetite, weight loss, upset stomach, chronic indigestion • *T. saginata* infections more commonly symptomatic because of the length of the tapeworm (up to 10 m compared with *T. solium*, 3 m) • **Cysticercosis**—humans may develop disease following ingestion of *T. solium* eggs; does not occur with *T. saginata* eggs; lifecycle similar as with animal hosts • Symptoms of cysticercosis determined by where the larvae encyst; most severe is in brain or eye; marked inflammatory reaction to larvae when they die in tissues
Diagnosis	• Detection of characteristic proglottids or eggs in feces • Worms can be differentiated by morphology of proglottids but eggs are identical • Cysticercosis diagnosed by presence of encysted larvae in tissues
Treatment, Prevention, Control	• Treatment with praziquantel; alternative is niclosamide • Prevention by proper cooking of beef and pork in regions where disease is endemic • Maintenance of good sanitary conditions

CLINICAL CASE

Neurocysticercosis

Chatel and colleagues[2] described a case of neurocysticercosis in an Italian traveler to Latin America. The patient was a 49-year-old man with a history of a 30-day stay in Latin America (El Salvador, Columbia, and Guatemala) 3 months before presentation with fever and myalgia. The clinical examination and routine laboratory test results were normal except for elevated creatine phosphokinase levels and mild eosinophilia. He received symptomatic antiinflammatory therapy, rapidly improved, and was discharged with a diagnosis of polymyositis. Two years later he was admitted to the hospital with retroocular headache and recurrent right hemianopsia. A neurologic examination revealed a left Babinski reflex with no motor or sensory dysfunctions. Laboratory tests were unremarkable, including a negative stool examination for ova and parasites. Cerebral magnetic resonance imaging showed the presence of several intraparenchymal, subarachnoidal, and intraventricular cysts (4–15 mm in diameter) with perilesional focal edema and ringlike enhancement. A specific antibody response to cysticercosis was demonstrated by enzyme-linked immunosorbent assay and immunoblotting techniques. The patient was treated with albendazole for two cycles of 8 days each. One year later he was in good health, and cerebral magnetic resonance imaging revealed significant reduction in the diameter of lesions. This case provides an interesting reminder of the minimal but real risks to travelers for acquiring Taenia solium *infections during foreign travel.*

DIPHYLLOBOTHRIUM LATUM

Epidemiology	• Worldwide distribution, particularly in western Europe, eastern Europe, Asia, and the United States • Broader geographic distribution related to regional or international transport of fish • Infection associated with eating raw or undercooked **fish**; freezing for 7 days or proper cooking will kill the parasite • Humans ingest undercooked fish with larvae in the tissues; larvae develop into mature adults in the small intestine and develop to up to 10 m in length; immature eggs are released from the proglottids and passed in feces • Eggs contaminating fresh waters require 2 to 4 weeks to develop into free-swimming larvae (coracidium) that are ingested by small crustaceans (copepods); these are ingested by large fish and the larvae migrate to the flesh where they develop into infectious plerocercoid larvae
Clinical Disease	• Most infections are **asymptomatic** • **Symptoms** include epigastric pain, abdominal cramping, nausea, vomiting, and weight loss • **Vitamin B_{12} deficiency** with anemia and neurologic symptoms
Diagnosis	• Detection of characteristic proglottids or eggs in feces
Treatment, Prevention, Control	• Treatment with praziquantel; alternative is niclosamide • Prevention by proper cooking of fish in regions where disease is endemic

CLINICAL CASE

Diphyllobothriasis

Lee and colleagues[1] reported a case of diphyllobothriasis in a young girl. A 7-year-old girl was seen in an outpatient clinic after the discharge of a chain of tapeworm proglottids measuring 42 cm in length. She had no history of eating raw fish, except once when she ate raw salmon flesh along with the rest of her family approximately 7 months earlier. The salmon was caught in a local river. She did not complain of any gastrointestinal discomfort, and all blood chemistry and hematologic studies were normal. The coprologic studies were positive for D. latum *eggs. The worm was identified as* D. latum *based on the biological characteristics of the proglottids: broad narrow external morphology, coiling of uterus, number of uterine loops, and position of the genital opening. A single dose of praziquantel 400 mg was given, but stool examination remained positive 1 week later. Another dose of 600 mg was given, and repeat stool examination 1 month later was negative. Among four family members who ate raw fish, just two—the girl and her mother—were identified as being infected. Consumption of raw salmon, especially those produced by aquaculture, is a risk for human diphyllobothriasis.*

The lifecycles and diseases caused by *H. nana* (mouse or dwarf tapeworm) and *Hymenolepis diminuta* (rat tapeworm) are similar, with humans serving as accidental primary hosts following ingestion of infected beetles in flours and cereals. A summary of *H. nana* is presented here.

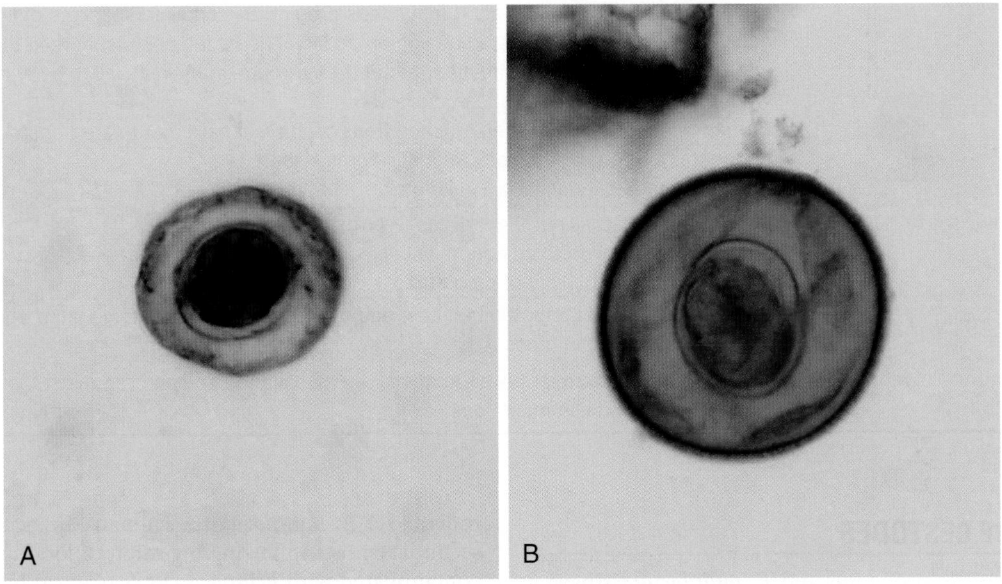

Eggs of (A) *Hymenolepis nana* and (B) *Hymenolepis diminuta*.

HYMENOLEPIS NANA	
Epidemiology	• Worldwide distribution • Most common tapeworm infection in North America; common parasite of mice • Human and mouse infections following ingestion of infective eggs in contaminated food; hatch in small intestine releasing larva that develop into the cysticercoid stage; attach to small intestine and mature into adult; eggs are infectious at the time of passing in feces; can be ingested directly or by **beetles** who can serve as an intermediate host for humans or rodents • Adult worms are small (<5 cm) and short lived, although autoinfections (direct ingestion of passed infectious eggs) can lead to hyperinfections
Clinical Disease	• Infections with small numbers of tapeworms are **asymptomatic** • Symptoms with large number of worms include diarrhea, abdominal pain, headache, and anorexia
Diagnosis	• Detection of characteristic eggs in feces
Treatment, Prevention, Control	• Treatment with praziquantel; alternative is nicosamide • Prevention by maintenance of sanitary conditions and personal hygiene

DIPYLIDIUM CANINUM	
Epidemiology	• Worldwide distribution • Parasite of dogs and cats with the flea as the intermediate host; human infections most common in children • Ingestion of a flea with infectious cysticercoid larvae initiates disease in a dog or cat; larvae develops into an adult that sheds proglottids containing packets of eggs; eggs are released and ingested by dog or cat larval fleas; the onchosphere in the egg is released in the flea intestine; penetrates through intestinal wall to body cavity, where it develops into a cysticercoid larva • Human infections occur when crushed **fleas** on the animal's mouth are transmitted accidentally when the animal licks a child or is kissed • Adult worms are about 15 cm in length
Clinical Disease	• Infections with small numbers of tapeworms are **asymptomatic** • Heavier infections produce abdominal discomfort, pruritus, and diarrhea; anal pruritus due to active mobility of proglottids
Diagnosis	• Detection of gravid proglottid in feces; egg packets containing embryonated eggs are rarely observed in feces
Treatment, Prevention, Control	• Treatment with praziquantel; alternatives are nicosamide and paromomycin • Deworm pets and eliminate fleas

TISSUE CESTODES

Echinococcus granulosus and *E. multilocularis* have a similar lifecycle varying primarily by the secondary hosts. Carnivores such as dogs, foxes, and coyotes are the primary host for *Echinococcus*, and the secondary hosts are sheep for *E. granulosus* and small rodents for *E. multilocularis*. Humans are accidental secondary hosts following ingestion of food or water contaminated with *Echinococcus* eggs in canine feces. Human disease primarily involves the liver and lungs, although dissemination to other organs (e.g., spleen, brain) can occur. The summary of *E. granulosus* is presented here.

ECHINOCOCCUS GRANULOSUS	
Epidemiology	• Present in sheep and cattle raising countries including Australia, New Zealand, southern Africa, and parts of Europe, South America, and North America • Infection acquired by dogs when they ingest the organs of animals with encysted parasite; develop into adults (less than 1 in) in the intestine and eggs shed in feces; sheep, cattle, goats, and pigs ingest eggs which hatch in the small intestine • Human infection following accidental ingestion of **eggs in food or water contaminated with dog feces**; the onchosphere is released and penetrates the human intestinal wall, enters the circulation and is carried to tissues, primarily the liver and lung (less commonly to central nervous system and bones)
Clinical Disease	• Human infection (**echinococcosis**) characterized by a slow-growing (5 to 20 years before symptomatic), tumor-like, unilocular cyst filled with tapeworm heads (hydatid sand) and fluid • Fluid potentially toxic if the cyst ruptures
Diagnosis	• Clinical, radiologic, and epidemiologic data confirmed at surgery • Serologic tests supportive but relatively insensitive
Treatment, Prevention, Control	• Surgical resection of the cyst is the treatment of choice plus albendazole • If in an inoperable location, treatment with albendazole; alternatives are mebendazole or praziquantel • Control of infections in dogs by preventing them from eating animal viscera and proper personal hygiene

CLINICAL CASE

Echinococcosis

Yeh and colleagues[3] described a 36-year-old pregnant woman at 21 weeks of gestation who presented with a 4-week history of a dry nonproductive cough. The patient denied any constitutional symptoms and had no new pets, environmental exposures, or sick contacts. It was her first pregnancy, and there were no complications. She had no medical conditions and did not smoke or drink alcohol. She was a financial consultant and enjoyed running and hiking. She had traveled to Australia, Central Asia, and sub-Saharan Africa in the past. The patient appeared well, with appropriate weight gain for the second trimester of her pregnancy. Her physical examination, including auscultation of her lungs, was normal. Her cough did not improve with use of an inhaled bronchodilator. Imaging studies were not performed because of her pregnancy. She had a normal uncomplicated vaginal delivery 4 months later. She continued to have a dry cough and presented to her physician months after delivery for a reevaluation of her cough. At that time, her physical graph revealed a soft-tissue mass, 7 cm in diameter, adjacent to the right heart border. High-resolution computed tomography (CT) scans of the chest confirmed the presence of a homogeneous and fluid-filled structure without septa, thought to be in the mediastinum. Subsequent echocardiography also confirmed a simple cystic structure with thin walls surrounding echo-free fluid that was indenting the right atrium. On the basis of the radiographic and echocardiography findings, the clinicians caring for the patient thought that the mass was most likely a benign pericardial cyst. Because she was not experiencing dyspnea, the patient declined surgical reaction. However, because of worsening cough over the next few months, she consulted a thoracic surgeon for elective resection. Intraoperative findings revealed an intraparenchymal pulmonary cyst in the right lung that was not attached to the pericardium or bronchus. The cyst was removed intact without gross spillage of the contents. Staining of the cyst wall with hematoxylin and eosin after cross sectioning showed an acellular laminated layer. Microscopic examination of the cyst contents showed protoscolices with hooklets and suckers in a background of histiocytes and eosinophilic debris, consistent with E. granulosus. *CT of the abdomen after removal of the thoracic cyst revealed no hepatobiliary disease. Postoperative screening for serum antibody against* Echinococcus *was positive. Praziquantel was administered for 10 days after surgery and albendazole for 1 month after surgery, with no complications. After this course of therapy, the patient had resolution of her cough and returned to her normal level of activity. There was no evidence of recurrent disease on CT follow-up 6 months after surgery.*

REFERENCES

1. Lee KW, Suhk HC, Pai KS, et al. *Diphyllobothrium latum* infection after eating domestic salmon flesh. *Korean J Parasitol.* 2001;39:319–321.
2. Chatel G, Gulletta M, Scolari C, et al. Neurocysticercosis in an Italian traveler to Latin America. *Am J Trop Med Hyg.* 1999;60:255–256.
3. Yeh WW, Saint S, Weinberger SE. Clinical problem-solving. A growing problem—a 36-year-old pregnant woman at 21 weeks of gestation presented with a 4-week history of a dry, nonproductive cough. *N Engl J Med.* 2007;357:489–494.

27

Arthropods

Arthropods serve an important role as vectors of many bacterial, viral, and parasitic diseases. The list below is a general summary of the most common human diseases associated with arthropod vectors.

Arthropod	Organism	Disease
Tick	*Anaplasma phagocytophilum*	Human anaplasmosis
	Borrelia burgdorferi	Lyme disease
	Borrelia, other species	Endemic relapsing fever
	Coxiella burnetii	Q fever
	Ehrlichia chaffeensis	Human monocytic ehrlichiosis
	Ehrlichia ewingii	Human granulocytic ehrlichiosis
	Francisella tularensis	Tularemia
	Orbivirus	Colorado tick fever
	Rickettsia rickettsii	Rocky Mountain spotted fever
Flea	*Dipylidium caninum*	Dog tapeworm
	Rickettsia prowazekii	Sporadic typhus
	Rickettsia typhi	Murine typhus
	Yersinia pestis	Plague
Lice	*Bartonella quintana*	Trench fever
	Borrelia recurrentis	Epidemic relapsing fever
	Rickettsia prowazekii	Epidemic typhus
Mite	*Orientia tsutsugamushi*	Scrub typhus
	Rickettsia akari	Rickettsialpox
Fly	*Bartonella bacilliformis*	Bartonellosis
	Hymenolepis nana	Dwarf tapeworm
	Leishmania species	Leishmaniasis
	Onchocerca volvulus	Onchocerciasis ("river blindness")
	Trypanosoma brucei	African trypanosomiasis
	Trypanosoma cruzi	Chagas disease
Mosquito	*Alphavirus*	Eastern equine encephalitis
		Venezuelan equine encephalitis
		Western equine encephalitis
	Brugia species	Malayan filariasis
	Bunyavirus	La Crosse encephalitis
	Dirofilaria immitis	Dirofilariasis
	Flavivirus	Dengue fever
		St. Louis encephalitis
		Yellow fever
	Plasmodium species	Malaria
	Wuchereria bancrofti	Bancroftian filariasis

SECTION VI Review Questions

QUESTIONS

1. One week after returning from a vacation in Mexico, a 24-year-old man developed a high fever for 3 days and then became jaundiced and fatigued for 1 week. Laboratory tests revealed the following: white blood cell count, 3200/mm^3; hemoglobin, 11.6 gm/dL; platelets, 112,000/mm^3; elevated liver function tests (aspartate aminotransferase, 2600 U/L; alanine aminotransferase, 3100 U/L); bilirubin, 12.6 mg/dL; creatinine, 1.3 mg/dL. Malaria smear was negative and his hepatitis serology results were: hepatitis A, immunoglobulin M positive and immunoglobulin G negative; hepatitis B surface antigen negative, hepatitis B core antibody negative; hepatitis C antibody negative. The patient's roommate remained in excellent health, with normal liver function tests and was seronegative for hepatitis A, B, and C. Which of the following would best protect the roommate from being infected by the patient?
   - **A.** Immune serum globulin
   - **B.** Hepatitis A vaccine
   - **C.** Hepatitis B hyperimmune globulin
   - **D.** Hepatitis B vaccine
   - **E.** Nothing is required

2. Collection of specimens for the diagnosis of which of the following diseases poses significant risks for physicians?
   - **A.** Histoplasmosis
   - **B.** Coccidiomycosis
   - **C.** Lyme disease borreliosis
   - **D.** Tularemia
   - **E.** Amebiasis

3. A 72-year-old diabetic male from Chicago, recently on etanercept for psoriasis, developed a fever on day 7 postresection of an adenocarcinoma of the descending colon. He is currently intubated and has a central venous line for hyperalimentation in his internal jugular vein. Two blood cultures were collected and after 2 days of incubation, yeast grew from the aerobic bottles of both cultures. What is the most likely identification of this fungus?

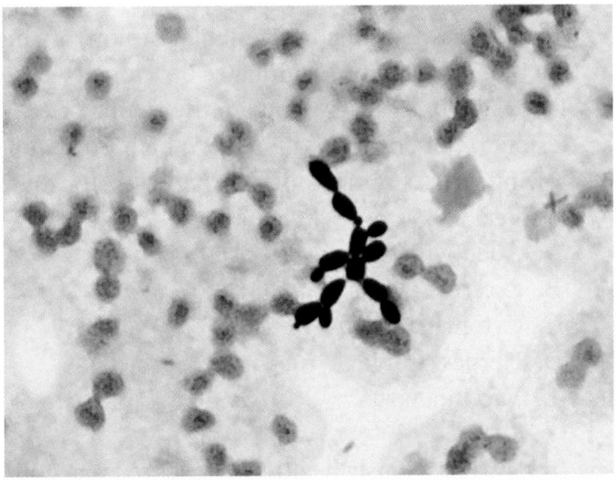

   - **A.** *Blastomyces dermatitidis*
   - **B.** *Candida parapsilosis*
   - **C.** *Cryptococcus neoformans*
   - **D.** *Histoplasma capsulatum*
   - **E.** *Malassezia furfur*

4. A patient with lupus treated with prednisone (60 mg/day for 6 weeks) developed bilateral pulmonary infiltrates. The organism was observed in the modified acid-fast stain of the bronchoalveolar lavage as long, branching, partially staining rods. Which one of the following is the most likely pathogen?

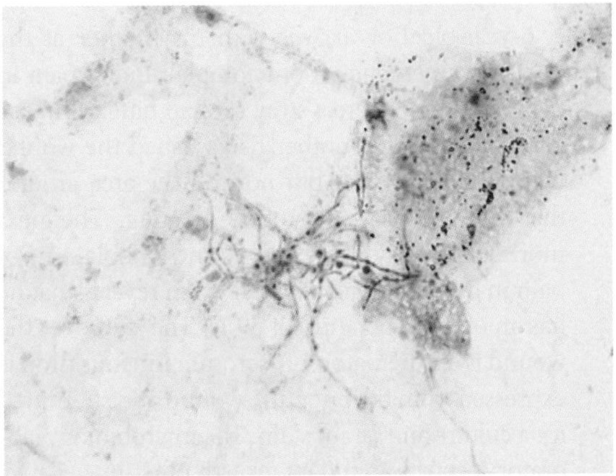

   - **A.** *Actinomyces israelii*
   - **B.** *Aspergillus fumigatus*

C. *Histoplasma capsulatum*
D. *Mycobacterium avium*
E. *Nocardia farcinica*

5. A wrestler developed a vesicular lesion on his shoulder. One of his teammates developed a similar lesion on his wrist and another had a crusted lesion at the border of his lips. Which of the following viruses is most likely responsible for these lesions?
A. Adenovirus
B. Coxsackievirus
C. Cytomegalovirus
D. Herpes simplex virus
E. Vaccinia virus

6. In July, a previously healthy 65-year-old man with a 40-year history of smoking developed severe bilateral pneumonia. He lived in Philadelphia his entire life and had no significant travel history. Sputum was collected and many neutrophils, but no organisms, were observed on Gram stain and acid-fast stain, and no growth was observed on routine bacterial or fungal culture. Which one of the following organisms is most likely responsible for this man's infection?
A. *Klebsiella pneumoniae*
B. *Legionella pneumophila*
C. *Mycobacterium tuberculosis*
D. *Histoplasma capsulatum*
E. Influenza A virus

7. A 6-year-old boy arrives with his mother at the pediatric emergency room complaining of pain in his right hand where a stray cat had bitten him the previous day. The mother had washed the wound with soap and water but noticed the area around the wound was red by that evening. The next morning, the boy awoke crying and complaining of pain in his hand. The physical exam reveals that he has an oral temperature of 39°C. The skin over the wound is erythematous. A serosanguineous drop is expressed from the puncture wound and submitted for a culture and Gram stain. The microbiology laboratory reports abundant growth of gram-negative coccobacilli. Which of the following organisms is most likely responsible for this infection?
A. *Capnocytophaga*
B. *Eikenella*
C. *Escherichia*
D. *Fusobacterium*
E. *Pasteurella*

8. A 32-year-old female farmer in Wisconsin presented to her family physician in June with a 3-week complaint of a low-grade fever, myalgias, a productive cough, and a skin lesion that developed during the previous week. The physician found an infiltrate on chest x-ray and collected sputum and a biopsy of the lesion for culture and microscopic stains (Gram, acid-fast). Faint-staining, large round cells, some with budding cells, were observed on the Gram stain and silver stain of the biopsy material (see figure) and the etiologic agent grew in culture after 2 weeks. The most likely diagnosis is:

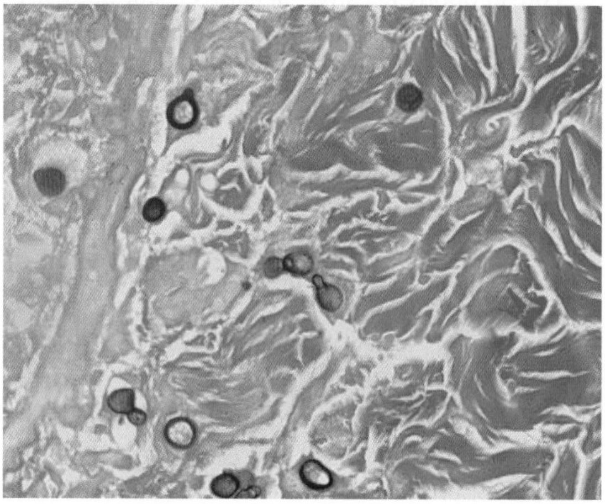

A. *Blastomyces dermatitidis*
B. *Candida albicans*
C. *Histoplasma capsulatum*
D. *Mycobacterium marinum*
E. *Sporothrix schenckii*

9. A 14-day-old baby is admitted to the hospital with a fever, hyperactivity, and a stiff neck. At the time of giving birth to the baby, the mother complained of flulike symptoms. Blood and cerebrospinal fluid were collected for culture. No organisms were seen on Gram stain but small, weakly beta-hemolytic colonies grew on the blood agar plates after 48 hours. The Gram stain of the colonies reveals small, gram-positive coccobacilli. The organism most likely responsible for this infection is:

A. *Escherichia coli*
B. *Listeria monocytogenes*
C. *Neisseria meningitidis*
D. Group B *Streptococcus*
E. *Streptococcus pneumoniae*

10. When waking her 6-year-old son for school, a mother observes that the boy is limping. She notices that his left knee is swollen, red, warm to the touch, and movement is painful. He states that he fell on the knee 2 days ago while playing with friends. The mother brings her son to see their pediatrician, who removes 15 mL of cloudy fluid from the knee. A Gram stain and culture of the fluid shows gram-positive cocci arranged in clusters (see figure). Which organism is most likely the cause of the boy's symptoms?

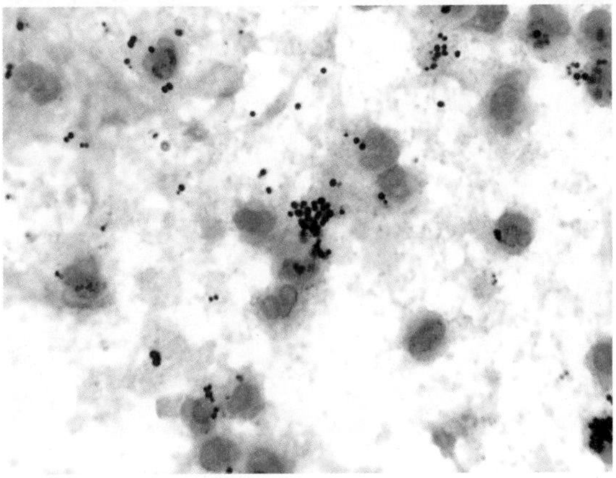

A. *Bacillus cereus*
B. *Enterococcus faecalis*
C. *Staphylococcus epidermidis*
D. *Staphylococcus aureus*
E. *Streptococcus pyogenes*

11. A 28-year-old sexually active woman presented to her gynecologist with a 3-day history of vaginal inflammation and a thick, whitish discharge. The discharge was examined microscopically and cultured on bacterial and fungal media. After 2 days the organisms in the picture were observed. Based on this observation, what is the most likely diagnosis for this infection?

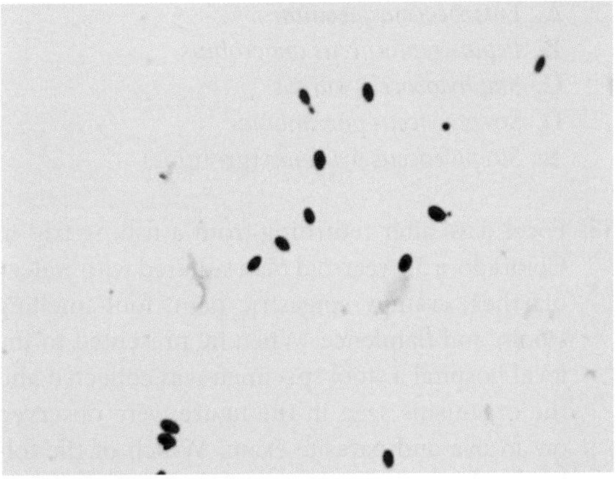

A. Gonorrhea
B. Chlamydial infection
C. Trichomoniasis
D. Bacterial vaginosis
E. Candidiasis

12. After an automobile accident, a 23-year-old woman requires an emergency splenectomy. Her subsequent recovery is uneventful. However, 4 weeks after the surgery, she is brought to the emergency department unconscious and nonresponsive. The physicians are unable to stabilize her and she expires 1 hour after she arrived. Blood is collected for culture, chemistry tests, and hematology tests. The technologist examining the peripheral blood smear observes abundant bacteria (see figure). Within 6 hours the blood cultures are also reported to be positive. Which organism is most likely responsible for this overwhelming infection?

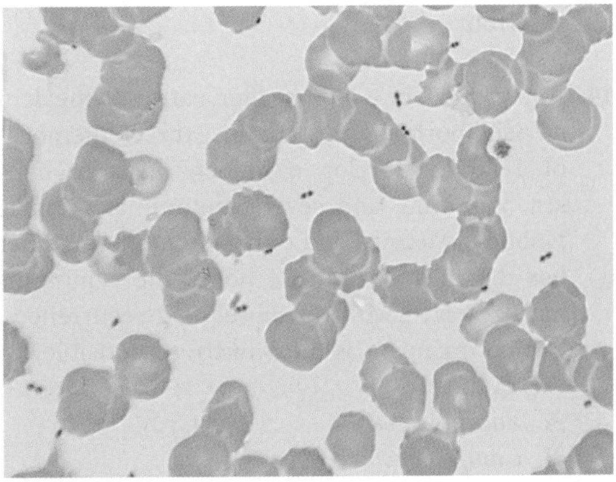

A. *Enterococcus faecium*
B. *Peptostreptococcus anaerobius*
C. *Staphylococcus aureus*
D. *Streptococcus pneumoniae*
E. *Streptococcus pyogenes* (group A)

13. For 4 days after returning from a fishing trip in Colorado, a 36-year-old man suffered with watery diarrhea, crampy epigastric pain, foul-smelling stools, and flatulence. When he presented to the local hospital a stool specimen was collected and the organisms seen in the figure were observed on an ova and parasite exam. Which of the following hosts is the most common reservoir for this parasite?

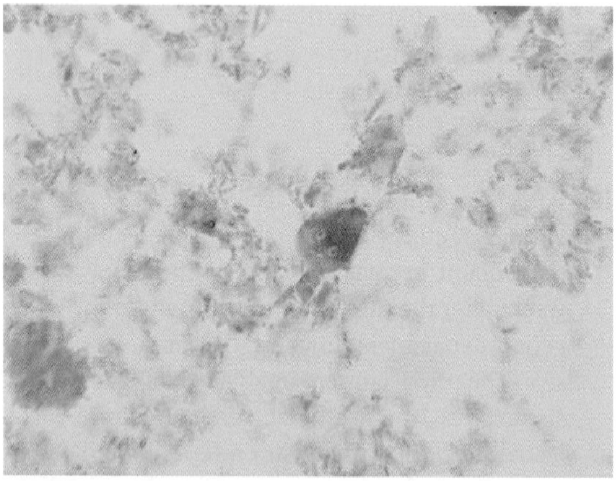

A. Beaver
B. Dog
C. Rabbit
D. Snake
E. Trout

14. Approximately 4 hours after eating a meal in a neighborhood restaurant, three members of a family develop a sudden onset of nausea, vomiting, and severe abdominal cramps. Nobody is febrile, and only one family member has diarrhea. Within 24 hours the symptoms have resolved with no subsequent recurrences. Which organism is most likely responsible for this outbreak?
A. *Bacillus cereus*
B. *Campylobacter jejuni*
C. Norovirus
D. Rotavirus
E. *Shigella sonnei*

15. A 52-year-old man develops peritonitis after rupture of his appendix. After surgery for repair of the rupture, the man is treated with clindamycin and ceftazidime. Approximately 5 days later the patient develops profuse diarrhea, abdominal cramps, and a fever of 38.5°C. During an additional 5 days the diarrhea worsens, with gross blood present in the stools and white plaques observed over the colonic mucosa (see figure). Which organism is most likely responsible for this patient's symptoms?

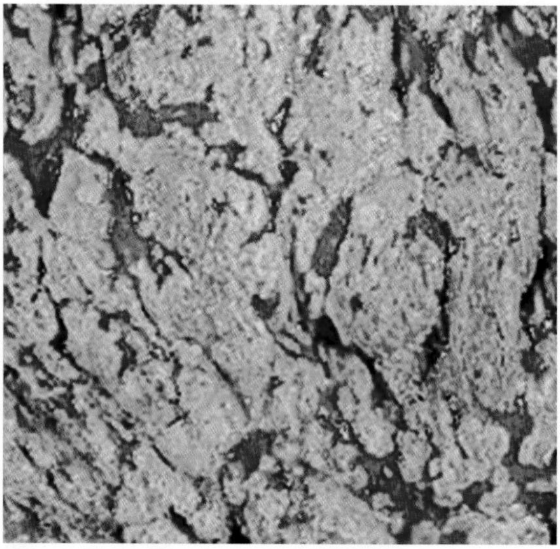

A. *Bacillus cereus*
B. *Clostridium difficile*
C. *Escherichia coli* O157
D. *Shigella sonnei*
E. *Staphylococcus aureus*

16. A 59-year-old woman presented to the emergency department with a 3-day history of eye swelling, a frontal headache, and low-grade fevers. The woman was slowly responsive to questions on physical examination. Laboratory tests showed the patient had an elevated white blood cell count with a predominance of neutrophils and a blood glucose level of 475 mg/dL. A computed tomography scan of the sinuses showed opacities in the ethmoid sinuses. A specimen from a sinus aspirate was collected for bacterial and fungal stains and cultures. A fungus was observed in the silver-stained material (see figure) and the mold grew in culture after 1 day. Which one of the following organisms is most likely responsible for this woman's infection?

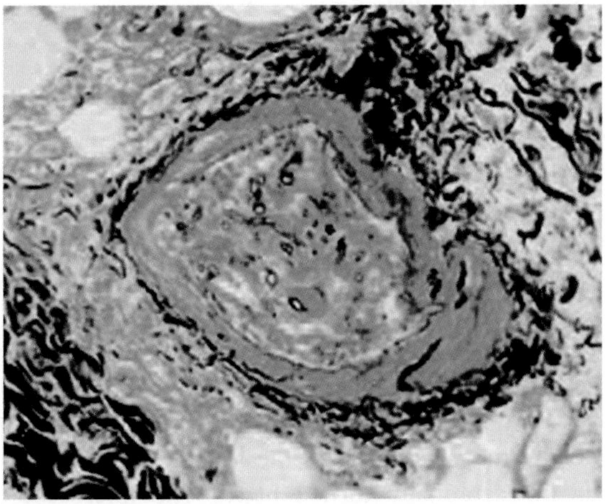

A. *Aspergillus*
B. *Bipolaris*
C. *Curvularia*
D. *Histoplasma*
E. *Rhizopus*

17. After 2 days of increasing pain during urination, a 20-year-old female college student goes to the student health center. Upon examination she complains of left flank tenderness and low-grade fevers. Her urine is cloudy and shows microscopic evidence of erythrocytes, pyuria, and abundant gram-positive bacteria. Her relevant past medical history is significant for no previous urinary tract infections, and she admits to being sexually active. Which organism is most likely responsible for this woman's infection?

A. *Candida albicans*
B. *Enterococcus faecalis*
C. *Neisseria gonorrhoeae*
D. *Staphylococcus aureus*
E. *Staphylococcus saprophyticus*

18. Approximately 4 weeks after a bone marrow transplant, a 42-year-old man returns to his physician with complaints of fevers and a productive sputum. The symptoms have developed during the preceding 5 days. A chest x-ray is obtained and a cavitary lesion is observed in the upper right lobe. While the patient is in the radiology department, he has a seizure. A computed tomography scan of his head shows a mass in the right parietal area of the brain. Cultures of the sputum collected at admission and of the brain and lung tissues are performed and, after 4 days, growth of weakly staining, filamentous gram-positive rods is observed. This same organism was observed in the direct Gram stain of the tissues (see figure). The organisms also stained weakly with the acid-fast stain. Which pathogen is most likely responsible for this man's condition?

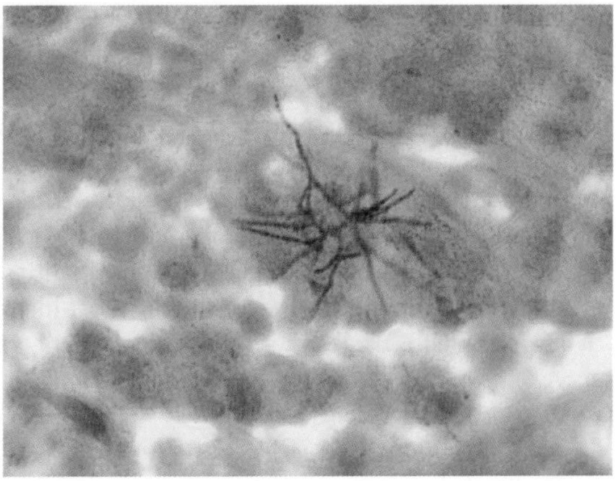

A. *Actinomyces israelii*
B. *Aspergillus fumigatus*
C. *Mycobacterium tuberculosis*
D. *Nocardia abscessus*
E. *Rhodococcus equi*

19. A 26-year-old woman living in Boston received a blood transfusion during the first trimester of her pregnancy. She had no significant travel history during her pregnancy. At birth her infant was small and appeared to have a disproportionately small head (microcephaly). Within 2 days the infant developed jaundice, hepatosplenomegaly, and a petechial rash. Urine samples were found to contain cells with "owl's eye" inclusion bodies. An x-ray of the infant's head at 1 week of age showed intracranial calcifications. The infant became increasing lethargic and experienced respiratory distress progressing to seizures. The infant eventually died. Which of the following is most likely responsible for this infection?

A. Cytomegalovirus
B. Herpes simplex virus
C. Rubella virus
D. *Toxoplasma gondii*
E. Zika virus

20. An 8-year-old boy fell while playing and abraded the skin over his thigh and hip. The injury did not appear serious and no effort was made to clean the wound or apply topical antibiotic creams. The wound over the hip worsened after 3 days, with inflammation and a small amount of purulence. That evening, the child developed a high-grade fever (40°C), headache, and a diffuse rash. By the time the child arrived at the hospital he was hypotensive, complained of severe myalgias, and had diarrhea. After 1 more day, his skin desquamated (including over the palms and soles), and he developed renal and hepatic abnormalities. Which of the following organisms is most likely responsible for this boy's infection?

A. *Bacillus cereus*
B. *Bacteroides fragilis*
C. *Clostridium perfringens*
D. *Staphylococcus aureus*
E. *Streptococcus anginosus*

21. A 34-year-old man told his wife that for the last 3 days he had been feeling progressively worse. His illness began with a headache, mild fever, and sweats. Over time the symptoms became more prominent, and his wife took him to the physician. The physician noted that the man had a temperature of 39°C, blood pressure of 137/85 mmHg, heart rate of 82 bpm, and respiratory rate of 25/min. This patient was previously in good health and returned from a trip to Mexico 3 weeks prior to this visit. While in Mexico the man ate only in high quality restaurants, although he did consume unpasteurized goat cheese. The physician ordered blood cultures for his patient and 3 days later the cultures were positive with very small gram-negative coccobacilli. Which one of the following organisms is most likely responsible for this patient's infection?

A. *Acinetobacter*
B. *Brucella*
C. *Escherichia*
D. *Francisella*
E. *Haemophilus*

22. A 45-year-old woman presented to her physician because she had several sores on her arm that had developed during the previous 2 weeks. The physician noted that the sores were ulcerative nodular lesions that followed the lymphatic system up her arm. Her axillary nodes were also enlarged. A specimen was aspirated from one of the lesions and a few oval, fusiform yeast cells were observed in culture. A slow-growing white mold grew in the fungal cultures of the lesions and the colonies gradually turned black. The microscopic morphology of the mold is shown in the figure. Which one of the following organisms is responsible for this woman's infection?

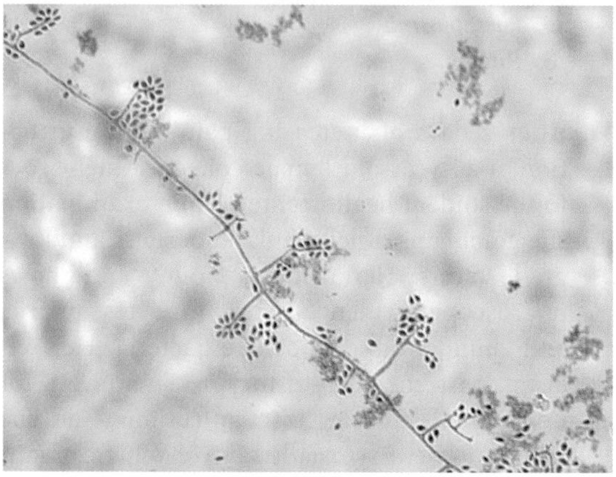

A. *Blastomyces dermatitidis*
B. *Candida albicans*
C. *Cryptococcus neoformans*
D. *Sporothrix schenckii*
E. *Trichophyton rubrum*

23. A 64-year-old man underwent intraabdominal surgery for colonic cancer. Five days after the surgery the patient developed peritonitis for which he was treated with ceftazidime, gentamicin, and metronidazole. Although he initially responded to this therapeutic regimen, on the third night of treatment he developed spiking fevers and abdominal tenderness. He was taken to surgery that night and 50 cc of purulent material was drained from his abdominal cavity. The material was submitted for Gram stain and culture, and blood was collected for culture. The organisms observed in the figure were grown from the aerobic and anaerobic blood cultures as well as from the purulent material. The most likely organism responsible for this infection is:

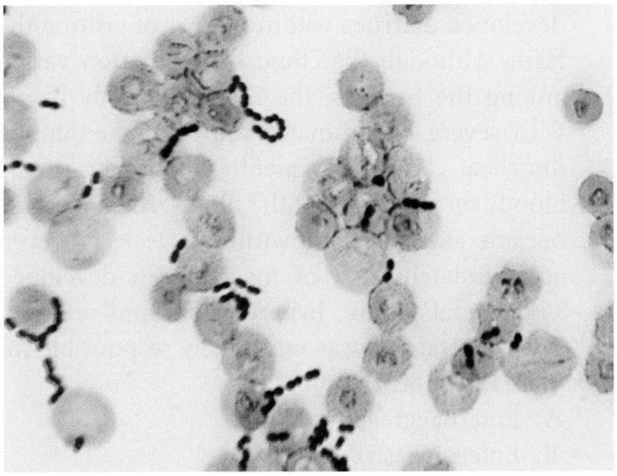

A. *Candida albicans*
B. *Enterococcus faecalis*
C. *Peptostreptococcus anaerobius*
D. *Staphylococcus aureus*
E. *Streptococcus pneumoniae*

24. A 19-year-old homosexual man was admitted for evaluation of a 2-week history of a nonproductive cough, fever, and shortness of breath. A chest radiograph was performed and demonstrated bilateral pulmonary infiltrates with both interstitial and alveolar markings. The man was HIV-positive and had a $CD4^+$ count that was less than 200 cells/mm^3. A bronchial alveolar lavage and biopsy were performed. Organisms measuring 4 to 5 µm were observed in the Gomori methenamine silver-stained section of the biopsy (see figure). Which organism is responsible for this man's infection?

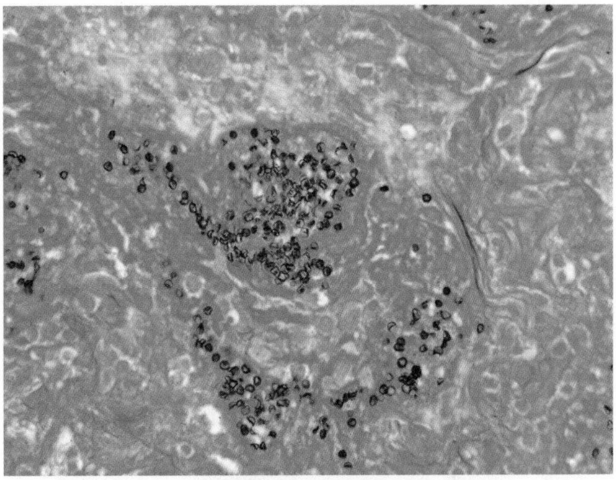

A. *Aspergillus fumigatus*
B. *Candida albicans*
C. *Cryptococcus neoformans*
D. *Histoplasma capsulatum*
E. *Pneumocystis jiroveci*

25. Approximately 36 hours after a neighborhood picnic 14 people developed diarrhea, with the majority complaining of abdominal cramps. Most had low-grade temperatures and 8 to 10 bowel movements a day. Bloody stools affected two people. Although symptoms resolved for most of these people within 1 week, two children and one adult had to be hospitalized. One additional adult developed joint pains in the hands, ankles, and knees that persisted for 1 week. Which one of the following organisms is the most likely cause of these infections?
A. *Bacillus cereus*
B. *Campylobacter jejuni*
C. Norovirus
D. *Salmonella* enteritidis
E. *Staphylococcus aureus*

26. Three days after a 23-year-old man returned from a camping trip in Mexico, he presented to the emergency department suffering from abdominal pain, nausea, fever, and bloody diarrhea. Stool specimens were collected and submitted to the laboratory for bacterial cultures and parasite exam. The bacterial cultures were negative but a parasite was observed (see figure). Which host is the primary reservoir for this parasite?

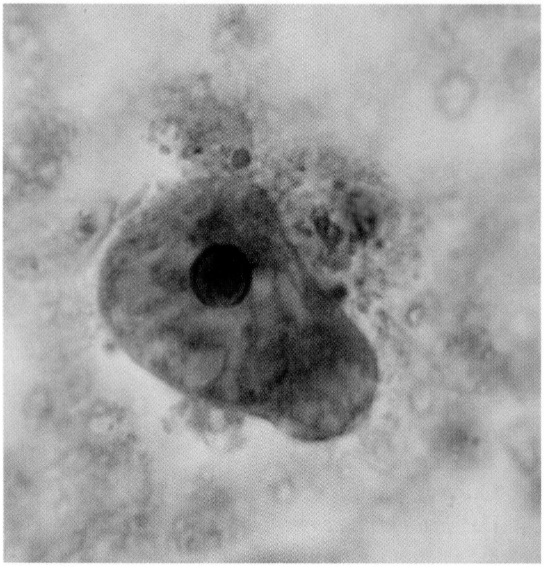

A. Cockroach
B. Dog
C. Fly
D. Human
E. Mosquito

27. A 74-year-old man was admitted to the hospital because of a 3-day history of high fever, myalgia, and chills accompanied by back pain and elimination of dark urine during the previous 12 hours. His temperature was 38.5°C, blood pressure was 120/70 mmHg, and respiratory rate was 30/min. Laboratory results included hemoglobin 131 g/L, hematocrit 0.41, serum urea 71 mg/dL, total bilirubin 4.1 mg/dL, lactic dehydrogenase 1250 U/L, and potassium 6.5 mEq/L. A urinalysis showed the presence of blood but less than five white blood cells per high-power field were seen. Within 6 hours of admission into the hospital the patient suffered a cardiac arrest and expired. Postmortem examination of tissues revealed microabscesses in the liver and gallbladder. Premortem blood cultures were positive within 6 hours of incubation for a gas-producing organism and cultures of the autopsy tissues grew the same organism. Which of the following organisms is most likely responsible for this patient's overwhelming infection?

A. *Bacteroides fragilis*
B. *Clostridium perfringens*
C. *Escherichia coli*
D. *Pseudomonas aeruginosa*
E. *Staphylococcus aureus*

28. In September 2000 an outbreak of *Escherichia coli* gastroenteritis occurred in Pennsylvania. Most of the infected patients had visited a popular dairy farm, where they had contact with the animals and where lunch and snacks were served. Patients developed diarrhea within 10 days of visiting the farm. Although the clinical presentation varied among the patients, the illness typically began with severe abdominal cramps and nonbloody diarrhea. Stools frequently became grossly bloody on day 2 or 3 of the illness. Most patients became asymptomatic within 1 week; however, approximately 10% of the children developed acute renal failure, hypertension, and seizures. Which organism was most likely responsible for these infections?

A. Enteroaggregative *E. coli*
B. Enteroinvasive *E. coli*
C. Enteropathogenic *E. coli*
D. Enterotoxigenic *E. coli*
E. Shiga toxin–producing *E. coli*

29. After returning from a trip to Arizona, a 30-year-old man experienced a respiratory illness with symptoms including a cough and fever. Approximately 1 week later he developed red, tender nodules on his shin. His physician collected sputum specimens for stains and cultures. After 3 days of incubation at room temperature, the fungal culture grew a white filamentous mold. The microscopic morphology of the mold is shown in the figure. Which of the following is most likely responsible for this infection?

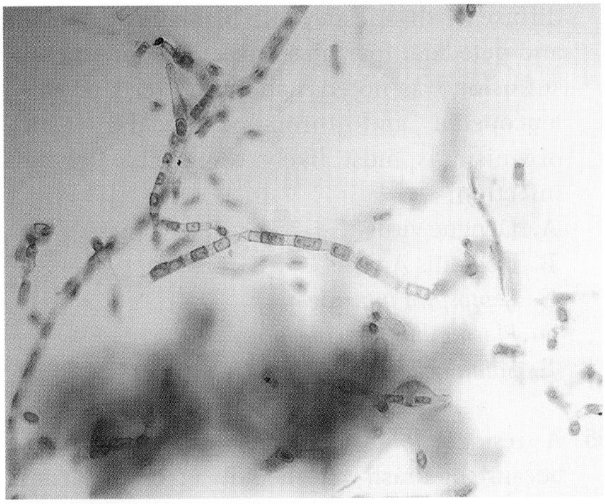

A. *Aspergillus fumigatus*
B. *Blastomyces dermatitidis*
C. *Coccidioides immitis*
D. *Histoplasma capsulatum*
E. *Sporothrix schenckii*

30. A 5-year-old boy complained to his mother that his throat hurt when he swallowed his food. The mother noted that the boy's throat was red and a whitish exudate had formed over his tonsils. The next day, a diffuse red rash developed on his chest. The mother took the boy to his pediatrician at which time the rash had spread over his neck, face, and limbs. The rash was most intense at folds of the skin. Which organism is most likely responsible for this infection?
A. *Bordetella pertussis*
B. Measles virus
C. Rubella virus
D. *Staphylococcus aureus*
E. *Streptococcus pyogenes*

31. A 23-year-old Peace Corps worker living in Africa for the previous year developed symptoms of nausea, vomiting, and diarrhea while visiting family in New York. Stool specimens were collected for bacterial culture and ova and parasite examination. The bacterial cultures were negative but the ova and parasite examination was positive for the organism shown in the figure. What is the most likely source of this woman's infection?

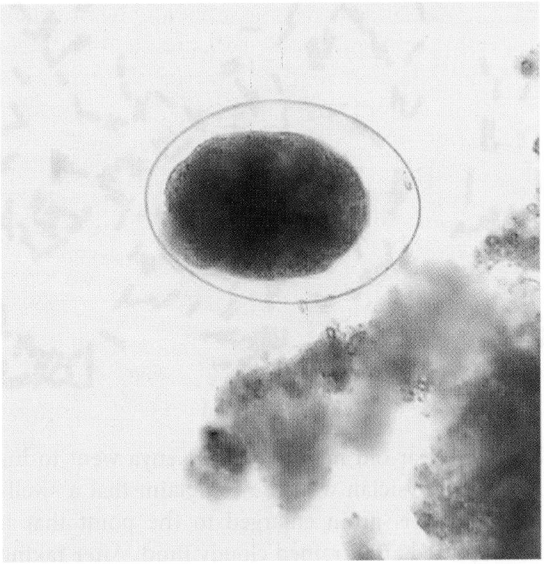

A. Consumption of uncooked pork
B. Consumption of contaminated raw vegetables
C. Direct skin penetration by infectious larvae
D. Oral exposure to the feces of an infected dog
E. Oral exposure to the feces of an infected human

32. A 42-year-old carpenter suffers a penetrating eye injury when a wooden splinter is deflected into his eye. Within 12 hours of the injury the eye is inflamed and painful. By the time the man goes to the emergency department, he has completely lost his vision in the eye. Drainage from the eye is collected on a swab and submitted for Gram stain and culture. Abundant gram-positive rods are observed on Gram stain (see figure) and within 12 hours of incubation, large b-hemolytic colonies are detected on the aerobic blood agar plates. Which organism is most likely responsible for this infection?
A. *Bacillus cereus*
B. *Bacteroides fragilis*
C. *Clostridium perfringens*
D. *Corynebacterium jeikeium*
E. *Nocardia farcinica*

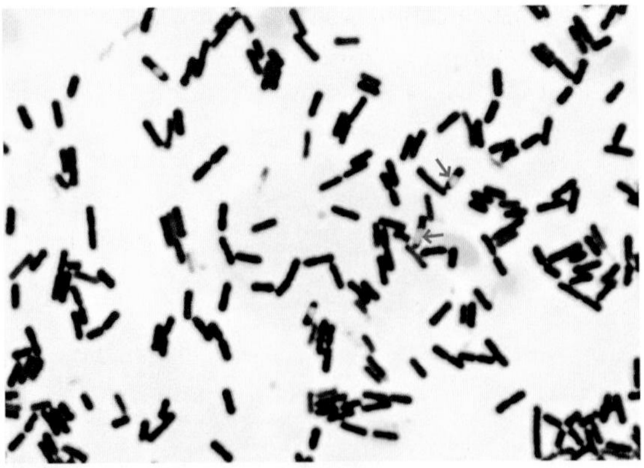

33. A 24-year-old man living in Kenya went to his local physician with the complaint that a swelling in his groin enlarged to the point that it ruptured and drained cloudy fluid. After taking a careful history, the physician discovered that the sexually active man had initially developed a small painless blister that ulcerated and then rapidly healed. Approximately 1 week later, the lymph nodes that drained the area had become enlarged. The area surrounding these swollen nodes became enlarged and tender. It was these lymph nodes that ruptured and drained purulent material. The patient felt feverish and had a headache and muscle aches. The physician made the diagnosis based on the clinical presentation and culture of the purulent material. Which organism was most likely responsible for this man's infection?

A. *Chlamydia trachomatis*
B. Herpes simplex virus
C. *Klebsiella granulomatis*
D. *Neisseria gonorrhoeae*
E. *Treponema pallidum*

34. A 32-year-old woman presented to her family physician with a 5-day history of fevers, headaches, retro-orbital pain, myalgias, and a rash. The symptoms began 3 days after she returned from a 1-month trip to Thailand. The rash developed initially on her face and then spread over her trunk and extremities. Before her travels, she received all the appropriate vaccinations and maintained malaria prophylaxis during her trip. Physical examination showed diffuse erythroderma with blanching erythema and petechial formation. Bilateral conjunctival suffusion was noted. Laboratory tests revealed leucopenia and thrombocytopenia. Which organism is most likely responsible for this infection?

A. Dengue virus
B. Hepatitis A virus
C. *Leptospira interrogans*
D. *Plasmodium falciparum*
E. *Salmonella* typhi

35. A resident of Wisconsin saw her physician because of a rash that she noticed on her arm. It began as a small papule and then enlarged during the next 10 days (see figure). When she presented this lesion to her physician the involved area was 30 cm in diameter, with a flat red border and an area of central clearing. She also had a headache, low-grade fever, and myalgias. Her activities during the weeks before the rash and symptoms developed included hunting with her dog, gardening, and swimming in a local lake. Which organism is most likely responsible for this infection?

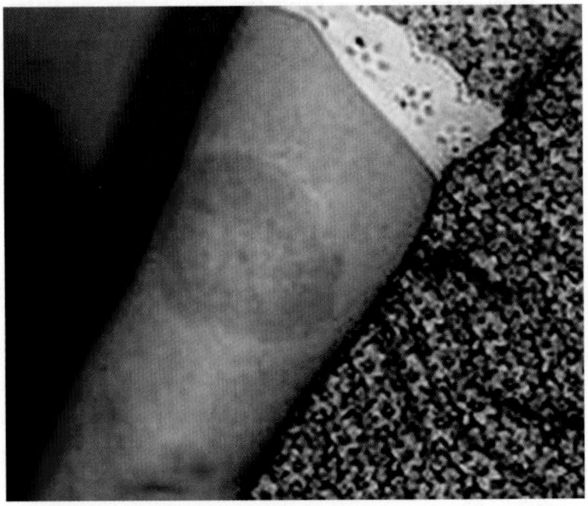

A. *Borrelia burgdorferi*
B. Brown recluse spider bite
C. *Malassezia furfur*
D. *Sporothrix schenckii*
E. *Trichophyton rubrum*

36. A 43-year-old sexually active, HIV-positive woman living in St. Petersburg went to her physician with a 4-day history of low-grade fevers, fatigue, and a painful sore throat. A gray-colored membrane was observed over both tonsils and extended over the uvula and soft palate. Adenopathy and cervical swelling were also present. When the physician attempted to remove the membrane for culture, he noticed that the underlying mucosa was edematous and bleeding. Which organism is most likely responsible for this infection?

A. *Bordetella pertussis*
B. *Candida albicans*
C. *Corynebacterium diphtheriae*
D. *Neisseria gonorrhoeae*
E. *Streptococcus pyogenes*

37. A 56-year-old businessman returned from China after a 1-year stay. On his return he developed diarrhea and abdominal pain in the right upper quadrant. Examination in the hospital revealed a palpable liver and laboratory tests documented an elevation in liver enzymes. When questioned about his diet he stated that he enjoyed eating many of the local delicacies, including raw fish and uncooked watercress. Parasite eggs were observed in the patient's stool (see figure). Which organism is most likely responsible for this patient's illness?

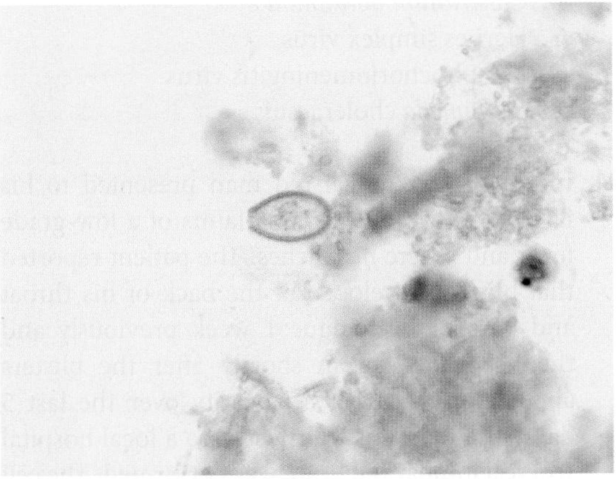

A. *Ancylostoma duodenale*
B. *Fasciola hepatica*
C. *Opisthorchis sinensis* (also known as *Clonorchis sinensis*)
D. *Paragonimus westermani*
E. *Schistosoma mansoni*

38. A 36-year-old woman with a history of rheumatic heart disease underwent dental extractions for severely decayed teeth. Prophylactic antibiotics were not administered because of a remote history of penicillin allergy. Approximately 6 weeks after the procedure, the woman developed fevers, chills, and night sweats. After 2 weeks of these symptoms, the patient saw her physician, who noted that she had experienced a 5-kg weight loss since her last visit. Which of the following organisms is most likely responsible for this patient's infection?

A. *Candida albicans*
B. *Staphylococcus aureus*
C. *Staphylococcus epidermidis*
D. *Streptococcus mutans*
E. *Streptococcus pneumoniae*

39. An 18-year-old male college student presented to the student health center with a sore throat, swollen cervical lymph nodes, fever, malaise, and hepatosplenomegaly. Which of the following agents is most likely responsible for this infection?

A. Adenovirus
B. Coxsackievirus
C. Epstein-Barr virus
D. Human metapneumovirus
E. *Streptococcus pyogenes*

40. Approximately 4 hours after eating a breakfast of scrambled eggs, ham, custard-filled Danish roll, and orange juice, a husband and wife developed nausea and started vomiting. They rapidly developed severe abdominal pain and diarrhea. The couple went to the local hospital and were found to be dehydrated, but had no evidence of fever, rash, or other signs. Which antibiotic should be used to treat these patients?

A. Amoxicillin
B. Ciprofloxacin
C. Oxacillin
D. Vancomycin
E. No antibiotic

41. Approximately 2 weeks after birth an infant developed watery discharge from both eyes. During the next few days this discharge became purulent and the conjunctiva became erythematous (see figure). The mother returned to the hospital with the infant and the pediatrician ordered culture and Gram stain of the discharge. No organisms were observed on Gram stain and the culture on blood agar and chocolate agar was negative. Which of the following drugs should be used to treat this infection?

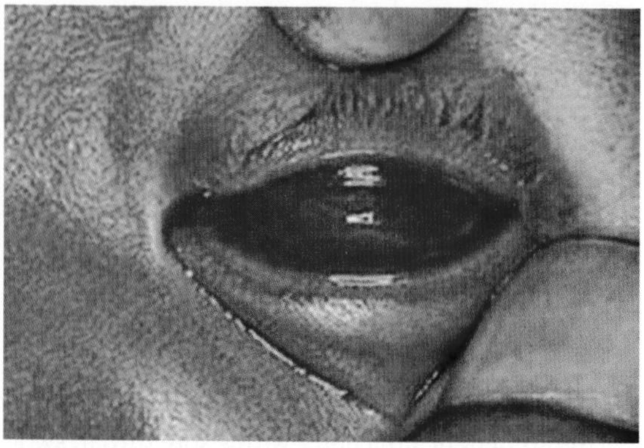

A. Acyclovir
B. Erythromycin
C. Imipenem
D. Penicillin
E. Tetracycline

42. Approximately 3 days after attending a wedding reception in St. Louis, Missouri, 32 guests became ill with symptoms that included diarrhea, anorexia, abdominal cramping, and a low-grade fever. Cultures for bacteria and viral pathogens were negative, but coccoid forms 8 to 10 μm in diameter were observed when the stool specimens were stained with an acid-fast stain. Which organism is most likely responsible for these infections?
A. *Candida*
B. *Cryptosporidium*
C. *Cyclospora*
D. *Cystoisospora*
E. *Microsporidia*

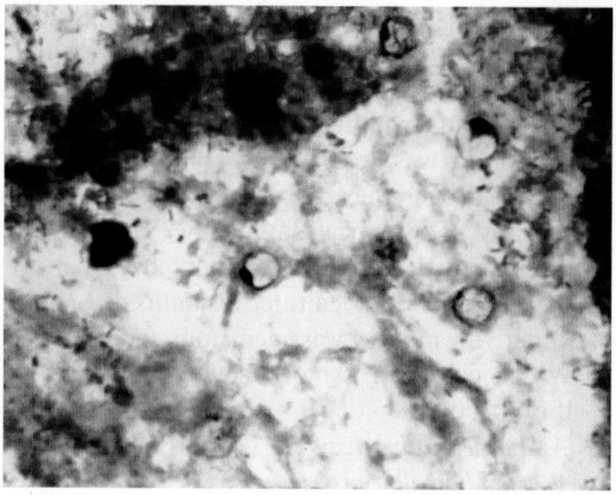

43. In late 2001 and early 2002, four infants residing in Staten Island, New York became ill with the same bacterial pathogen. The infants were between the ages of 3 weeks and 18 weeks. All had been in good health following uneventful pregnancies. Two infants were breast-fed and two were formula-fed. Upon presentation to the hospital, all infants were irritable, lethargic, and constipated. Two infants had sluggishly reactive pupils, and two were described as having loss of facial expression. Three of the infants required mechanical ventilation. Specimens of blood, stool, urine, and cerebrospinal fluid were collected for microbiological testing. Which organism was most likely responsible for these infections?
A. *Campylobacter jejuni*
B. *Clostridium botulinum*
C. Herpes simplex virus
D. Lymphochoriomeningitis virus
E. *Salmonella* choleraesuis

44. In August, a 26-year-old man presented to his family physician with complaints of a low-grade fever and severe headaches. The patient reported that blisters developed at the back of his throat and base of his tongue 1 week previously and the headaches began shortly after the blisters appeared, increasing in severity over the last 5 days. The man was transferred to a local hospital where a lumbar puncture was performed. The cell counts and chemistry for the cerebrospinal fluid were: 177 cells with 81% lymphocytes, a normal

glucose (54 mg/dL) and elevated protein (60 mg/dL). No organisms were observed on Gram stain and bacterial and fungal cultures were negative. After 2 weeks the patient's headaches gradually decreased in frequency and intensity. The most likely cause of this patient's symptoms is which of the following organisms?

A. Coxsackievirus A
B. *Cryptococcus neoformans*
C. Herpes simplex virus
D. *Naegleria fowleri*
E. *Streptococcus pneumoniae*

45. During a military conflict in Somalia, soldiers developed a febrile illness characterized by the abrupt onset of fever with rigors, severe headache, myalgias, arthralgias, lethargy, photophobia, and coughing. A petechial rash developed 4 days into the illness and then faded 1 to 2 days later when the symptoms waned. Splenomegaly and hepatomegaly were also present. After 10 days the symptoms recurred. The tentative diagnosis for these soldiers was relapsing fever, which was confirmed by serology. Which vector is most likely responsible for transmission of this disease?

A. Flea
B. Hard tick
C. Louse
D. Mite
E. Mosquito

46. Three patients presented to an inner city hospital with infections subsequently demonstrated to be caused by the same organism. The first patient, a 23-year-old prostitute, presented with a temperature of 38.5°C, hypotension, icterus, pulmonary rales, and muscle tenderness. The second patient, a 38-year-old male, had a temperature of 38.5°C, icterus, mild upper quadrant tenderness, and muscle tenderness. The third patient, a 28-year-old male, had flulike symptoms, a low-grade fever, and muscle tenderness. The first and third patients had cut their feet on glass in a city alley, whereas the second patient cut his hand on glass in an alley. The patients had not been in contact with each other and no one had a significant travel history. Two of the patients developed acute renal failure in the second week of hospitalization; one patient developed meningitis. A fourth patient was subsequently reported to the public health department with a similar illness. One common feature for all four patients was a history of swimming in a city reservoir 7 to 10 days before their illness developed. Which organism is most likely responsible for these illnesses?

A. Hepatitis A virus
B. *Leptospira interrogans*
C. *Mycobacterium marinum*
D. *Naegleria fowleri*
E. *Vibrio vulnificus*

47. A 22-year-old man presents to the emergency department with complaints of eye pain and blurred vision during the preceding day. He did not remember an eye injury but had been wearing contact lenses for an extended period when the eye pain started. The patient also admitted to cleaning his contact lenses with tap water. Examination of the eye revealed ulceration of the cornea. Bacterial cultures of the eye were negative; however, Giemsa stains of the eye scrapings revealed an organism (see figure). Which of the following organisms is most likely responsible for this infection?

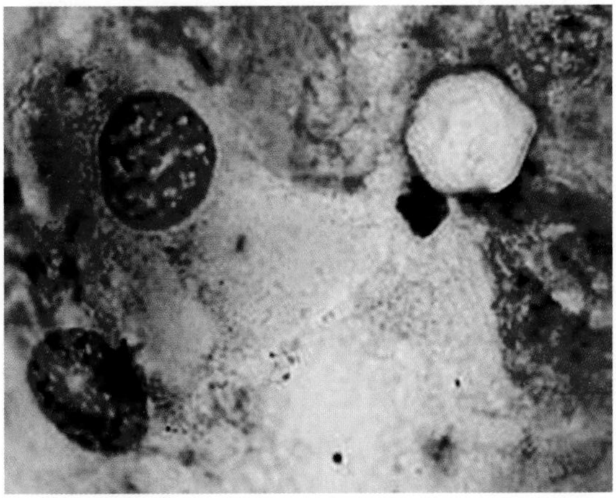

A. *Acanthamoeba*
B. *Dientamoeba*
C. *Entamoeba*

D. *Isospora*
E. *Microsporidia*

48. A 60-year-old woman living in Connecticut presented to her physician with a 5-day history of high fevers (up to 40°C), headaches, myalgias, and malaise. She remembered that 12 days before the start of her illness she removed two engorged ticks from her legs. Leukopenia and thrombocytopenia were documented at the time she was admitted into the hospital. During the course of her illness, no evidence of a rash developed. The fever, however, was persistent despite intravenous treatment with ceftazidime and vancomycin, and she became increasingly confused and somnolent. Bacterial cultures of blood, cerebrospinal fluid, and stool were negative. Giemsa stains of her peripheral blood demonstrated intracellular organisms in the granulocytic cells. Which organism is most likely responsible for this infection?
A. *Anaplasma phagocytophilum*
B. *Babesia microti*
C. *Coxiella burnetii*
D. *Plasmodium vivax*
E. *Rickettsia rickettsii*

49. A 20-year-old male college student was brought to the student health center by his girlfriend. Upon physical examination the patient was found to be obtunded, with a temperature of 39°C, blood pressure 104/52 mmHg, and heart rate of 148 bpm. He had a stiff neck and generalized petechial rash with two areas of purpura. Cerebrospinal fluid was collected. The opening pressure was 180 mm H_2O, white blood cells 4300/mm^3 with 91% neutrophils, glucose 10 mg/dL, and protein 755 mg/dL. A Gram stain and culture of the cerebrospinal fluid was performed with both tests positive for the organism seen in the figure. Which organism is most likely responsible for this patient's infection?
A. *Cryptococcus neoformans*
B. *Haemophilus influenzae*
C. *Listeria monocytogenes*
D. *Neisseria meningitidis*
E. *Streptococcus pneumoniae*

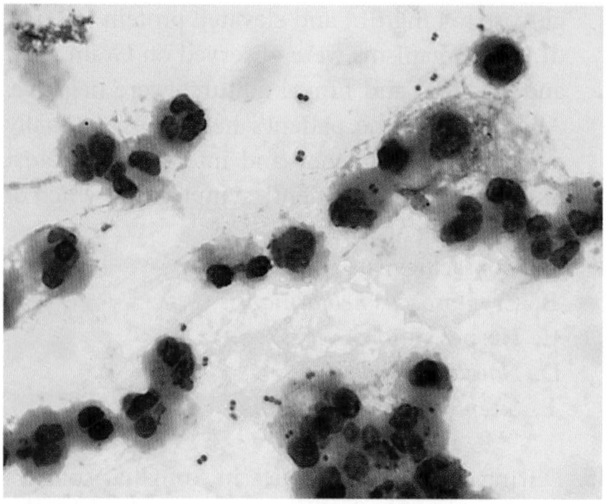

50. A 61-year-old man presents to his physician with diarrhea, abdominal pain, and a nonproductive cough. The diagnosis of multiple myeloma was made 2 years prior to this episode, and 1 month before his current illness began, he underwent a bone marrow transplant. Induced sputum and blood are collected for bacterial culture and stool specimens are collected for bacterial culture and ova and parasite examination. The sputum and stool cultures are negative but the blood culture is positive for *Escherichia coli*. The ova and parasite examination is also positive for an organism (see figure). Which parasite is most likely responsible for this patient's illness?

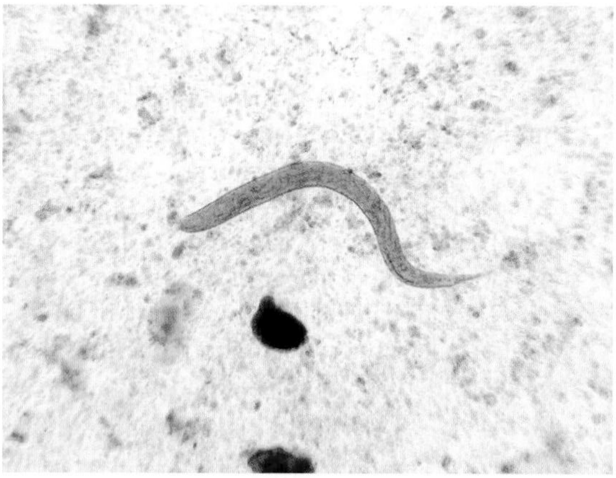

A. *Ancylostoma*
B. *Ascaris*
C. *Necator*
D. *Strongyloides*
E. *Trichinella*

ANSWERS

1. Correct answer: B. Hepatitis A vaccine.
The patient had serologic and clinical evidence of an acute hepatitis A virus infection. This virus is spread person-to-person by fecal contamination. Although immune serum has been used historically to control spread of infections, hepatitis A vaccine is now preferred.

2. Correct answer: D. Tularemia.
Francisella tularensis (the etiologic agent of tularemia) is highly infectious, capable of penetrating unbroken skin. This is a significant health hazard for both physicians and laboratory personnel. *Histoplasma* and *Coccidioides* are significant risks for laboratory personnel when the mold form of these fungi grow in the laboratory; however, the yeast form of *Histoplasma* and the spherule form of *Coccidioides* which are present in the patient's clinical specimens are not infectious. The diagnosis of *Borrelia burgdorferi* infections is primarily by serology and *Entamoeba histolytica* in stool specimens is not considered a health risk if the specimens are appropriately handled.

3. Correct answer: B. *Candida parapsilosis.*
Each of the fungi listed in this question exist as yeasts in the patient; however, only *C. parapsilosis* can grow in blood cultures in 2 days. This yeast is also associated with hyperalimentation, so isolation in this immunocompromised patient is not unusual. *Malassezia furfur* is also associated with hyperalimentation but it would not be isolated in traditional blood cultures because it requires lipids for growth. *Cryptococcus neoformans* is recovered in blood cultures but it typically requires 3 to 5 days before growth is detected. Both *Blastomyces dermatitidis* and *Histoplasma capsulatum* can grow in blood cultures but must be incubated for 2 weeks or longer.

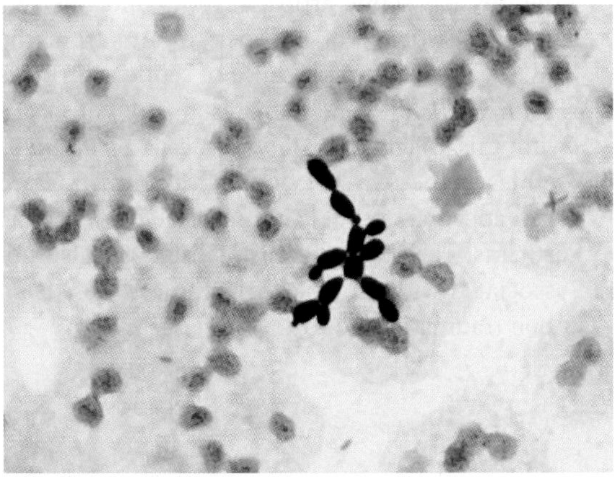

Candida parapsilosis.

4. Correct answer: E. *Nocardia farcinica.*
Only *Nocardia* and *Mycobacterium* will stain with the modified acid-fast stain. *Nocardia* characteristically forms long, branching, partially staining acid-fast rods. Mycobacteria are typically shorter with minimal branching and stain uniformly. *Actinomyces* can resemble *Nocardia* with long, branching rods but these organisms do not stain acid-fast.

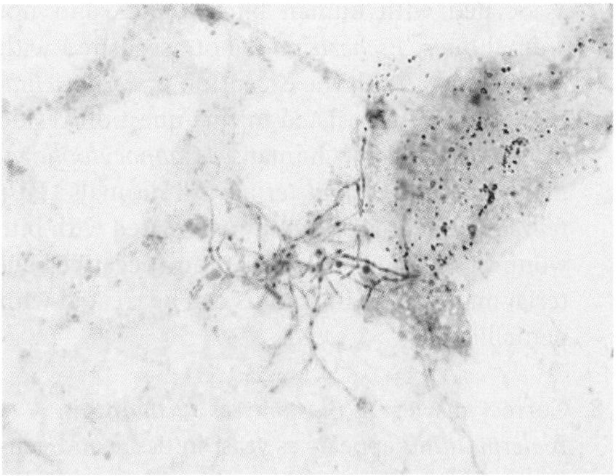

Nocardia farcinica.

5. Correct answer: D. Herpes simplex virus.
The lesions are characteristic of herpes gladiatorum and oral herpes, diseases caused by herpes simplex virus. The disease is spread when one person's vesicular lesion (usually orofacial) comes into contact with another person's skin. Similar lesions are not produced by the other viruses listed in this question.

6. Correct answer: B. *Legionella pneumophila.*
L. pneumophila does not stain well with the Gram stain so microscopy is typically negative. Traditional media also does not support the growth of *Legionella* so cultures are also negative.

Specialized media supplemented with cysteine and iron are required. *Klebsiella* will be observed on the Gram stain and grows readily on conventional bacterial media. *Mycobacterium* will stain with the acid-fast stain. *Histoplasma* would not be observed in the Gram stain or acid-fast stain, but will grow in fungal cultures. Influenza virus infections are typically not observed during the warm months of the year.

7. Correct answer: E. *Pasteurella.*
Pasteurella multocida is commonly associated with animal bite wounds, particularly cat bites. Cats can inflict a deep puncture wound that is difficult to clean adequately. *Capnocytophaga* are also associated with animal bites but these are long, thin, gram-negative bacilli. *Fusobacterium* is also long and thin, but is a strict anaerobe. *Eikenella* resembles *Pasteurella* but is associated with human bite wounds and not animal bites. *Escherichia* is not associated with bite wounds. With the exception of *Escherichia*, the other bacteria listed in this question reside in the mouths of humans (*Capnocytophaga*, *Eikenella*, and *Fusobacterium*) or animals (*Pasteurella*) and are commonly associated with bite wounds. Although these are gram-negative bacteria, many of the infections can be treated with penicillin.

8. Correct answer: A. *Blastomyces dermatitidis.*
B. dermatitidis appears as yeast in tissue and generally grows after 2 weeks in culture as a mold. *Histoplasma capsulatum* has a similar growth pattern although the yeast cells are typically much smaller than *Blastomyces.* Additionally, blastomycosis is characterized by the predilection to disseminate, producing characteristic skin lesions. Infection with *Sporothrix schenckii* is also characterized by the development of skin lesions but these are primary infections associated with the introduction of the fungus directly through skin penetration. *Candida albicans* can cause skin lesions but it would grow more rapidly in culture. *Mycobacterium marinum* characteristically causes skin lesions but these are also associated with direct penetration of the skin; also, the acid-fast stain would be positive for mycobacterial infections.

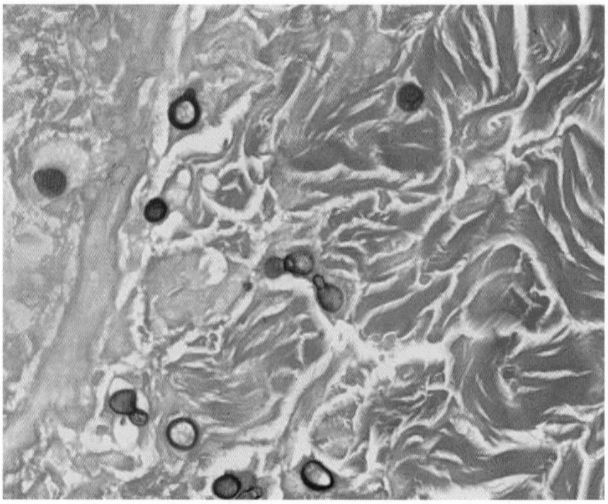

Blastomyces dermatitidis.

9. Correct answer: B. *Listeria monocytogenes.*
Although *L. monocytogenes* is most likely the bacterium that caused the meningitis, all five of the listed bacteria can cause meningitis. *Escherichia coli* and group B *Streptococcus* (*Streptococcus agalactiae*) are primarily restricted to babies less than 1 month of age; however, *E. coli* is a gram-negative rod and *S. agalactiae* is a gram-positive coccus. The other three bacteria can cause meningitis in all age groups although *Neisseria meningitidis* is most common in young adults, while *Listeria* and *Streptococcus pneumoniae* are primarily observed in the young and the very old. Only *Listeria* is a small gram-positive rod and the organism grows slowly both in the patient and in culture.

10. Correct answer: D. *Staphylococcus aureus.*
The boy has septic arthritis. In a child this age, with no evidence of an open wound from the fall, the most common cause of septic arthritis is *S. aureus.* The Gram stain results are consistent with this diagnosis. *Staphylococcus epidermidis* resides on the skin surface and has a similar Gram stain appearance, but is not associated with septic arthritis. The other organisms listed are also not associated with septic arthritis unless there is an open traumatic wound.

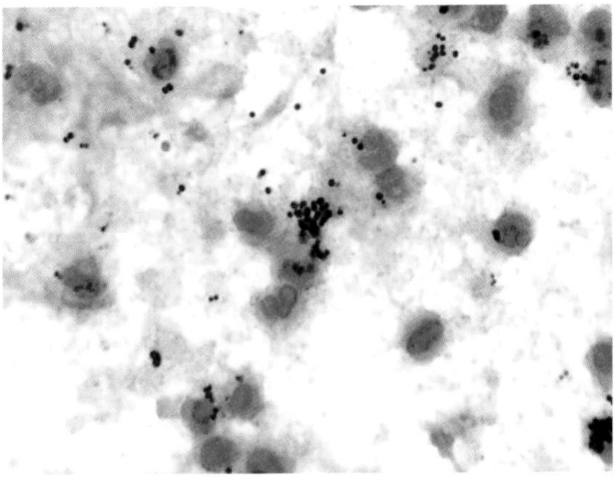

Staphylococcus aureus.

11. Correct answer: E. Candidiasis.
The organisms observed in the microscopic examination are yeast cells, so a *Candida* infection is the most likely diagnosis. *Neisseria gonorrhoeae* would appear as gram-negative diplococci. *Chlamydia trachomatis* are intracellular bacteria and would appear as iodine-staining inclusions in the infected cell. *Trichomonas vaginalis* is a flagellated parasite. Bacterial vaginosis represents an alteration of the vaginal microbiome, with a shift from a predominance of gram-positive rods (i.e., lactobacilli) to a mixture of anaerobic species.

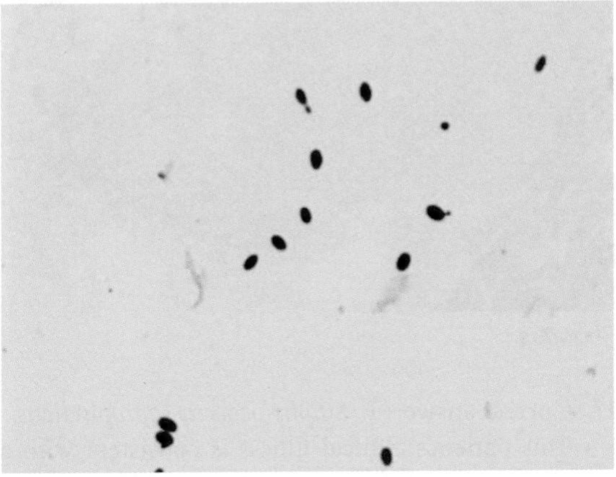

Candidiasis.

12. Correct answer: D. *Streptococcus pneumoniae.*
Patients that are asplenic are at increased risk of developing overwhelming infections with encapsulated organisms. The spleen is responsible for producing opsonizing antibodies, required for the removal of encapsulated organisms such as *S. pneumoniae, Haemophilus influenzae,* and *Neisseria meningitidis.* In the absence of a functional spleen, infection with these organisms can reach a magnitude that allows the organisms to be observed directly in blood specimens. The vast majority of these infections are caused by *S. pneumoniae.* Observation of gram-positive cocci in pairs in the blood confirms the diagnosis.

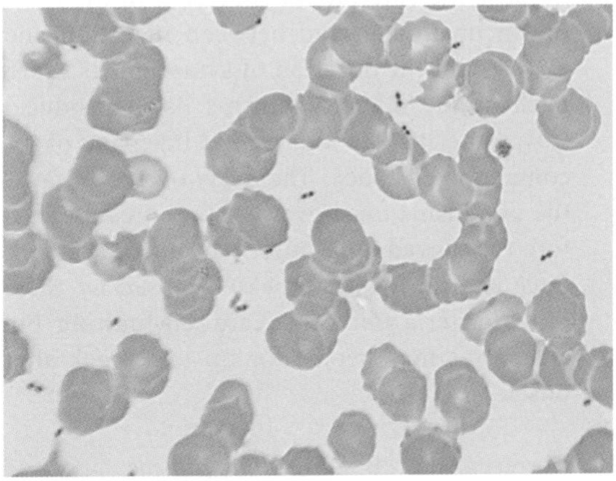

Streptococcus pneumoniae.

13. Correct answer: A. Beaver.
The organism in the figure is *Giardia lamblia. Giardia* has a worldwide distribution, with streams and lakes contaminated in mountainous areas. The sylvan distribution is maintained in reservoir animals such as beavers and muskrats. In this setting, giardiasis is acquired through the consumption of inadequately-treated contaminated water. The other animals listed in the answers to this question (dog, rabbit, snake, and trout) have not been implicated in disease caused by this parasite.

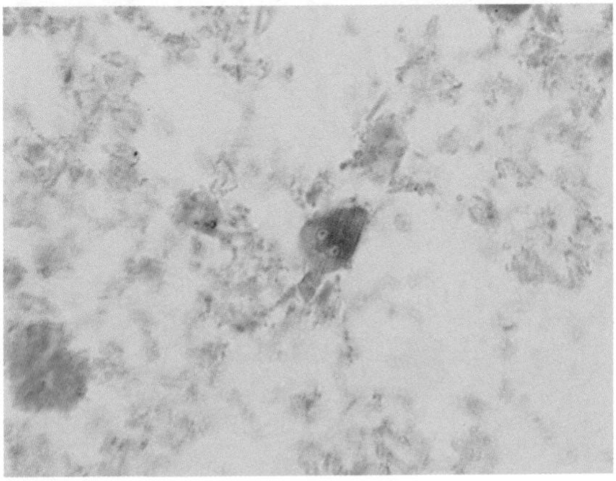

Giardia lamblia.

14. Correct answer: A. *Bacillus cereus.*
The clinical presentation of this disease is consistent with food poisoning caused by *B. cereus.* Disease is mediated by a heat-stable enterotoxin. *B. cereus* can grow in contaminated foods, releasing the enterotoxin. Subsequent reheating of the food does not inactivate the enterotoxin. Because the enterotoxin is present in the food, the incubation period between ingestion and disease and the duration of symptoms is short. Each of the other organisms listed produces gastroenteritis 1 to 3 days after ingestion of the contaminated foods. The delay occurs because the organisms must grow in the intestines before they invade the intestinal mucosa or produce enteric toxins. Diseases caused by these other bacteria and viruses are self-limiting, but symptoms may persist for up to 1 week after onset.

15. Correct answer: B. *Clostridium difficile.*
All five organisms in the answers to this question can cause gastrointestinal disease; however, the important clue is that the symptoms developed after the patient started antibiotics. β-lactam antibiotics and clindamycin are most commonly associated with disease caused by *C. difficile.* The antibiotics suppress the bacteria normally present in the gastrointestinal tract and allow proliferation of *C. difficile*, which may have been present in the intestine or acquired during hospitalization. The presence of white plaques over the colonic mucosa is consistent with the more severe form of disease, pseudomembranous colitis. The early stage of *C. difficile* disease is referred to as "antibiotic-associated diarrhea".

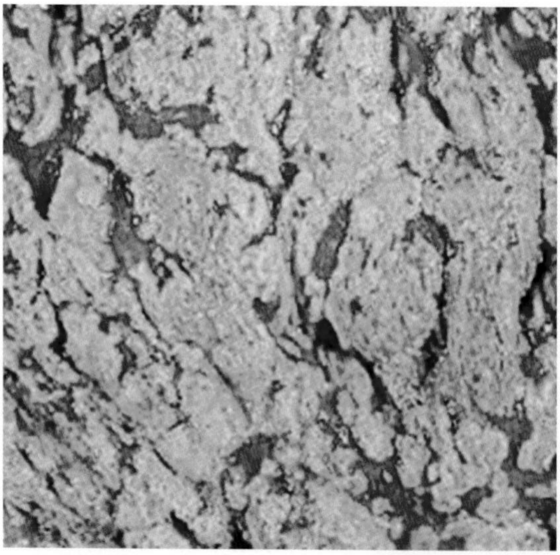
Pseudomembraneous colitis caused by *Clostridium difficile.*

16. Correct answer: E. *Rhizopus.*
The organism in the figure is a nonseptate mold (a zygomycetes). The only mold listed in this question that is nonseptate is *Rhizopus.* Other zygomycetes that cause human disease include *Absidia, Cunninghamella, Mucor, Rhizomucor*, and *Saksenaea.* These molds are ubiquitous and exposure for most people is inconsequential. Some individuals, such as patients with uncontrolled diabetes mellitus, are at increased risk for infections. Rhinocerebral mucormycosis (invasion of a zygomycetes into the sinuses and then to the orbit or brain) is a particular concern in diabetic patients in acidosis. This disease is fatal unless promptly treated.

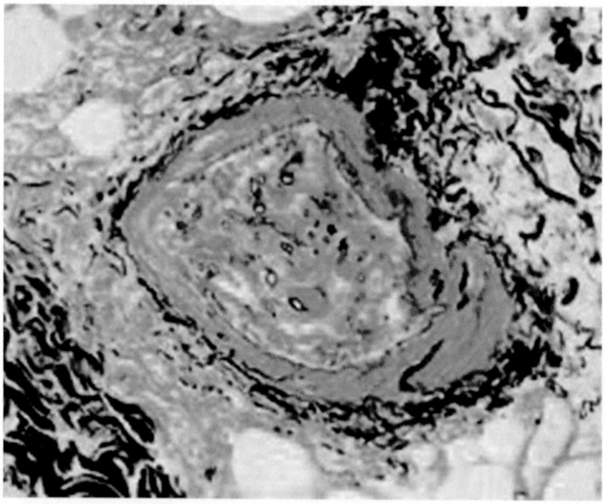
Rhizopus.

17. Correct answer: E. *Staphylococcus saprophyticus.*
This patient's clinical illness is consistent with a urinary tract infection (UTI). It could be restricted to the bladder (cystitis) or more likely involve the kidneys (acute pyelonephritis). The latter is indicated by the flank pain (over the kidney) and fever. *S. saprophyticus* causes UTIs primarily in young, sexually active women. This organism can also produce upper tract infection with urinary tract stone formation due to production of

urease by the bacteria, leading to alkalization of the urine and mineral precipitation. The Gram stain is consistent with a *Staphylococcus* infection. This would also be consistent with *Staphylococcus aureus* but UTIs with this organism are less common unless the patient is also bacteremic with *S. aureus*. *Enterococcus faecalis* is also a gram-positive coccus that can cause UTIs but typically this is in patients who have been treated with broad-spectrum antibiotics and are either catheterized or have a history of urinary tract manipulations. *Candida albicans* will stain gram-positive but is much larger than bacteria and would not be mistaken for bacteria. *Neisseria gonorrhoeae* is a gram-negative diplococci.

18. Correct answer: D. *Nocardia abscessus.*
An infection with *N. abscessus* typically presents as a bronchopulmonary infection, with dissemination to the central nervous system or subcutaneous tissues as a common complication. These bacteria are gram-positive but characteristically stain poorly. *Nocardia* have mycolic acids in their cell wall and are weakly acid-fast. *Actinomyces israelii* can resemble *Nocardia* but does not stain with the acid-fast stain. *Mycobacterium tuberculosis* is strongly acid-fast but does not form long filaments. *Rhodococcus equi* is partially acid-fast and does cause cavitary pulmonary disease, but does not typically disseminate to the brain and the morphology resembles cocci (as implied by the name) or short rods. *Aspergillus fumigatus* is a mold that produces cavitary pulmonary disease.

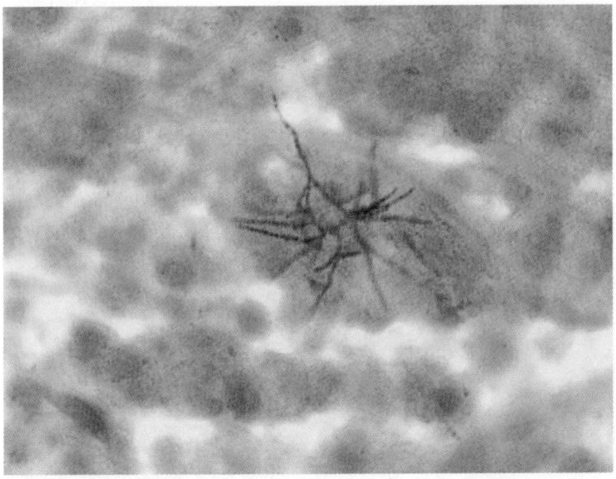

Nocardia abscessus.

19. Correct answer: A. Cytomegalovirus.
The most frequent causes of congenital infection are the so-called TORCH agents (*Toxoplasma*, rubella virus, cytomegalovirus, and herpes simplex virus). Cytomegalovirus, the only agent associated with owl's eye inclusion bodies, is the most common viral cause of congenital malformation. The mother likely suffered a primary asymptomatic cytomegalovirus infection as a result of her blood transfusion and transmitted the virus to her baby. Infants infected with herpes simplex virus may have vesicular lesions but would not have calcifications. Infants infected with rubella virus usually suffer from cataracts and deafness. Congenital infections with Zika virus are well-documented but this woman did not live in an area where viral transmission through an infected mosquito has been documented.

20. Correct answer: D. *Staphylococcus aureus.*
This boy had toxic shock syndrome produced by *S. aureus*. Toxic shock syndrome is characterized by multiorgan dysfunction, skin desquamation, and shock. *Bacteroides fragilis* and *Clostridium perfringens* can produce overwhelming disease (myonecrosis) that can be rapidly fatal but would not present with a rash or desquamation. *Bacillus cereus* is associated with diarrheal disease and eye infections following trauma. *Streptococcus anginosus* is associated with focal abscess formation.

21. Correct answer: B. *Brucella.*
This man had an infection with *Brucella*, most likely with *Brucella melitensis*, which is associated with contaminated dairy products. This is a slow-growing, gram-negative coccobacillus. *Francisella* and *Haemophilus* can also resemble this organism on Gram stain, although neither is associated with goat cheese. *Francisella* infections most commonly follow exposure to infected ticks or rabbits, and *Haemophilus* infections are typically in the very young or elderly. *Acinetobacter* and *Escherichia* would not be confused for *Brucella* on Gram stain.

22. Correct answer: D. *Sporothrix schenckii.*
This woman has an infection with the dimorphic fungus *S. schenckii*. The mold lives in soil rich in

organic material. Most infections are acquired when the fungus is introduced into the cutaneous tissues by mild trauma, usually associated with gardening. At body temperature the fungus replicates as a yeast and has been referred to as "cigar-shaped". Typically, relatively few yeast cells are observed in the clinical specimens. At 25°C to 30°C the fungus grows as a dematiaceous or pigmented mold. The delicate "rosette" arrangement of the conidia (round, fruiting structures on the thin hyphae) is characteristic of *Sporothrix* (suggesting the dangers of rose gardening). *Candida* and *Cryptococcus* exist only in the yeast form and *Trichophyton* only as a mold. *Blastomyces* is a dimorphic fungus but the yeast and mold forms do not resemble *Sporothrix*.

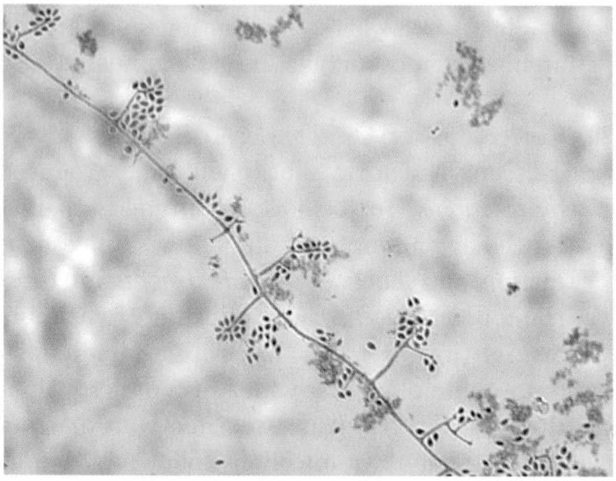

Sporothrix schenckii.

23. Correct answer: B. *Enterococcus faecalis.*
Organisms responsible for peritonitis have demonstrated an ability to produce disease in the intestinal tract (i.e., they have specific, relevant virulence factors). Even though many different species of bacteria are present in the intestines, relatively few produce peritonitis. *Enterococcus* organisms, both *E. faecalis* and *Enterococcus faecium*, can cause peritonitis. The Gram stain result for the patient is consistent with this organism. Two additional organisms that commonly cause peritonitis are *Escherichia coli* (which is treated effectively with ceftazidime) and *Bacteroides fragilis* (which is treated with metronidazole). Yeasts such as *Candida albicans* could also be responsible for infection in this setting; however, the organism would not grow anaerobically. *Peptostreptococcus anaerobius* is associated with polymicrobic abdominal infections, but this organism would not grow aerobically. Streptococci and staphylococci are uncommon causes of peritonitis in this setting. As can be seen in the figure, the Gram stain of *Enterococcus* can be confused with *Streptococcus pneumoniae.*

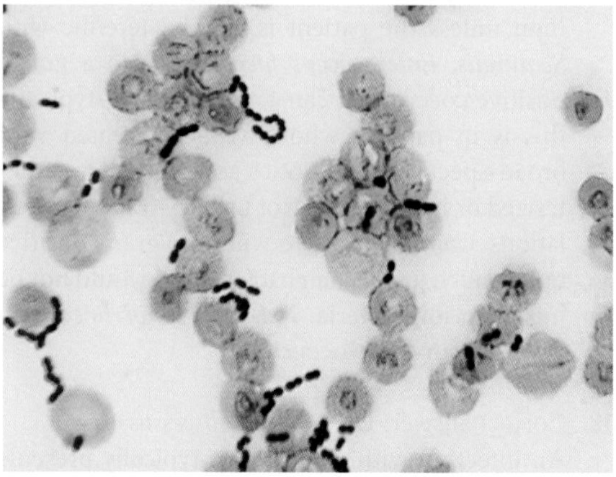

Enterococcus faecalis.

24. Correct answer: E. *Pneumocystis jiroveci.*
This patient had *Pneumocystis* pneumonia, a common infection in HIV-AIDS patients. *P. jiroveci*, like all yeasts, will stain with silver stains. This fungus must be distinguished from *Candida albicans* and the yeast forms of other fungi. *C. albicans* rarely causes pulmonary infections, so this organism is less likely than *P. jiroveci* to be responsible for the patient's infection. *Aspergillus fumigatus* does not form yeastlike cells. *Cryptococcus neoformans* causes pulmonary infections, particularly in immunocompromised patients; however, the cells are slightly larger and are typically surrounded by a capsule. The yeast form of *Histoplasma* is smaller and typically intracellular.

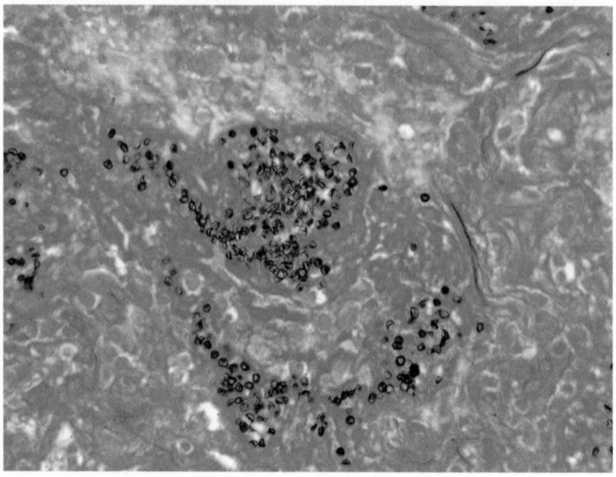

Pneumocystis jiroveci.

25. Correct answer: B. *Campylobacter jejuni.*
All of the organisms listed in this question can cause diarrheal disease. *Bacillus cereus* and *Staphylococcus aureus* are intoxications, with their toxins ingested with previously contaminated foods. The most common presentation for disease caused by these two organisms is a rapid onset of symptoms (typically 4 hours), acute diarrhea and abdominal cramps, and resolution within 24 hours. Norovirus is the most common virus associated with diarrheal disease, and *Campylobacter* and *Salmonella* are the most common bacteria. Although each can produce similar symptoms, the reactive arthritis observed in one patient is primarily a complication of *Campylobacter* infections.

26. Correct answer: D. Human.
The parasite observed in the figure is the trophozoite form of *Entamoeba histolytica*, the etiologic agent of amebiasis. Patients infected with *E. histolytica* pass noninfectious trophozoites and infectious cysts in their stools. The trophozoites cannot survive in the external environment or when transported through the stomach. Therefore the main source of water and food contamination is the asymptomatic carrier who passes cysts. Cockroaches and flies can serve as vectors of this parasite by transferring the cysts from human feces to food or water. Dogs do not serve as reservoirs, and mosquitoes have not been implicated as vectors.

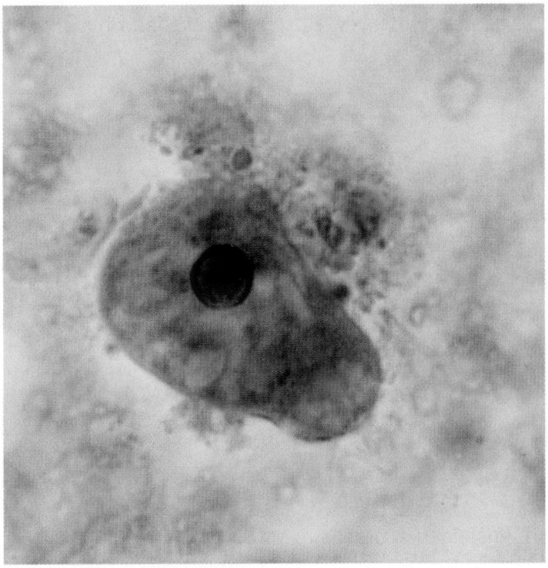

Entamoeba histolytica.

27. Correct answer: B. *Clostridium perfringens.*
Massive hemolysis is a rare but well-recognized complication of a *C. perfringens* infection, which this patient had. It is surprising that this complication is not seen more commonly, in light of the variety of hemolytic toxins produced by this organism. The most important is alpha toxin, a lecithinase that lyses erythrocytes, platelets, leukocytes, and endothelial cells. This toxin can produce enhanced vascular permeability and results in massive hemolysis and bleeding. Although the other organisms listed in this question produce hemolytic toxins, none have been associated with the massive hemolysis that was seen in this patient.

28. Correct answer: E. Shiga toxin–producing *Escherichia coli.*
All five groups of *E. coli* in the answer to this question have been implicated as causes of gastroenteritis. Infections with enterotoxigenic *E. coli*, enteropathogenic *E. coli*, and enteroaggregative *E. coli* are generally restricted to the small intestine, whereas infections with Shiga toxin–producing *E. coli* and enteroinvasive *E. coli* primarily involve the colon. The patients in this report had colitis, with or without blood. Ten percent of the patients (children) developed hemolytic uremic syndrome, which is characterized by acute renal failure, microangiopathic hemolytic anemia, thrombocytopenia, hypertension, and central nervous system manifestations. Shiga toxin–producing *E. coli* (formerly called enterohemorrhagic *E. coli*), but not enteroinvasive *E. coli*, is frequently associated with hemolytic uremic syndrome in children.

29. Correct answer: C. *Coccidioides immitis.*
This man had coccidioidomycosis. This fungus is endemic in the southwestern states of the United States, with infections common in Arizona. Most exposures result in an asymptomatic infection; however, progressive pulmonary disease and meningitis can occur. The mold form of this dimorphic fungus grows in nature and is highly contagious. The arthroconidia (barrel-shaped spores seen in the figure) can be readily dispersed in winds and drift for hundreds of miles. Inhalation of these spores can initiate infection. The form of the fungus seen in patients is that of a thick-walled spherule filled with endospores.

None of the other fungi listed in the answers to this question can produce arthroconidia.

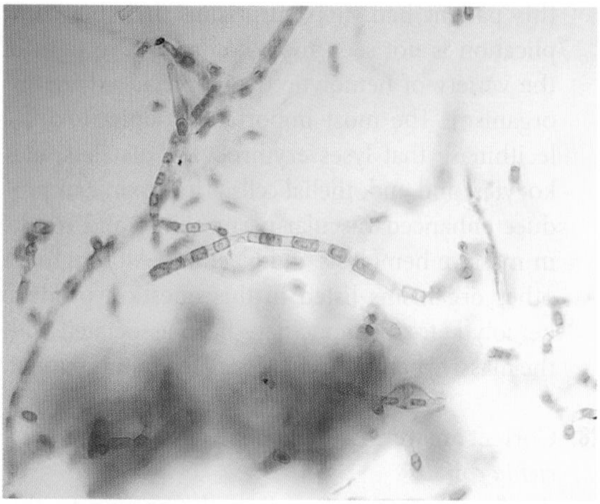

Coccidioides immitis.

30. Correct answer: E. *Streptococcus pyogenes.*
This is a classic presentation of scarlet fever caused by *S. pyogenes* (group A *Streptococcus*). Infection initially develops as pharyngitis, although a wound infection may occur. The distribution of the rash and the more intense inflammation along the skin folds (Pastia sign) is characteristic of the scarlatiniform rash. *Bordetella pertussis* produces a primary infection of the throat and emits a toxin that mediates the systemic signs of disease (pertussis or whooping cough); however, the clinical presentation of the rash is not consistent with *B. pertussis.* Measles and rubella viruses can initiate infection as an upper respiratory tract infection that disseminates as characterized by a rash, but the rash is a maculopapular rash and does not resemble scarlet fever. *Staphylococcus aureus* can also present as a rash in toxic shock syndrome but it is typically followed by desquamation, and the clinical illness is much more severe with multiorgan failure.

31. Correct answer: C. Direct skin penetration by infectious larvae.
This woman was infected with a hookworm, either *Ancylostoma duodenale* or *Necator americanus.* The eggs of these two parasites are indistinguishable. Eggs are shed in the feces of an infected patient. If the eggs are deposited on shady, well-drained soil, they can hatch and mature into infectious larvae. The larvae then penetrate unbroken skin (usually bare feet), migrate to the lungs, and find their way to the small intestine. *Strongyloides* is the other important nematode that initiates infections in humans by penetrating the skin.

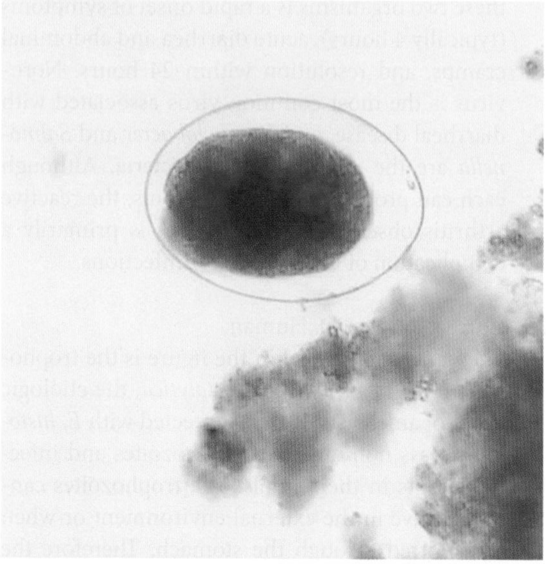

Hookworm.

32. Correct answer: A. *Bacillus cereus.*
Both *B. cereus* and *Clostridium perfringens* are spore-forming organisms found in nature, can cause rapidly progressive diseases, and can produce large, β-hemolytic colonies on blood agar plates. However, *B. cereus* grows aerobically and

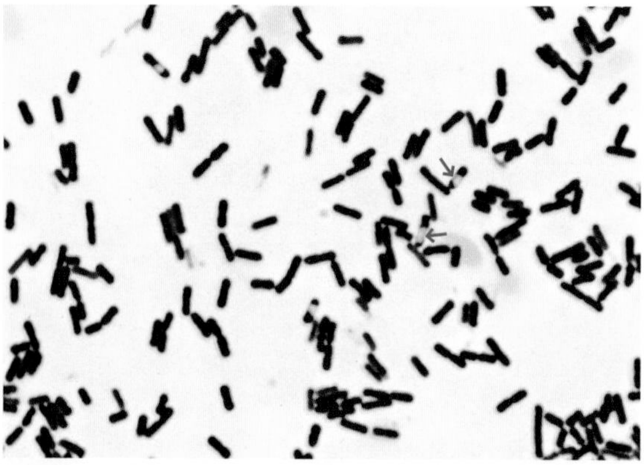

Bacillus cereus. The clear areas in the gram-positive rods are unstained spores (arrows).

C. perfringens is an anaerobic organism. *Corynebacterium jeikeium* colonizes the skin surfaces and, although it could be isolated in an eye specimen, it would not be associated with this type of infection. *Nocardia farcinica* is also found in nature and is gram-positive, but is not associated with rapidly progressive eye infections. *Bacteroides fragilis* is an anaerobic gram-negative rod.

33. Correct answer: A. *Chlamydia trachomatis.*
The patient had lymphogranuloma venereum caused by *C. trachomatis.* The infection is endemic in Africa, Asia, and South America and is sporadically reported in North America, Australia, and Europe. The disease is caused by four specific serotypes of *C. trachomatis*: serotypes L1, L2, L2a, and L3. Adenopathy ("bubo") with ulcer formation is characteristic of the disease. Herpes simplex virus produces a painful ulcer at the site of initial infection. The swollen, ulcerating lymph nodes seen in lymphogranuloma venereum are not characteristic of herpes infections. *Klebsiella granulomatis* is not culturable. *Neisseria gonorrhoeae* can be cultured on chocolate agar and specialized media (e.g., Thayer-Martin) but does not present as described in this patient. *Treponema pallidum* (the etiologic agent of syphilis) produces a painless ulcer, is not characterized by ulcerating lymph nodes, and does not grow in culture. *C. trachomatis* can be cultured in tissue culture cells (an intracellular pathogen); however, the most common test is nucleic acid amplification.

34. Correct answer: A. Dengue virus.
Infections with dengue virus can range from asymptomatic to a life-threatening hemorrhagic fever. Most infections are characterized by a 4- to 7-day incubation period followed by an acute onset of fever, headache, retro-orbital pain, myalgias, and rash. Disease is typically self-limiting after a 6- or 7-day course, although progression to dengue hemorrhagic fever and shock syndrome can occur. Infection with hepatitis A virus, *Leptospira interrogans, Plasmodium falciparum,* and *Salmonella* Typhi can all produce febrile illnesses in travelers to developing countries. Hepatitis A can initially present as a mild flulike illness with fever, headache, myalgias, and malaise. Symptoms will progress to development of dark urine followed by pale stools and yellow discoloration of the skin and mucous membranes. Development of a rash is not characteristic. Symptomatic *L. interrogans* infections are typically characterized by high fevers, myalgias, and headaches. Conjunctival suffusion may be present. A rash is not commonly seen. *P. falciparum* would present as a febrile illness with nausea, vomiting, and diarrhea. This disease is unlikely with the history of compliant malaria prophylaxis. *S. typhi* infections are characterized by fever, headache, myalgias, and malaise. Although a rash may develop, it is not a prominent feature of the infection.

35. Correct answer: A. *Borrelia burgdorferi.*
This woman's symptoms are a classic description of erythema migrans, a rash that develops in the primary stage of Lyme disease. The rash initially develops at the site of the tick bite. The rash will disappear after a few weeks and other transient lesions may subsequently appear. It is common to have no history of a tick bite at the time of presentation because infection most commonly develops following exposure to the nymph stage of the hard. The hard tick in this stage is the size of a poppy seed and likely would not be noticed. A spider bite would have a more aggressive stage of development with localized necrosis. *Malassezia furfur* and *Trichophyton rubrum* produce localized skin manifestations but not the systemic symptoms observed in this woman. *Sporothrix* produces ulcerative, nodular lesions along the lymphatics (not like this woman's presentation) and systemic symptoms.

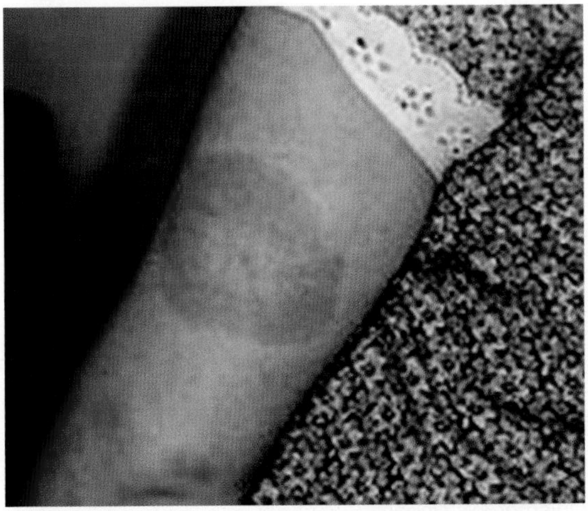

Erythema migrans skin lesion caused by *Borrelia burgdorferi.*

36. Correct answer: C. *Corynebacterium diphtheriae.* This patient's disease is respiratory diphtheria, which is characterized by an abrupt onset of malaise, a sore throat, exudative pharyngitis, and a low-grade fever. A firm, adherent pseudomembrane consisting of bacteria, lymphocytes, plasma cells, and fibrin will develop over the tonsils and adjacent structure. *Bordetella pertussis*, *Neisseria gonorrhoeae*, and *Streptococcus pyogenes* can produce pharyngitis, but none of these organisms are associated with pseudomembrane formation. *Candida albicans* produces oral thrush, most commonly observed in immunocompromised patients such as HIV-AIDS patients. Again, a pseudomembrane would not be observed with *Candida* infections. Diphtheria has been eliminated in many countries with childhood vaccination but is still seen in some countries where vaccination is not widespread.

37. Correct answer: C. *Opisthorchis sinensis* (also known as *Clonorchis sinensis*).
O. sinensis is the Chinese liver fluke. This patient's travel history and diet indicate that he could have been infected with this organism or *Fasciola hepatica*, the sheep liver fluke. *O. sinensis* is associated with consumption of infected raw fish and *F. hepatica* with uncooked watercress. The diagnosis is made by examination of the stool for characteristic eggs. The eggs of *O. sinensis* are much smaller than the *F. hepatica* eggs. The other parasites listed in the question are not associated with hepatitis and their eggs would not be confused with *O. sinensis* eggs.

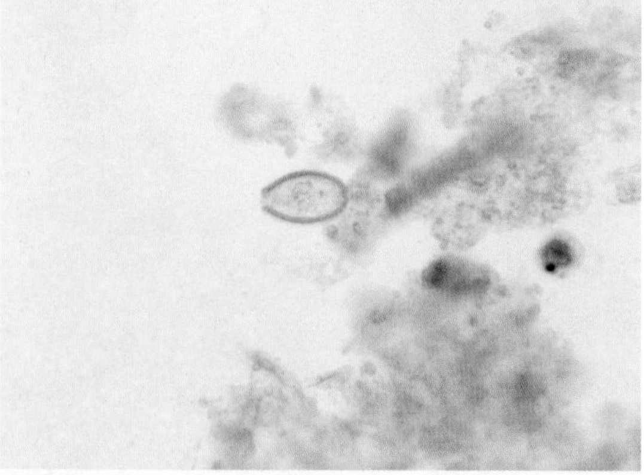

Opisthorchis sinensis.

38. Correct answer: D. *Streptococcus mutans.*
This patient had subacute bacterial endocarditis, which is characterized by an indolent onset and vague symptoms of poor health developing over weeks to months. *S. mutans* is a member of the viridans group of streptococci and is a normal resident of the upper respiratory tract. It has the ability to adhere to the surface of teeth as well as damaged heart valves. It is recognized that patients with preexisting damaged heart valves (e.g., rheumatic heart disease) are at significant risk for developing valvular infections unless prophylactic antibiotics are administered before dental procedures. The other organisms listed in the answers to this question are members of the upper respiratory tract and could theoretically be responsible for endocarditis. However, *Candida albicans* is an uncommon cause of endocarditis; *Staphylococcus aureus* is more commonly associated with a rapidly developing course of disease (i.e., acute endocarditis); *Staphylococcus epidermidis* is associated with subacute diseases but those typically involving a surgical cardiac procedure such as placement of an artificial heart valve; and *Streptococcus pneumoniae* is an uncommon cause of endocarditis and almost always presents in an acute form.

39. Correct answer: C. Epstein-Barr virus.
The patient's clinical history is consistent with Epstein-Barr virus infection or infectious mononucleosis. Adenovirus is a common cause of pharyngitis, with or without conjunctivitis, but would not be associated with hepatosplenomegaly. Coxsackievirus and human metapneumovirus are common causes of upper respiratory tract infections ("common colds") and *Streptococcus pyogenes* is the most common cause of bacterial pharyngitis, but none of these organisms would produce hepatosplenomegaly.

40. Correct answer: E. No antibiotic.
The most likely cause of this food poisoning is *Staphylococcus aureus.* Staphylococcal food poisoning is produced by preformed toxins present in food. Viable bacteria may not be in the food at the time it is consumed because reheating the

food after preparation can kill the staphylococci without affecting the heat-stable toxin or its activity. For this reason, antibiotic therapy would not alter the clinical course of this condition and is not recommended.

41. Correct answer: B. Erythromycin.
This child had inclusion conjunctivitis caused by *Chlamydia trachomatis.* The infection is acquired at birth during passage through an infected birth canal. After a 2- to 3-week incubation period, the infant develops symptoms as described in this case. Pneumonitis may also develop. *C. trachomatis* lacks a peptidoglycan layer in the cell wall, so β-lactams antibiotics (e.g., penicillin, imipenem) are ineffective in treating infections caused by this organism. Erythromycin and newer macrolide antibiotics (e.g., azithromycin) are the drugs of choice for treating this infection. Tetracyclines are not recommended for infants and resistance has been found against this antibiotic. Acyclovir is an antiviral drug used to treat herpes virus infections which is not what this infant had.

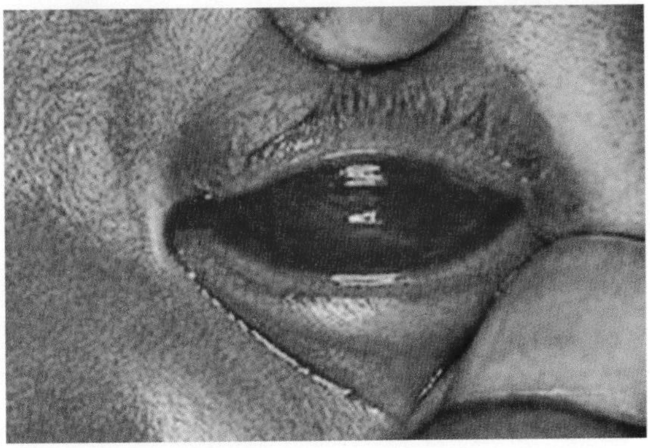

Inclusion conjunctivitis caused by *Chlamydia trachomatis.*

42. Correct answer: C. *Cyclospora.*
Of the organisms listed in the answers to this question, all are acid-fast except *Candida.* The easiest way to differentiate the acid-fast parasites is by their size: microsporidia are 1 to 2 μm in diameter; *Cryptosporidium* is 4 to 6 μm; *Cyclospora* is 8 to 10 μm; and *Cystoisospora* is 10 to 19 μm wide and 20 to 30 μm long.

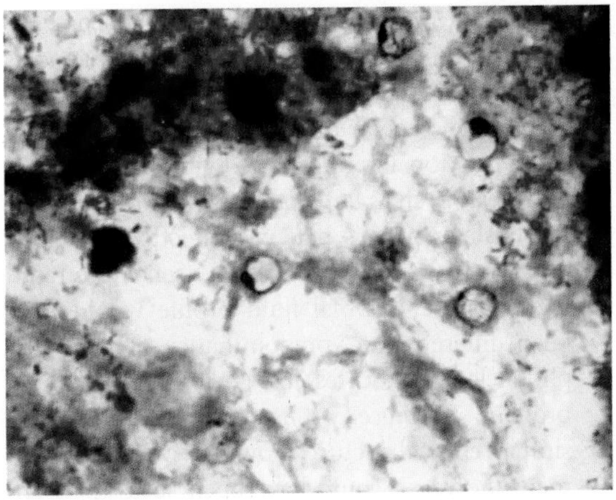

Cyclospora.

43. Correct answer: B. *Clostridium botulinum.*
This case describes a somewhat unusual outbreak of infant botulism because none of the children had a history of ingestion of honey or other contaminated food products. Consumption of honey is not recommended for infants less than 6 months of age because it can be contaminated with spores from *C. botulinum.* The infants lived in an area where construction was underway and they were exposed to dust contaminated with *C. botulinum* spores. *C. botulinum* is commonly isolated from soil samples. Although the epidemiology of this outbreak is unusual, the clinical presentation is common and should have alerted the medical staff. Botulism should be suspected in infants less than 1 year of age who are constipated and have weakness in sucking, swallowing, or crying. Progressive muscle weakness and respiratory failure are symptoms of advanced disease. All of these infants' symptoms were effects of the botulinum toxin that blocks neurotransmission at peripheral cholinergic synapses by preventing release of the neurotransmitter acetylcholine. Although each of the other pathogens listed in this question can cause disease in neonates, none would produce this clinical picture.

44. Correct answer: A. Coxsackievirus A.
This patient had aseptic meningitis. Enteroviruses including the coxsackieviruses are the most common cause of viral meningitis during the summer months. The blisters in the patient's

throat and mouth are consistent with a preceding coxsackievirus A infection. Specific diagnosis of coxsackievirus A infection is most commonly made by molecular methods such as polymerase chain reaction amplification of viral nucleic acids. If bacteria such as *Streptococcus pneumoniae* were responsible for this patient's infection, the progression of disease would have been more rapid and the cerebrospinal fluid profile would have been different (i.e., predominance of polymorphonuclear leukocytes, low glucose, and elevated protein). *Cryptococcus neoformans* can cause a similar clinical picture; however, without treatment the yeast would have been seen on Gram stain and would have grown on both the bacterial and fungal media. Herpes simplex virus can produce vesicular lesions and aseptic meningitis as seen in this patient; however, this diagnosis is less likely because the patient would have been much sicker. *Naegleria fowleri* can cause a primary meningoencephalitis; however, the disease is rapidly fatal and the ameba would be observed in the cerebrospinal fluid upon careful examination.

45. Correct answer: C. Louse.
These soldiers had louse-borne epidemic relapsing fever caused by *Borrelia recurrentis*. This disease is spread person-to-person by infected lice, with humans the only reservoirs. Lice ingest the *B. recurrentis* during a blood meal, and the bacteria multiply in the hemolymph of the parasite. Infection is transmitted when the louse is crushed on the skin surface (bacteria are not present in the saliva or feces of the lice). Fleas, mites, and mosquitos are not infected with *B. recurrentis*. Soft ticks are the vectors of endemic relapsing fever, and hard ticks are the vectors of Lyme disease.

46. Correct answer: B. *Leptospira interrogans*.
Leptospirosis is typically an asymptomatic infection. For patients who develop clinically apparent disease, the onset of symptoms generally develops 1 to 2 weeks after exposure to the bacteria. The initial presentation is a flulike illness with fever and myalgias. These may remit after 1 week or progress to a more advanced disease, such as meningitis or a generalized illness with headache, rash, vascular collapse, thrombocytopenia, hemorrhage, and hepatic and renal dysfunction. The reservoirs for *Leptospira* infections are rodents, particularly rats, as well as dogs and farm animals. The bacteria can colonize the renal tubules of infected animals and be shed in urine. Human infections are most commonly acquired by contact with contaminated water (e.g., standing water, lakes).

47. Correct answer: A. *Acanthamoeba*.
Acanthamoeba species can produce a devastating keratitis that is difficult to treat and frequently leads to enucleation of the eye. The keratitis is usually associated with eye trauma that occurred before contact with contaminated soil, dust, or water. In this patient's situation, the eye trauma is likely related to contact lens use that can abrade the surface of the cornea. The use of contaminated water to clean the contact lenses can introduce the amoeba onto them. The other parasites listed in the answers to this question are not associated with eye infections.

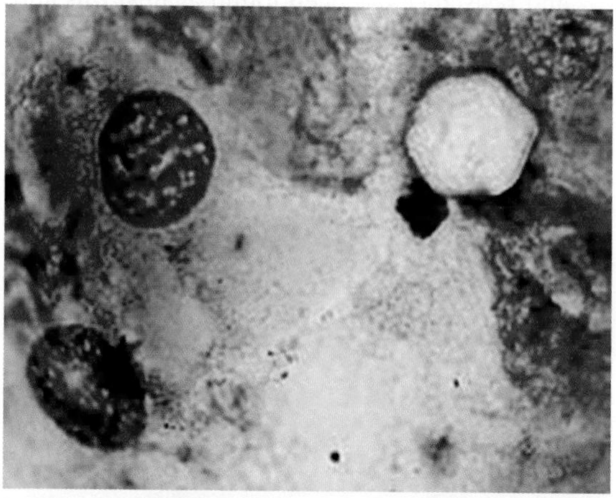

Acanthamoeba.

48. Correct answer: A. *Anaplasma phagocytophilum*.
A. phagocytophilum (formerly *Ehrlichia phagocytophila*) is the etiologic agent of human anaplasmosis (previously called human granulocytic ehrlichiosis). Clinically, it is difficult to differentiate *A. phagocytophilum* infections from *Rickettsia rickettsii* infections, although a rash is less commonly seen in *A. phagocytophilum* infections. In addition, ticks are the vectors for *A. phagocytophilum* and *R. rickettsii*, the etiologic agent of Rocky Mountain spotted fever. The observation of intracellular bacteria (i.e., morula) in peripheral blood granulocytes is useful for

distinguishing between these two organisms. Infected blood cells are observed more frequently with human anaplasmosis than with monocytic ehrlichiosis. Despite this positive result, the diagnostic tests of choice for anaplasmosis are nucleic acid amplification and serology. *Coxiella burnetii* is a related intracellular organism that causes infections most commonly by the airborne route (although ticks can be responsible for some infections). *Babesia microti* and *Plasmodium vivax* cause blood infections but infect erythrocytes and not granulocytes.

49. Correct answer: D. *Neisseria meningitidis.*
All of the organisms listed in the answers to this question can cause meningitis. The clinical picture is consistent with bacterial meningitis, so it is unlikely that *Cryptococcus neoformans* would cause meningitis in a previously healthy person. Furthermore, the Gram stain is inconsistent with *Cryptococcus* (a fungus). The most common causes of meningitis in college students are *N. meningitidis* and *Streptococcus pneumoniae. N. meningitidis* is a gram-negative diplococci with sides flattened against each cocci, and *S. pneumoniae* is a gram-positive diplococci with the cells arranged end-to-end. The Gram stain and clinical presentation for this patient is consistent with *N. meningitidis. Haemophilus influenzae* is a gram-negative rod that causes meningitis in unvaccinated children ages 3 months to 5 years. *Listeria monocytogenes* is a gram-positive rod that causes meningitis in the very young and the elderly.

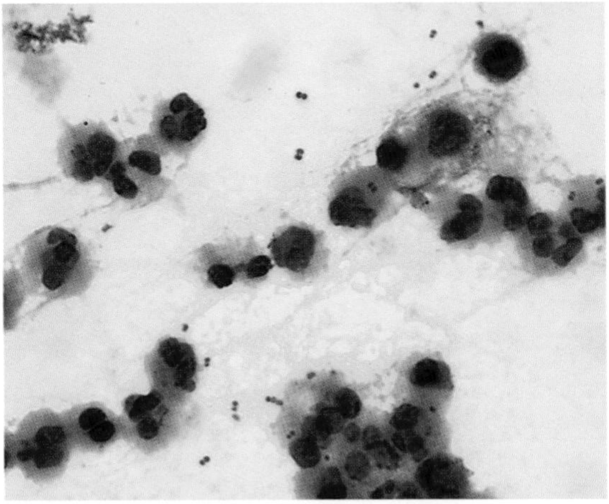

Neisseria meningitidis.

50. Correct answer: D. *Strongyloides.*
This patient has an infection with *Strongyloides stercoralis.* The larvae of the parasite are able to penetrate skin, enter the circulatory system, and pass through the lungs. The worms are coughed up, swallowed, and then develop into adults in the small intestine. Eggs are deposited in the intestinal mucosa, where they hatch, releasing the larvae. Larvae and not eggs are detected in the stool specimens. Autoinfections can occur in immunocompromised patients. In this situation, the larvae in the stool develop into the infectious filariform larvae and repenetrate the intestines, initiating their migratory path from the circulatory system to the lungs, and then to the small intestine. Autoinfections are characterized by perforation of the intestines when the larvae penetrate the intestinal wall to the circulatory system and pneumonitis when the worms migrate through the lungs. Passage through the intestinal wall is the likely reason for bacteremia with *Escherichia.* Hookworms have the same developmental cycle, but eggs and not larvae are found in the stool specimens. Larvae for *Ascaris* or *Trichinella* would not be observed in clinical specimens.

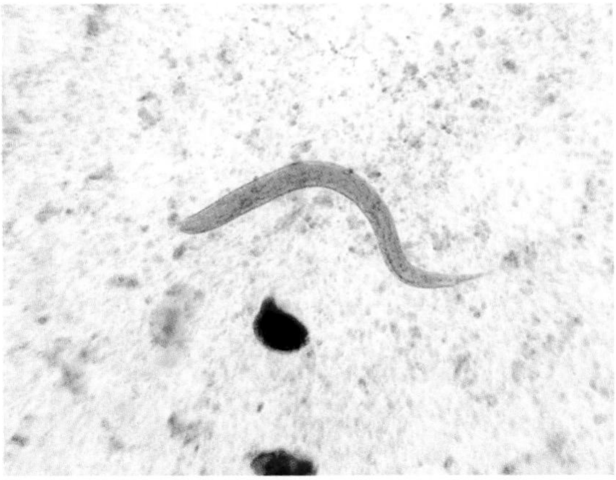

Strongyloides stercoralis.

INDEX

Page numbers followed by *f* indicate figures, *b* indicate boxes, and *t* indicate tables.